Springer Series on Behavior Therapy and Behavioral Medicine

Series Editors: Cyril M. Franks, Ph.D., and Frederick J. Evans, Ph.D.
Advisory Board: John Paul Brady, M.D., Robert P. Liberman, M.D., Neal E. Miller, Ph.D., and Stanley Rachman, Ph.D.

Michael D. LeBow, Ph.D., is Professor of Psychology at the University of Manitoba and directs the Manitoba Obesity Control Center. This is his sixth book. He has written extensively on the topic of behavior therapy, particularly behavior therapy in obesity research and treatment.

Dr. LeBow completed his Ph.D. at the University of Utah, Salt Lake City, in 1969. For two years he was on the faculty of Dartmouth Medical School in Hanover, New Hampshire.

Currently he divides his time between the Psychology Department and the Psychological Service Center, a multi-disciplinary training facility for graduate students in clinical psychology. Supervision, teaching, research, writing, and direct clinical service to individuals and families occupy his working hours.

Child Obesity

A New Frontier of Behavior Therapy

Michael D. LeBow, Ph.D.

Foreword by Cyril M. Franks, Ph.D.

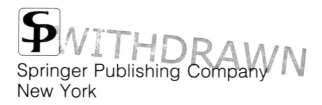

Springer Publishing Company
New York

Springer Publishing Company, Inc.
200 Park Avenue South
New York, New York 10003

84 85 86 87 88 / 10 9 8 7 6 5 4 3 2 1

Library of Congress Cataloging in Publication Data

LeBow, Michael D.
   Child obesity.
   (Springer series on behavior therapy and behavioral medicine; 12)
   Bibliography: p.
   Includes index.
   1. Obesity in children—Psychology aspects—Addresses, essays, lectures. 2. Reducing—Psychological aspects—Addresses, essays, lectures. 3. Behavior therapy—Addresses, essays, lectures. I. Title. II. Series. [DNLM: 1.Obesity—In infancy and childhood. 2. Obesity Therapy. 3. Behavior therapy—In infancy and childhood. W1 SP685NB v. 12 / WD 210 L449c
RJ399.C6L35   1983   618.92'398'06   83–10190
ISBN 0–8261–3780–6
ISSN 0278–6729

Printed in the United States of America

To Bill and Matthew

Contents

Appendixes   187

Foreword

It has been said on more than one occasion that behavior therapy has a long past but a short history. Although the practice of reinforcement, if not the knowledge of principles, stems back to antiquity, the emergence of behavior therapy as scientifically validated treatment did not see the light of day until the late 1950s. Within three decades, what was once viewed as a radical alternative has become part of the establishment. Behavior therapy began as little more than a limited extension of conditioning techniques based largely upon animal research. It progressed to include the correction of a few circumscribed maladaptive habits in humans. Now, it has evolved into a widely accepted intervention strategy with general applicability across a broad spectrum of individual and societal problems. How this came about would be subject matter for an entire book, but it suffices here to affirm the point and draw attention to progress made. Of immediate relevance are current notions about the nature of behavior therapy and the implications of these notions for theory and practice.

The truism that each phase in the progression of a new discipline brings with it a new set of problems is exemplified by recent developments in behavior therapy. The particular set of problems with which we are struggling at this time pertains to the definition of behavior therapy, its identity, and its unique contributions to the mental health field. When behavior therapists are not conducting surveys or reviewing the literature, they are busily defining their domain and agonizing over their right to exist. Definitions range from the narrowly doctrinal to the expansively epistemological and each has its own strengths and weaknesses. The more precise the definition, the easier it is to say what is and what is not behavior therapy. The broader the definition, the harder it is to be exclusive and to differentiate behavior therapy from nonbehavioral systems. Prevailing definitions, such as the one currently advocated by the Association for the Advancement of Behavior Therapy (AABT), attempt to steer a middle course between precise articulation of boundaries, on the one hand, and a general comprehensiveness that excludes virtually nothing, on the other. In so doing, distinctions between behavior therapy and other therapeutic systems become blurred, and it is increasingly difficult to pinpoint what it is about behavior therapy that makes it unique.

If behavior therapy is to remain an identifiable entity—and there is no compelling reason, either philosophically or pragmatically, why this must be so—then it is important that we try to identify its unique characteristics. In earlier times, behavior therapists pointed with pride to alleged therapeutic successes, to the power of conditioning as an explanatory concept, to the new techniques that had been invented or discovered, to the brevity of treatment, to the longlasting changes that were brought about by these methods, and to the many new areas into which behavioral interventions could be introduced successfully. As behavior therapists grew older and wiser, they came to realize that, while still very commendable, successes were less dramatic than had been believed, many techniques were of limited applicability, maintenance was an elusive phenomenon, and conditioning *per se* probably could not account satisfactorily for everything that occurred during the intervention process.

Gradually, at times painfully, came the realization that the advantages of behavior therapy rest upon something more substantial than the "I-am-better-than-you comparisons" of the formative years with psychotherapy. The advantages of behavior therapy, and thereby its unique contribution, lie more in conceptual strengths than specific attainments, in the methodology, in the rigor of its approach, and in its concern with such matters as accountability and outcome evaluation.

Contemporary behavior therapy is best characterized as an approach based upon a set of theoretical methodological assumptions common to most but not all behavior therapists rather than either a compendium of specific techniques or a unitary system. Its hallmarks are replication, outcome evaluation, and account-ability; openness toward testable alternatives; appeal to data rather than authority or doctrine; the absence of any universally accepted set of therapeutic techniques or even intervention strategies; emphasis upon current rather than historical determinants of behavior; overt behavior change as the main criterion by which treatment is to be evaluated, and the specification of treatment goals in objective terms; and a growing concern with social as well as conventional validity.

It is upon this foundation that child obesity is examined in LeBow's book. For obvious reasons, childhood obesity is a disorder that readily lends itself to technique innovations, the search for brief procedures, and the proclamation of new fads of questionable treatment value. It is tempting for unwary behavior therapists who still think in terms of therapeutic rather than conceptual potency to fall into these traps. LeBow, a seasoned campaigner in both behavior therapy and child obesity, neatly sidesteps most of these hazards. He demonstrates a compre-hensive knowledge of childhood obesity and its many intricacies; he recognizes the strengths and weaknesses of behavior therapy—its accomplishments and its limitations. LeBow takes a penetrating and critical look at childhood obesity from the vantage point of the sophisticated behavior therapist of the 1980s.

The hope for successful intervention within this little understood problem area rests upon individuals such as LeBow who are prepared to proceed systematically yet cautiously in their continuing quest for knowledge and effective clinical strategies. While both practical and theoretical answers are to be found in this book, of equal significance is LeBow's straightforward discussion of what has yet to be accomplished. LeBow not only poses questions that need to be answered, he suggests methods that assist in formulating answers. At this stage in our knowledge, this is probably a more significant contribution than any glib how-to manual or dogmatic exposition of theory.

For the practitioner confronted with the need to do something about the problems of childhood obesity *now,* this volume offers many suggestions. It is an excellent practical manual with a variety of useful suggestions for assessment and intervention. The thoroughness of this book and the knowledge and thought that LeBow has put into its many pages will ensure its prominence as a major resource for years to come.

Cyril M. Franks
Graduate School of Applied and Professional Psychology
Rutgers University

Preface

For those afflicted by it and for those attempting to treat it, childhood obesity is a confusing, intractable, and punishing condition. I address this book to practitioners and their students who try to alleviate this problem. I also address this book to researchers and their students who undertake searches that aim at not only improving the ways to alleviate it but also explaining the phenomenon better and uncovering the backgrounds and characteristics of the afflicted youngsters. Sometimes, fortunately, the skills and goals of the therapist and the scientist are effectively blended, the product being the obesity researcher–practitioner.

The main subject in this volume is behavior therapy for childhood obesity. This is a new field, one that I hope becomes more encouraging to scientists and more helpful to patients than has the behavior therapy for adult obesity. This book examines much literature pertinent to obesity among children. I focus primarily on youngsters from 5 to 12 years of age. On occasion, however, I include 13-year-olds in the discussions, either because they present problems like those of younger children or because the handling of data in some critical studies makes it quite difficult to do otherwise. Further, on occasion I discuss infants and toddlers, particularly those studies that examine connections between very early-age and later-age obesity.

Chapters 1 and 2 address the description, measurement, nonbehavioral treatment, epidemiology, and natural history of childhood obesity. The next three chapters examine behavior therapy principles, problems, approaches, and applications relevant to caring for obese children. Chapter 6 discloses and discusses obstacles to treatment that researchers and practitioners should remain aware of when designing and offering remedial programs. Finally, the two remaining chapters to some extent recapitulate and expand on what has been previously discussed: Chapter 7 does so while it focuses on adolescence; while Chapter 8 asks current research questions about obese children, their treatment, the settings and agents of their treatment and prevention. The appendixes provide nutritional, calorie expenditure, interview, and normative data (for example, weight, skinfold). References and the index help to guide the reader to further information.

Various individuals and organizations assisted me while I wrote this book, some of whom are credited in the acknowledgments. I wish here to thank others, notably the authors of the studies I read, whose discoveries I hope to have accurately portrayed and, within this group, those whom I personally contacted for their recent works and advice. These individuals are Drs. K. D. Brownell, T. J. Coates, P. J. Collipp, and A. W. Voors. Thank you for taking the time to answer my questions.

I also would like to express appreciation to Dr. Cyril Franks for interesting me in doing this book and, more generally, for reinforcing my previous scholarly efforts.

Further I thank Ms. Marlene Krenn for her diligence as a library researcher and Ms. Barbara Watkins of Springer Publishing Company for her editorial guidance. And I thank Ms. Barbara LeBow for her pointed criticisms and several typings of the manuscript. Her support, example, and intelligence helped to create the environment conducive to the book's completion.

Note of Caution

Before treating an obese child or adolescent, consult the youth's family physician or pediatrician (see Appendix F).

CHAPTER 1

Describing, Approaching, and Detecting Obesity in Children

They may be easy to recognize, and they may not be. They may be thought of as weak in character and physical strength by those close to them, and they may not be. They may be feeling afflicted and beset upon, and they may not be. They may be malnourished, and they may not be. They may, for a time, be taller and more skeletally mature than their peers, and they may not be. They may be responsive to professional help, and they may not be. Obesity among children is confusing, difficult to characterize, and difficult to define (Khan, 1981).

Why Does a Child Become a Fat Child? *etiology*

The question perplexes. It puzzles the obese youngster, his parents, pediatricians, and obesity researchers who search for solutions to the condition. Much research work attempts to answer the question, why does the child become fat (Collipp, 1980a), but as yet no satisfactory response has been found. Childhood obesity is a multifaceted problem affected by genetic, physiologic, social, and economic variables, different constellations playing greater or lesser roles for different obese children. I sadly predict that, for many years to come, this will remain one of the most mysterious, intractable, and omnipresent disturbances of the young in our society.

We can, nonetheless, quite simply describe how it arises and describe, in a general sense, how to go about treating it. We can do so by invoking the concept of energy (caloric energy), balance of energy, and imbalance of energy (calorie imbalance). Calories are units of heat, units of energy.

But when you have a surplus of energy you are not necessarily more vigorous, more ready to do something (Deutsch, 1976). Increasing your energy supply does not make you more energetic. For one health reason or another, you may be unable to utilize the energy. Moreover, you do not eat calories, though for simplicity we talk as if you do. You eat food that supplies fuel that can, under the right circumstances, be used for growth (see Morgan, 1980), repair, survival, and activity; the chemical energy ultimately derived from food can be transformed into the mechanical energy needed for activity (Mathews & Fox, 1976).

In this volume, as in many current treatises on nutrition, exercise, and obesity, when the word calories is written, kilocalories (or one calorie multiplied by 1000) is meant. A kilocalorie is the heat needed to increase one kilogram of water one degree centigrade (Mayer, 1972); in SI (Système International d'Unites) *joules* replaces calories—one kilocalorie is 4.184 kilojoules.

Calorie imbalance means that the amount of energy consumed does not equal the amount of energy expended. There are two inequalities, two types of calorie imbalance, and several possible reasons each of these arises that will be discussed. Positive energy imbalance, the first inequality and the one that descriptively answers the question as to why a child becomes fat, occurs when consumption exceeds expenditure. This imbalance comes about and lasts long enough to make the child obese due, perhaps, to overeating. The overeating results from either consuming extreme amounts of rich foods or from having a body that is very efficient; that is, calories from food are captured and stored more efficiently than normally, and therefore, though total intake is moderate, a surplus of calories forms anyway. Also, it may arise and last long enough to make the child obese due to underexercising or to a combination of overeating and underexercising. Whatever the source of the excess energy, it will be stored as fat (triglyceride) in adipocytes—in adipose cells already present, or in new adipocytes that develop (Salans, 1974) or both (Hirsch & Knittle, 1970, Chapter 2). In any case, the adipose tissue enlarges. We can say that a positive energy equation exists or has existed whereby the intake of calories has been greater than the expenditure of them, meaning the ratio of calorie intake to calorie outgo has been and perhaps continues to be greater than one. In other words, the child is fat because at some time he has been in a state of positive energy imbalance of a sufficient degree for a sufficient period. Often factors that led up to the situations producing this state and the role of resulting internal events in perpetuating it are unclear.

The opposite of positive energy imbalance, with its opposite conditions and opposite effects, is negative energy imbalance. Calorie intake is less than calorie outgo. A negative energy equation that describes this situation is written below.

Calorie deficit = Calorie expenditure − Calorie Intake

when

$$\frac{\text{Calorie intake}}{\text{Calorie expenditure}} < 1$$

The equation says that the deficit in calories equals the difference between the expenditure and intake of them, when expenditure exceeds intake. Negative energy imbalance, like positive energy imbalance, is achieved by changing the value of one or both terms on the manipulable side of the equation—the child eats less, moves more, or does both. For many of the obese children that practitioners treat, achieving a negative energy state and then maintaining it for a time is the objective of treatment. But, as indicated by the literature recounted in this book, the objective frequently is not reached. Not only is it difficult to attain, but the attempt to attain it can be perilous (See Chapter 6).

Avenues to the Negative Energy Equation

Causing a state of negative energy imbalance amounts to changing the relationship of calorie intake to calorie outgo. Focusing on the calorie intake term means giving the child less to eat, fewer calories. This can be done by reducing the constituents of the basic food groups—vegetables and fruits, breads and cereals, milk, and meat (see Collipp, 1980c, pp 336–339 for amounts and suggestions). Practitioners vary as to which specific foods they seek to reduce and how much energy intake reduction they view as necessary (see for example Tables 6.1 and 6.2).

The worth of the changes they make can be evaluated along a few dimensions. One dimension is the degree to which the recommended dietary allowances for a child (see Appendix A) are altered. In general, the optimal diet for a youngster, whether or not he needs to become thinner, includes a continuing source of water, macronutrients, and micronutrients. Macronutrients are comprised of carbohydrates, protein, and fat, with calorie equivalents per gram being roughly four for protein, four for carbohydrate, and nine for fat; micronutrients are comprised of vitamins A, D, E, and K (fat soluble), B and C (water soluble), and minerals (iron, calcium, for example).

Dwyer (1980), in a most informative piece on diets for children and adolescents, makes several recommendations useful to obese juveniles and their parents. She advises cutting down, not cutting out, high energy, low nutrient foods (such as candy) "by keep(ing) the sugarbowl off of the table," reducing snacks, substituting fruit juices for soda pop, and saving treats (for example, apple pie and cake) for Saturdays and Sundays instead of serving them throughout the week. She also advises reducing the intake of fat by choosing leaner cuts of meat and by fading out whole milk while fading in skim; this fading in and out can be accomplished by progressively increasing the ratio of nonfat to whole milk when making fluid from powder. Other tips include reducing the availability of problem foods in the home, increasing the presence of desirable foods, and carefully watching what goes into the child's lunch box. Thus, Dwyer provides both dietary and behavioral advice. Her article pertains to the diets of all children and adolescents, not just those who are obese.

About obese children, however, two questions arise concerning avenues toward creating therapeutic energy imbalance by altering calorie intake. These are: How is it done? How successful is it?

Dieting

Researchers and practitioners have tried to get obese children to diet using hospitalization, psychotherapy, and counseling in summer camps, schools, and doctor's offices. As the strategies for doing so have varied, so have the lengths of time the diets have been in effect, and so have the degrees of restriction imposed.

Moderate Restrictions.   Alley and colleagues (1968), for example, simply gave 50 obese juveniles a 1000 kcal/day diet (Jones, 1972); 49 of these outpatients were above the 90th percentile in weight. Alley and colleagues also gave 19 of their group appetite suppressants. The authors' sample consisted of 24 males, ages 7 to 19, and 26 females, ages 6 to 19; about 60 percent of the sample was 13 and under. Monthly checkups (see also Asher, 1966; Howard, Dub, & McMahon, 1971) or checkups at longer intervals were carried out for one to five years. Results—body weight change—revealed that 14 of the patients lost from 2.3 kg to nearly 30 kg and that 12 stayed about the same, growing in height; the others (48 percent) gained. Finally, more boys than girls failed to reduce. Recognizing the importance of accounting for height change on weight change, the authors applied a ponderal index to their data, their formula being height (inches) divided by the cube root of weight (pounds). After analyzing their data in this way, they concluded their success rate to be 54 percent. This estimate may have been unduly conservative as K. A. Edwards (1978) later showed. Using a different yardstick, the weight index, he recomputed the data, and found in one of his analyses a 25 percent higher success rate.

Deschamps and co-workers (1978) also treated outpatients; the youngsters, 17 obese girls and 20 obese boys, ranged in ages from 6 to 16. In contrast to Alley and colleagues, however, these researchers used somewhat more liberal calorie allowances—1200 to 1500 kcal/day (cited in Simić, 1980). Patients stayed on the diet, which was 40 to 50 percent carbohydrate, 30 to 35 percent fat, and 15 to 20 percent protein, for 3 to 24 months, depending on how much they needed to reduce. Weight losses, interpreted in terms of change in degree of weight excess, varied. Thirty-two of the patients, mostly children, did well; mean excess fell by 2.3 standard deviations. Five patients gained; perhaps because, as reported, they did not heed the dietary tutelage. In addition to looking at body weight, Deschamps and co-workers followed insulin response changes. The majority of the weight losers, to a great extent the younger patients, switched from elevated insulin responses at the start of treatment to more acceptable values by the end. Seven, however, showed increases over treatment; they switched the other way.

More Severe Restrictions.   Similarly, tracking the effects of dieting on a broad spectrum of body variables (Figure 6.1), Widhalm and Schernthaner (1979) studied 25 older children, mean age 12.8; of concern was the type of diets fed to the children. Diets were isocaloric, about 735 kcal/day, but 12 youths received a regimen a good deal lower in fat and higher in carbohydrate than did the others;

there was a difference of over 20 percent in fat and 15 percent in carbohydrate between the diets, whereas protein content varied less than 6 percent. Weight losses failed to mirror dietary differences. Overall, patients who were 35 percent overweight on the average at the start, lost a mean of nearly five kg; therefore treatment, though neither statistically nor clinically significant, had some impact. Five kg in three weeks is an acceptable rate of loss.

Although weight changes failed to differentiate between the groups, blood lipid profiles taken after intervention did. Those patients given the lower-fat diet exhibited a significant reduction in serum cholesterol, mainly LDL (low-density-lipoprotein) cholesterol. Widhalm, Maxa, and Zyman (1978) likewise reported that 14 girls and boys, ages 11 to 13, who dieted at a summer camp lost almost five kg and sustained a significant reduction (over 20 percent) in serum cholesterol. Again, LDL cholesterol decreased; unfortunately, so did HDL (high-density-lipoprotein) cholesterol (see also Weninger, Widhalm, Strobl, & Schernthaner, 1980); high levels of HDL cholesterol are believed to lower the risk of atherosclerosis (Streja, Steiner, & Kwiterovich, 1978).

The Widhalm and Schernthaner diets are low in calories. Even lower, of course, is total starvation—zero calorie diets; these, however, are only infrequently used in childhood obesity treatment. They are not widely recommended. Collipp (1980c), discussing the "Long Island Child Life Program," reported that 18 obese (50 percent overweight) children between the ages of 8 and 16 were fasted for 12 days in a hospital. Energy intakes each day were under 40 kcal. Weight losses ranged from 6 to 13 percent with a mean of 10 percent. One of the great dangers of starvation treatment is that the child may sustain significant losses of lean tissue; and one of the major disappointments, as seen in the studies on adults and adolescents at any rate, is that positive results are transient (Drenick, 1981; Drenick & Johnson, 1978; Nathan & Pisula, 1970). Collipp's report permits neither an evaluation of danger nor one of disappointment.

Less extreme than total fasting and aimed at preventing excessive losses in lean tissue is protein-sparing modified fasting (Bistrian & Sherman, 1978; Blackburn, 1978). Merritt, Bistrian, Blackburn, and Suskind (1980) illustrate this approach in a recent study of 16 (6 girls, 10 boys) extremely obese 9 to 16-year-olds (see also Merritt, Blackburn, Bistrian, Palumbo, & Suskind, 1981). The only food these youths, averaging just under 13 years of age, received for four weeks after being evaluated was lean meat—1.4 to 3 grams per day, per kilogram of ideal body weight. Results for the entire group (comparisons on younger versus older patients were absent) showed greater weight losses earlier in treatment. For the month, the mean reduction was over seven kilograms. Change in percent overweight was marked, falling 17 points, from an average of 181 percent at the start to 164 percent at the finish; lean body mass reductions were moderate (see Merritt, Schlaman, Bistrian, & Suskind, 1978). Notably, while on the program, patients were followed closely; for example, weights were regularly checked, blood samples were drawn, and urinalyses were performed.

Such surveillance is necessary. The modified fasting approach is, as the authors note, still experimental. In view of the widespread controversy about its appropriateness for adults, it is only logical to advise caution in using it for children (Golden, 1979). Merritt and colleagues would agree, yet they are most hopeful about its potential, seeing short-term semistarvation as a reasonable alternative to protracted, albeit milder, calorie intake restriction (see also Merritt, 1978).

Drugs

Pediatricians and family physicians sometimes prescribe anorectic agents for obese children. They do so in order to help the youngsters they treat to follow dietary plans; often, the professional has evidence that counselling to lessen calorie intake has failed. The children gain or simply stay the same weight. Can drugs help when used this way, as adjuncts, as dieting helpers?

Opinion Is Divided.   Baritussio, Enzi, Rigon, Molinori, Fnelmen, & Crebaldi (1978), for example, tested the effects on weight loss of 20 mg fenfluramine given t.i.d. (three times a day) or 1 mg mazindol given b.i.d. (twice a day) to groups of children undergoing an 800 kcal/day diet comprising 20 percent fat, 35 percent carbohydrate, and 45 percent protein; fenfluramine causes little if any central nervous system stimulation, whereas mazindol does, but unlike the amphetamines acts primarily on the limbic system (Grollman, 1980). The authors also included a third group—diet only—in their investigation. Fourteen boys and seven girls, ages 9 to 13 and from 30 to 90 percent overweight at the outset, participated in this eight-day experiment conducted in a hospital. Those in the mazindol-plus-diet condition significantly outperformed those in the fenfluramine-plus-diet group, whereas the diet-only subjects fell in between. Average loss in the fenfluramine group was 1.2 kg; average loss in the mazindol group was 2.5 kg.

Israsena, Israngkura, and Srivuthana (1980) also scrutinized the effects of fenfluramine in a dietary program, but their study was appreciably longer and was conducted with outpatients. The diet they used was set at between 800 kcal and 1200 kcal/day, with carbohydrate calories equalling the sum of calories from both other macronutrients; in addition, they prescribed exercise. Ninety youngsters, all at least 20 percent overweight, some more than 90 percent overweight, received this calorie-reduction approach for two months; the children ranged in age from 1.5 to 15 years, but over half were under 10. Fifty-four percent finished. Almost 41 percent of the finishers lost from .3 kg to 4.5 kg, whereas 39 percent lost nothing, and 20 percent gained from .5 kg to 1.3 kg; height changes, if any, were undisclosed.

More than half of the finishers were still 30 percent or more overweight by treatment's end and so were offered further care. This included 20 mg fenfluramine administered one to three times daily. Using a double-blind trial lasting four months, Israsena and co-workers evaluated the effects of this drug against a placebo. They compared those 16 individuals who completed the trial—placebo versus fenfluramine subjects. Significant differences emerged. The active drug group posted the better weight losses. Nevertheless, the magnitude of reduction was small, about 1.8 kg; as in the diet-only segment of this study, however, height change data were missing, making it difficult to interpret the weight changes found.

There were unwanted side effects reported for some of the patients in the fenfluramine cohort. Yet these side effects were thought to be of minor importance and not in opposition to the authors' essential belief: Fenfluramine administration is helpful in treating obese children, particularly in treating those having a hard time following a calorie reduction plan (see also Bacon & Lowrey, 1967).

But Coates and Thoresen (1978) hold that such drugs add little. Alley and co-workers' (1968) report mentioned previously supports their view. Drug treatment for the 19 patients receiving it did not appreciably change their weights (see also Jacobelli, Simeoni, Vecci, & Agostino, 1979; Rayner & Court, 1975). Coates and Thoresen go on to note more generally the dangers of amphetamines: abuse and dependence. In addition, they articulate problems with such nonamphetamines as chlortermine: Controlled evaluations fail to show immediate and long-term success (see Lorber cited in Lancet, 1978), and reliable data on following the drug prescriptions are, like the data on following dieting prescriptions, absent.

Grollman (1980) is more emphatic in decrying the resort to drugs as adjuncts to calorie intake reduction approaches. After discussing the drugs that are available, he states: " . . . the use of most effective agents is contraindicated in children under the age of 12" (p. 396) (see also Golden, 1979). Grollman also paints a bleak picture about the effectiveness and safety of using hormones (for example, thyroid, pituitary, human chorionic gonadotropin, progesterone) in treatment. Rivlin's (1975) stance is not too dissimilar; he advises "caution and restraint" in applying these agents.

Surgery

Surgery (such as Jejunoileal bypass, gastric bypass) is drastic. The weight loss from it results from caloric restriction as much as malabsorption (Bray, 1976; Lancet, 1978). This surgery is a last-resort way to treat extremely obese juveniles (Polich, Stauter, Kirkpatrick, & Larson, 1978).

Criteria for measuring how obese is too obese vary. Polich and co-workers recommend 300 percent overweight as the minimum before recommending surgery. Randolph, Weintraub, and Rigg (1974) advise avoidance of surgery unless the patient remains over twice ideal weight for two years; among other criteria, they stress the need for cooperation from patient and parent that is assured before surgery as well as a history of failure with dieting approaches. Because surgery is so drastic an intervention, one that may produce undesired physical sequelae such as wound infection, growth interference, and protracted vomiting, it is done infrequently (Schwartz, 1979) and not without censure from surgeons themselves (see Ravitch, 1980).

In addition, results of this type of surgery have been mixed. Anderson, Soper, and Scott (1980) report on 41 patients who were surgically treated for obesity; thirty, of normal intelligence, averaged 17 years of age, and eleven (four girls, seven boys), retarded with Prader-Willi syndrome (see Chapter 2), averaged 13 years of age. Outcomes for the retarded children only, the younger group, will be mentioned in this chapter. Nearly all received the gastric bypass; one underwent gastroplasty (see Tapper, 1980). Criteria for surgery were capacity for normal physical activity, basic healthiness, and weight two times over the ideal; the criterion of heaviness was waived for some because Prader-Willi children will grow heavier if left untreated. In any event, the mean preoperative degree of excess weight was 231 percent. One year after surgery this figure fell 53 percent. Four years later it dropped an additional 2 percent. Thus, by the five year follow-up there was a 55 percent reduction in the original excess. This amount is, however, an average. As the authors note, their sample had failures as well as successes. A single death, over four years after surgery, occurred but was determined to be unrelated to the operation; one wound infection, the only one that occurred, was, however, related to the surgery. Nonetheless, in view of the increase in weight expected for these children, and in view of the possibly correlated shortened life expectancy, Anderson and colleagues feel optimistic about the prospects of surgical intervention.

Modifying Calorie Outgo

Although there are several ways to alter calorie intake, there is today only one way for practitioners to alter calorie expenditure: increase physical activity. Children do, of course, expend calories growing (Rose & Mayer, 1968) and living (metabolism), but physical activity is manipulable. Practitioners can modify this component of energy expenditure. And there are advantages to doing so (see Beck, Epstein, Wing, & Ossip, 1980; Brownell & Stunkard, 1980b; Court, 1977; Dwyer, Blonde, & Mayer, 1972; Mayer, 1980, Ch. 6), yet, to date, calorie restriction has received greater attention in obesity control programs for children.

Seltzer and Mayer (1970) provide a well-known exception. They showed that numerous obese youngsters in an elementary school environment profited from having their lives made more active. These children were encouraged to do such things as play soccer and volleyball, and to race for approximately one hour daily; probably as a result these youngsters held heaviness and fat increases down (see also Collipp, 1980c). They became lighter and thinner (LeBow, 1977), more so than did untreated and partially treated obese youngsters (Mayer, 1980); differences were significant for the primary school boys only; although the girls, as well as many of the older (junior high school) participants, evidenced similar trends.

Progress endured for about four years (Mayer, 1975). In part, federal funding cutbacks, however, led the school system to stop the program; a general relapse ensued, as evidenced in a checkup conducted three years later (Mayer, 1975).

Nutrition education was included in this multidisciplinary effort to help obese youngsters forestall encroaching obesity, but there was no specific diet prescribed. Combinations of formal dieting and increasing physical activity have occurred, however, in other programs; these programs have tried to simultaneously alter both terms of the negative energy equation when trying to bring about the therapeutic result (for example, Kahle, Walker, Eisenman, Behall, Hallfrisch, & Reiser, 1982; Widhalm, Maxa, & Zyman, 1978; and Ylitalo, 1981).

The Still Elusive Result

Regardless of which avenue the researcher–practitioner believes best, progress, if it occurs at all, is likely to be short-lived (Lloyd, Wolff, & Whelen, 1961; Mayer, 1975; Merritt, 1978). Anderson and colleagues' (1980) findings, though not overwhelmingly positive, are an exception to this caveat; but as Randolph (1980) notes, more data and longer follow-ups are required before radical intervention for the severely obese, the only group for which it is intended, is warranted. In general, considering all the methods discussed above, successes in treatment coexist with failures in treatment. Rarely is it clear why the results that do happen, happen. Sadly, in conclusion, none of the aforenamed avenues to creating the negative energy equation can promise the obese pediatric patient both a safe and successful journey along the road to thinness.

Measuring Obesity

Determining Fatness

Knowing if a child is fat by observing his shape requires no real training. But, as stated, not every fat child is easy to recognize, and measuring the degree of fatness and fatness-change requires more than cursory observation. Investigators, therefore, apply various techniques to do the job. One technique involves determining body weight. The assumption is that those who are too fat are too heavy, which sounds reasonable. Undoubtedly the assumption is true for some, as Mayer (1968) affirms, but as he also argues, it is false for others (Morris & Chinn, 1981; Seltzer & Mayer, 1965).

Consider two 11-year-old boys each weighing 50 kg and each standing 142 cm. One is the kind of child who plays hockey in winter, soccer in spring, swims in the summer, enjoys regular bouts of football in the fall, and loves tag, running, and hide-and-seek. He hates being still for too long; he is a mover. The other child also loves athletic contests, but his pleasure comes from watching them played on the television. He avoids contact sports. He seeks spectator sports. He plays infrequently; he is not a mover. Although these two boys are equal in weight and in height, they do not closely resemble each other in behavior. Their figures also differ. They wear different-sized pants because the sedentary boy is a good deal more corpulent than is the active boy. Their moderatly high weights, though equal, reflect different levels of fatness.

Body weight is a measure of fat and non-fat components (such as, muscle) and so may mirror the excessiveness of one or the other. A number of weight indexes are available, but research on which among them is most suitable is scanty (see Cole, Donnet, & Stanfield, 1981; DuRant & Linder, 1981); regardless of which index is used, however, when judging fatness from heaviness in children it should be remembered that the weight measure reflects the youngster's age, sex, height, and build.

Overweight, a term we have used before, is weight in excess of some ideal, some standard. The degree of excess thought of as obesity in adults and sometimes in children, too, is 20 percent (Rowe, 1980). Yet a few researchers and practitioners working in the childhood obesity area set it higher; Khan (1981), for example, puts it at over 30 pecent for those youngsters over six-years-old; he lowers it to 20 percent for those under six; Court (1979) says 20 percent is "frankly obese" (see also Neumann, 1977). Garn, Clark, and Guire (1975) challenge the validity of this 20 percent cutoff. They demonstrate that this figure, if applied to the young, might result in underestimating fatness, and if applied to the adolescent might do the opposite. Garn and associates measured degrees of fatness in samples of children, adolescents, and adults; ages, according to the authors' graph, were two years to well over seventy and fatness was reaching at least the 85th percentile on triceps skinfold (see below). The question posed was whether the measures of overweight and overfat were isomorphic. In other words, the authors asked if the overfat, as they defined fatness, were the overweight, as they defined overweight (20 percent overweight). Simply put, did fatness and heaviness correspond at the levels selected? According to Garn and co-workers, they did with adults but they did not with children and they did not with adolescents. Many obese teenagers tended to be heavier than the 20 percent overweight standard. Many obese children, in contrast, tended to be lighter.

As these data suggest, if researchers rely only on weight to select their subjects they risk excluding numbers of fat children who are not 20 percent overweight and including numbers of heavy adolescents who are not overfat. Thus, when choosing fat juveniles for a scientific enterprise, including a study on the prevalence of obesity in a population, researchers may need to use different weight standards for different age groups or, better still, they may need to make both weight and fatness assessments. Body weight, by itself, seems not to be a precise chronicler of juvenile obesity, especially as it exists in the mild to moderate ranges, for the heavy are not always that fat, and the fat are not always that heavy. But what about evaluating the effects of a treatment on those who are already said to be obese? How can change in weight show the worth of therapy?

Weight Differences

Change in weight can demonstrate the worth of therapy by showing that manipulations carried out produce desired effects. If procedures believed to produce weight losses do produce weight losses, then, provided there are proper controls in the design of the experiment, the procedures may be said to be effective. But their meaningfulness, the clinical benefits produced, remains in doubt until it is demonstrated that the weight losses are related to other positive changes, such as fat loss, blood pressure decrease, aerobic fitness increase, self-perception improvement, and school performance improvement (see Chapter 6).

One reason behaviorists have applied their methods to overweight adults is because weight-change has been considered to be a dependent variable that is both reliable and simple to obtain. It is both indeed. But its clinical import during the early days of the behavioral control of obesity—the first 10 years—has been cast aside. For children undergoing long-term care, body weight-change often is, when used by itself, an insufficient marker of progress. It is only one evaluator of a therapy, albeit a major one. No doubt its place as an important yardstick of a treatment's value is assured. Let us, therefore, look at several weight-change indices.

It is change from $time_1$, usually the start of treatment, to $time_2$, the end of treatment, to $time_n$ follow-up(s), that researchers and practitioners want to express. Several ways to do so are available. Investigators might choose to employ the weight-divided-by-height ratio; a ponderal index (see Alley et al., 1968); the body mass (Quetelet) index—that is, weight divided by height squared (see Dugdale & Lovell, 1981); or the weight-for-length index in which current weight to height is divided by expected (standard) weight to height (DuRant & Linder, 1981). Indices vary in complexity.

Kilograms-lost. This is the simplest way to express a downward change in weight. One kilogram equals 2.2 pounds; one pound equals .454 kg. Kilograms-lost is written as follows:

kilograms-lost = kg at $time_1$ - kg at $time_2$

(If the weight at $time_2$ exceeds the weight at $time_1$, there has, of course, been a gain.)

An 80 kg boy reducing to 70 kg after 30 long weeks of treatment loses 10 kg. He should feel proud of his success. Another boy, on the same regimen, starting treatment weighing 60 kg and also losing 10 kg, should likewise boast of his success with impunity. Both may have similar feelings of accomplishment, and both may receive similar compliments from family and friends, but their therapist may legitimately feel differently about their triumphs. Should the therapist wish to compare the lads according to who did better, kilograms-lost would be a poor index. One reason for this is that the accomplishments by themselves, 10 kg reductions, fail to consider the dissimilarity of the two boys' starting weights—a 20 kg dissimilarity. This difference in heaviness could have made a difference in results. Starting weights may have influenced progress. Thus, even though the heavier boy made quite an effort to reduce 10 kg, his effort was perhaps not as great as his lighter but equally tall and seemingly triumphant peer. Because the lighter have less available weight to lose (Bellack & Rozensky, 1975), they may have to struggle more to do as well as do the heavier. The lighter boy may have to make more dramatic lifestyle changes to reduce as much as the heavier. In calorie measurements, the lighter among us require less to maintain their weights and expend less doing the same exercises; in other words, in order to lose at the same rate as the heavier person, the lighter person has to take in fewer calories and has to work harder to expend as many calories.

Some Alternative Measures of Change.   Recognizing the problem of bias just articulated, the therapist might choose to determine percent of body weight lost (Gormally, Buese-Moscati, Clyman, & Forbes, 1977).

$$\text{Percent body weight lost} = \frac{\text{kg lost}}{\text{kg at time}_1} \times 100$$

Thus, the 80 kg boy who reduces 10 kg loses 12.5 percent of his body weight. His colleague, the 60 kg boy who reduces 10 kg, loses 16.6 percent of his body weight.

$$
\begin{array}{lcc}
 & \text{Boy One} & \text{Boy Two} \\
\text{Percent body weight lost} = & \dfrac{10\ \text{kg}}{80\ \text{kg}} \times 100 & \dfrac{10\ \text{kg}}{60\ \text{kg}} \times 100 \\
= & 12.5\% & 16.6\%
\end{array}
$$

Consequently, it seems that the second boy, lighter than the first one to begin with, reduced 4.1 percent more weight than did the heavier child even though each lost the same amount—10 kg. Interpreting success by measuring only percent of body weight lost shifts the bias. Now, it is against the heavier lad.

In addition to bias, a problem with each of the two preceding indexes is that they ignore variables of height, age, and sex. Granted, in the illustrations I said the two children were of equal height and the same gender. If, however, their ages differed when treatment began, the relative extent of their dilemmas could have differed too. Clinically, it is imperative to ask if treatment reduces the problem and to what extent it does so. For the overweight child, the weight aspect of this imperative translates into how much of the excess weight is eliminated by treatment's end and afterward. An index that attempts to answer is percent overweight lost, below.

$$\text{Percent overweight lost} = \frac{\text{kg lost}}{\text{kg overweight}} \times 100$$

Accordingly, if the 80 kg boy discussed above is 20 kg overweight, his progress can be expressed as a 50 percent loss in percent overweight.

$$\text{Percent overweight lost} = \frac{10 \text{ kg}}{20 \text{ kg}} \times 100 = 50 \text{ percent}$$

Notice, as the numerator of this ratio (results of treatment) approaches the denominator (the original excess), the percentage of overweight lost approaches one hundred. This yardstick, however, is not problem free either (Merritt, 1978). In contrast to what no change in weight means for an adult, no change in weight may still indicate some progress for a child. The youngster is, for instance, growing linearly; the adult is not. Therefore, the child's degree of overweight may change in time, even if his weight stays constant. The percent overweight lost measure fails to reflect the overweight, overtime change that may occur without alterations in actual weight.

One index that does consider overweight change across time, is written as the difference between two ratios.

$$\text{Change in percent overweight} = \left[\frac{\text{kg at time}_1}{\text{ideal kg at time}_1} - \frac{\text{kg at time}_2}{\text{ideal kg at time}_2}\right] \times 100$$

If the 80 kg boy is 20 kg overweight, his ideal weight at the start of treatment is 60 kg. Let's say that ideal weight for him at the end of treatment is 65 kg. If he loses 10 kg, he sustains a 25 percent reduction in overweight. His degree of overweight, in other words, has changed by 25 percent from time$_1$ to time $_2$; any two times (for example, the start of treatment and follow-up) can be used. The 60 kg boy, to go on with the illustration, is only 15 kg overweight at the beginning of treatment and not overweight at all after losing 10 kg by its end. Therefore, he has changed 33 percent in overweight. Arithmetically:

$$\begin{array}{c} \text{Boy One} \\ \text{Change in percent overweight} = \left[\frac{80 \text{ kg}}{60 \text{ kg}} - \frac{80 \text{ kg} - 10 \text{ kg}}{65 \text{ kg}}\right] \times 100 \\ = (1.33 - 1.08) \times 100 \\ = 25\% \end{array}$$

$$\begin{array}{c} \text{Boy Two} \\ \text{Change in percent overweight} = \left[\frac{60 \text{ kg}}{45 \text{ kg}} - \frac{60 \text{ kg} - 10 \text{ kg}}{50 \text{ kg}}\right] \times 100 \\ = (1.33 - 1.00) \times 100 \\ = 33\% \end{array}$$

There is an eight percent difference between the two patients in percent overweight change. Both boys lose the same number of kilograms, but the lighter one changes more in percentage overweight, overtime. Of the two children, he may be the better off at the finish of treatment because he is no longer overweight at all. However, whether or not he has outperformed the heavier child, whether the methods of therapy have been better suited to him, is debatable.

Comparing actual to expected weight at some designated time following intervention in order to say what the weight alterations, post-treatment to follow-up, mean is similar to indexing change in percent overweight. Kingsley and Shapiro (1977), for instance, compared the weight changes they expected, obtained by using weight tables, to those they actually witnessed. They made the comparison in order to learn about the extent of gaining above expectancy; they found normal increases over time. In other words, they found that after-intervention-gaining was not indicative of relapse.

Apropos of this type of evaluation, Edwards (1978) offered the weight index. He computed it by subtracting the ratio of standard weight to standard height from a child's present weight-to-height ratio. Standards are the population of youngsters of the same age, sex, and height as the treated youngster; Edwards used norms modified from Guthrie (1975). The ratio is written in the way following:

$$\text{Weight index} = \frac{\text{Present weight}}{\text{Present height}} - \frac{\text{Standard weight}}{\text{Standard height}}$$

A result of zero means that growth in height and weight of any one child is, as Edwards noted, perfect at the time the measurement is made. Despite failure to consider lean body weight versus fat weight (Foreyt & Goodrick, 1981), and despite being a derived measure that does not substitute for naming starting and ending weights and heights (Coates & Thoresen, 1980), the weight index has value. Edwards demonstrated its value (Alley et al., 1968; also see Application 5, Chapter 5).

The Change Towards Ideal.   The previous three formulas require setting desirable (ideal) weights. Determining a specific ideal weight, however, is not easy. Actually, it may be even harder to determine a child's ideal weight than that of an adult because the variability among growing children is so pronounced (Khan, 1981). Mahoney (1975b) offers linear equations for adults that give approximations to Department of Agriculture norms of desirable weights. He suggests that a man's ideal weight could be determined by multiplying height in inches by four and then subtracting 130. A woman's ideal weight could be similarly determined except the height multiplier is 3.5 and the subtrahend is 110. Johnson (1979) reviews a formula for determining ideal weights of children. He advises allowing 4.5 kg in weight per 30.5 cm in height up to 121.9 cm and then add 2.3 kg for each 2.54 cm up to 152.4 cm.

A more popular method than those above is to set ideal weights from published standards—charts supplying norms. For adults, those most frequently used are the *Metropolitan Life Insurance Tables of 1959;* these are derived from the *Build and Blood Pressure Study* of the same year; a new data base now exists (Society of Actuaries, 1980). The procedure is to select an ideal weight from the table of desirable weights for men and women 25 years of age and older. This is simple and straightforward, yet the results may give patient and therapist unrealistic and inaccurate objectives. One reason they may do so is that the charted weights derive from a nonrandom sample of the population (Seltzer, 1965; Seltzer & Mayer, 1967); norms may understate ideal weights resulting in erroneous mortality estimates (Andres, 1980). Another reason is that the tables give no directions for categorizing patients' frame sizes; desirable weights vary with not only height but size of frame.

There are also standards charts for children. Weil (1977) cites six of these charts noting that none is problem-free. Most often, the NCHS (National Center for Health Statistics) norms are the ones used (Rowe, 1980). They supply cross-sectional data obtained between 1963 and 1974 on youths, two to eighteen years of age. Among the drawbacks with the NCHS charts are failure to discriminate the fat and non-fat components of body weight (DuRant & Linder, 1981; Rowe, 1980), failure to account for geographical setting and race (Rowe, 1980), and failure to say, as suggested earlier (Garn et al., 1975), which weight level is excessive (Rowe, 1980). Furthermore, the percentile rankings given by the NCHS tables fail to reflect the weight changes of those youngsters who are extremely heavy (DuRant & Linder, 1981). Nevertheless, the charts usually allow researchers and practitioners to track the progress of most of the patients they see. (I have, therefore, included an updated version of these norms in Appendix D.)

Using NCHS growth curves, Foreyt and Goodrick (1981) set goal weight as the median weight of youngsters who are, in height, sex, and age, like the child to be treated; percent overweight is then computed as the ratio of starting weight to goal weight, goal weight could change over time, multiplied by one hundred. At the present level of our knowledge, this is a useful practice.

Another useful practice is to provide as much raw data as possible when publishing research or presenting case presentations. Needed are weights, heights, and ages at times$_1$ - n on each boy and girl receiving an intervention. Rate of loss data and dropout figures also need to be readily available, as should precise descriptions of which height–weight standards are used and how overweight, ideal weight, and change of overweight are determined. Information must be comprehensive if investigators and clinicians are to compare treatments (see Bellack & Rozensky, 1975; Gormally et al., 1977).

As seen, a vast array of weight measures exist. All of them can determine how much lighter a child is after therapy, but none indicate how much thinner he has become; that is the purpose of the measures described below.

Fatness Differences

Like tracking changes in weight, the problem of tracking changes in fatness is addressed by serial measurement—measurement before, during, and after treatment. The problem of deciding if a child is too fat in the first place (see Barker, 1976; Siddamma & Venkatramaiah, 1977), and if he is still too fat after part or all of treatment has been attempted is, to some degree, the problem of finding norms. The question of "too fat" is parried by "too fat for what," and this response is often answered by something close to "fatter than peers."

Each of the problems, therefore, involves measurement. The most precise way to assess fatness—how fat anyone of a specific age and race is—is through autopsy, not a tool of the therapist, to be sure. Less drastic and less direct are injecting fat-soluble gases (for example, cyclopropane); weighing in and out of water, making certain to correct for residual air in the lungs and intestines (densitometry); applying the total body potassium method; using ultrasound; and employing soft-tissue radiography (see Garrow, 1982). These techniques are, however, complex, time consuming, and some are seen as unsuitable for children (VanGelderen, 1976).

Nonetheless, mounting a program of fatness-change requires that investigators and clinicians measure fatness; as discussed, heaviness is not necessarily fatness, lightness is not necessarily the absence of fatness, and weighing is not *the* solution. Therefore, a simple way to estimate fatness changes over time is needed. One method, indirect and criticized for its poor reliability when applied to the individual (Steel, 1977; Stuart, Mitchell, & Jensen, 1981) and for not being as good as using areas of fat in estimating body fat (Frisancho, 1981) is the skinfold determination method (see Lohman, 1981; Owen, 1982).

Skinfold Determinations. The working assumption underlying the skinfold measurement is that a constant proportion of fat (50 percent, for example) is laid down just beneath the skin (Seltzer & Mayer, 1965); there is disagreement, however, regarding the extent this amount varies as a function of age, sex, and degree of obesity (see Bray, 1976; Durnin & Womersley, 1974). Standards for the triceps and subscapular sites, two often-measured sites (Schwartz, 1979), are available (Tanner & Whitehouse, 1975). Mainly, however, it is the triceps site for which values exist (Frisancho, 1974; 1981; Lauer, Connor, Leaverton, Reiter, & Clarke, 1975; Seltzer & Mayer, 1965; Appendix E); yet tables unbiased with respect to major variables, such as race, are hard to come by (DuRant & Linder, 1981). Abstracted from Seltzer and Mayer (1965), Table 1.1 contains a frequently employed set of norms (Foreyt & Goodrick, 1981). It portrays the minimum triceps skinfolds signifying obesity in Caucasian boys and girls from five to eighteen years of age.

To measure skinfolds one needs uniform procedures. Seltzer and Mayer (1965) offer the following instructions:

Table 1.1
Obesity Standards in Caucasian American Juveniles

Age (Years)	Minimum triceps skinfold thickness indicating obesity (mm)	
	Males	Females
5	12	14
6	12	15
7	13	16
8	14	17
9	15	18
10	16	20
11	17	21
12	18	22
13	18	23
14	17	23
15	16	24
16	15	25
17	14	26
18	15	27

The skinfold measurement to be obtained is the (doubled) thickness of the pinched 'folded' skin plus the attached subcutaneous adipose tissue. The person making the measurement pinches up a full fold of skin and subcutaneous tissue with the thumb and forefinger of his left hand at a distance about 1 cm from the site at which the calipers are to be placed, pulling the fold away from the underlying muscle. The fold is pinched up firmly and held while the measurement is being taken. The calipers are applied to the fold about 1 cm below the fingers, so that the pressure on the fold at the point measured is exerted by the faces of the caliper and not by the fingers. The handle of the caliper is released to permit the full force of the caliper arm pressure, and the dial is read to the nearest 0.5 mm. Caliper application should be made at least twice for stable readings. If the folds are extremely thick, dial readings should be made three seconds after applying the caliper pressure.[*]

[*]From C. C. Seltzer and J. Mayer, "A simple criterion of obesity," *Postgraduate Medicine, 38* (1965), p. A104. Copyright © 1965 by McGraw-Hill. Reprinted by permission of the publisher.

Grimes and Franzini (1977) add the following specific directives for the triceps and subscapular sites:

Triceps Site. Taken over the mid-point of the muscle belly, midway between the olecranon (elbow) and the tip of the acromion (the highest point of the shoulder), with the upper arm hanging vertically (Edwards et al., 1955). Note: If the examiner suspects that the triceps muscle has been pinched up with the fatfold, the subject should stiffen the arm (to define the muscle) and then relax it for the measurement. The mid-point of this site should be measured and marked with a felt pen, since subcutaneous fat varies considerably in this area.

Subscapular Site. Taken 3–5 cm on a line from the inferior angle (bottom tip) of the scapula (the flat triangular bone in the back of the shoulder) at an angle of about 45° to the vertical with the patient's shoulder and arm relaxed. Seltzer and Mayer (1965) suggest that this skinfold be taken 'in a line slightly inclined in the natural cleavage of the skin.'[*]

Furthermore, researchers and practitioners should use a caliper that exerts a constant pressure at the measurement site equalling 10 g/mm^2 (Seltzer & Mayer, 1965); either the Lange, manufactured in the United States, or the Harpenden, manufactured in England, will suffice (see also Rowe, 1980 for a description of Ross Laboratories' Adipometer). Practice in using these devices is essential. So also is replication of the procedures employed essential when making serial assessments over time on one or more children. When using published standards, choose the side of the body from which the standards are derived; Durnin and Womersley (1974), however, report no major effect resulting from side of body in their study of adults. Furthermore, it is wise to mark the place to be pinched before applying the caliper; use a tape and felt-tip pen. Also, it is advisable to take multiple measurements at each assessment. Grimes and Franzini advise a third measurement only if the first two disagree by more than 5 percent, but note that too many attempts to gauge the same site may result in low values; moreover they recommend, as do Seltzer & Mayer, waiting a short period after the caliper is applied to obtain accurate readings—counting 1000, 2000, 3000 eliminates the necessity of having a clock.

Agreement is needed on how to measure skinfolds in children and adolescents to make comparisons among studies possible. Also needed are tables that sum up various skinfolds into estimates of percentage body weight that is fat (for example, Durnin & Womersley, 1974, for adults). Such data would permit the development of obesity modification scores for youngsters analogous to the relative fatness change score (Relfatch), which has been reported by Mahoney, Rogers, Straw, and Mahoney (1977), for use with adults.

[*]From W. B. Grimes and L. R. Franzini, "Skinfold measurement techniques for estimating percentage body fat," *Journal of Behavior Therapy and Experimental Psychiatry*, 8 (1977), p. 67. Copyright © 1977 by Pergamon Press, Inc. Reprinted by permission of the publisher.

At present, in order to estimate change in fatness, investigators may tabulate the actual skinfold thickness differences over several intervals separated by no, one, or more interventions. These measurements should be supplemented by others, such as circumference changes in thighs, arms, hips, and waist (Bray, Greenway, Molitch, Dahms, Atkinson, & Hamilton, 1978; also see Table 5.4), assessed using reliable tape measures.

On the whole, the practices discussed above are relatively easy to carry out. Yet as indicated, they are usually not seen in obesity-change programs. Fatness determinations are lacking in treatment regimens for both adults and children. To rectify this deficit, researchers and practitioners will have to more routinely couple fatness-change measurements with the weight-change ones that they customarily provide. This will move us one step closer to a comprehensive understanding of the kinds of effects a particular treatment is capable of producing.

CHAPTER 2

The Epidemiology and Natural History of Childhood Obesity

Chapter 1 described and measured fatness and heaviness in children and surveyed some of the treatments. In this chapter, while I remain cognizant of the fact that standards of measurement influence what is said about obesity in children, I will examine prevalence, connections, and concomitants. In the studies to follow the terms obese and overweight are often used synonomously, overweight becoming the measure of overfatness; usually, however, it is obesity that is of the greatest interest.

Prevalence

How many obese youngsters are there? Estimates vary. Thus, Jones (1972) says that 10 percent of British school children are too heavy; Craddock (1978) puts the figure at 5 to 15 percent. Lloyd and Wolff (1980) set it at somewhere between 2 and 6 percent; Grinker (1981) estimates 10 to 13 percent for children in the United States; Khan (1981) cites 10 to 40 percent; Powers (1980), 6 to 15 percent; and Ferguson (1981), 25 percent. Ditschunheit, Jons, and Englehardt (1978), measuring 7000 West German school children, report that almost 8 percent are overweight; boys outnumber girls. Simić (1980), quoting his own work with several thousand Yugoslavian youngsters from the country and the city, finds rates of overweight to be close to 5 percent (see Buchberger, 1977 for rural and urban Swiss children). Other studies, some on infants (see Myres & Yeung, 1979 for a summary), children and adolescents may be found to similarly vary in proposed estimates (for example, Abraham & Nordsieck, 1960; Fisch, Bilek, & Ulstrom, 1975; Hathaway & Sargent, 1962; Howard et al., 1971; Laurer, Connor, Leaverton, Reiter, & Clarke, 1975; Takahashi, 1979).

Why the variability? In general, it is because study populations and obesity definitions vary. Thus, differences may emerge because of how rich or poor the children's families are (Arteaga, DosSantos, & Dutra de Oliviera, 1982); what race the children are; whether they are physically handicapped (Guy, 1978); where they live (Garn, Clark, & Guire, 1975); where they have emigrated (Ramirez &

Mueller, 1980); age, sex, and whether relative weight is the measure used (DuRant, Martin, Linder, & Weston, 1980; Kohrs, Wang, Ekland, Paulsen, & O'Neal, 1979); whether skinfold is the measure (Stunkard, d'Aquili, Fox, & Filion, 1972); or whether it is a combination of the two (Sgaramella, Jayakar, Galante, & Pennetti, 1979; Thomson & Cruickshank, 1979); and, finally, differences may emerge because different cutoff points, criteria for obesity, are employed.

Regarding criteria, obese using one set of standards is not always defined as obese by another (Garn et al., 1975). Investigating a sample of British school children ages 6 to 14, Colley (1974) reported the percentages of youngsters at each age having triceps skinfolds greater than 20 mm and those having triceps skinfolds greater than 25 mm; he measured 1241 boys and 1181 girls. For each skinfold-thickness criterion, higher percentages of girls in comparison to boys (except 7-year-old girls using the 25 mm criterion) exceeded the cutoff points; sex differences in fatness became larger as age increased (see Brownell & Stunkard, 1980a). Over 4 percent of the 10-year-old boys exceeded the 20 mm criterion; under 4 percent exceeded the 25 mm criterion. More dramatic were the differences for 10-year-old girls. Just over 16 percent exceeded the lower obesity criterion, but only 3.8 percent exceeded the higher level. Hence, in this study, as would be expected in general, the higher the cutoff point for obesity, the lower the prevalence of obesity.

Likewise, Stunkard and associates (1972) found different rates of prevalence with different obesity criteria. They took fatness measurements—triceps skinfolds—on more than 3300 Caucasian children, ages 5 to 18. One criterion of obesity, an empirically derived reading, represented the top 10 percent of each sex with the thickest fatfolds obtained with Lange calipers; for boys this was 18 mm whereas for girls it was 23 mm. The second criterion involved the norms of Seltzer and Mayer (1965), presented in Table 1.1. Judging obesity in the 6-year-old group by the first criterion—the percentile criterion—the authors discovered that 8 percent of the girls from the lower socioeconomic classes were obese; none from the upper classes were. By the second criterion, however, 21 percent more of the lower class girls and 3 percent more of those in the upper class were obese. Similarly, prevalence of obesity in boys from different socioeconomic groupings differed with the different obesity standards applied. For the 6-year-olds, about 11 percent from the lower classes and none from the upper were obese when the percentile criterion was used. By the Seltzer and Mayer criterion, however, about 40 percent from the lower classes and 25 percent from the upper classes were obese.

In sum, prevalence rates will vary with the use of different investigative practices, different definitions of the problem, and different characteristics of the populations. The epidemiology of childhood obesity, as a topic of research, is fraught with such differences.

Connections

The multiple causes of obesity bespeak the mix of the factors about to be discussed. In this discussion correlational analysis is used, for causal linkages in the natural history of childhood obesity are rarely statable; indeed it is only when we are dealing with the scarcer forms of obesity, for example those wherein genetic factors clearly predominate, that we may move noticeably closer to causation.

Class, Race and Family Connections

Where do we find the fat children in society? The answer is unclear. Demographic data that link prevalence with affluence locate the obese child sometimes in poor families, but not too poor, and sometimes in middle-income families. Stunkard and colleagues (Goldblatt, Moore, & Stunkard, 1965; Moore, Stunkard, & Srole, 1962) have pioneered in documenting the association between social class and obesity; they show in the Midtown Manhattan Study (Srole, Langner, Michael, Opler, & Rennie, 1962) a relationship between these variables that is strongest for the adult female. The obese, as measured by weight for height, have a lower socioeconomic status (income, occupation, rent) than do the nonobese.

Stunkard et al. (1972), as discussed above, essentially replicated this finding in Caucasian children. Using triceps skinfold estimates of fatness, the aforenamed percentile and Seltzer and Mayer (Table 1.1) criteria of obesity, and a measure of socioeconomic status based on the father's occupation, Stunkard and co-workers demonstrated that by the age of 6, dramatic differences were prevalent; this was especially so for girls. For them, obesity was nine times more prevalent in the lower socioeconomic groupings (see also Ginsberg-Fellner, Jagendorf, Carmel, & Harris, 1981).

But these girls, and boys, too—boys showed similar but less marked class–obesity associations—resided in eastern U.S. cities. Poverty for these youngsters might not be considered poverty for others. Garb, Garb, and Stunkard (1975) developed this idea in their study of 613, 6 to 12-year-old Navaho children on whom they collected triceps skinfold information. They analyzed results for the 527 youngsters who, on the basis of a seven point index of acculturation, fell into the higher and lower classes—criteria of income, occupation, and education were inapplicable. Using the acculturation measure of social class affiliation, they found that the less acculturated—those children living at subsistence levels—were the less fat; the poorer, then, were the thinner.

According to Garb and colleagues, these data do not gainsay the earlier findings on social class and obesity. Rather, they add to them. Postulating a skewed and inverted U-shape relationship to describe the prevalence of obesity, the authors imply that the very poor are like the very rich, and that the acculturated Navaho resembles the lower-class city child (see also Arteaga et al., 1982).

Garn and associates would agree that the poor are the thinner, but unlike the

Stunkard and co-workers' (1972) study, the thinner for Garn and associates are predominantly lower-class urban-dwelling children. Data from the Ten State Nutrition Study (TSNS) (Garn & Clarke, 1975)—a cross-sectional survey of over 40,000 persons, 16,000 of whom are in the pediatric age range—the Preschool Nutrition Survey (Garn et al., 1975), and the Techumseh Community Health Survey (Garn, Hopkins, & Ryan, 1981) articulate class-fatness relationships; they compare triceps skinfold of children with per capita income and income-to-needs ratios of families. TSNS data strongly indicate that greater numbers of obese, taller, and heavier youngsters are more affluent than are their opposites; fatter children come from median-income families. Regardless of income levels, girls are more corpulent than are boys at all ages, but as the girls grow older, income levels appear to become part of a changing picture. During adolescence the poorer seem to become fatter and, although the data are cross-sectional, there is a strong suggestion that they stay that way during adulthood. Not so the richer. As adults, they are thinner. Garn and associates call this phenomenon an "income related reversal of relative fatness."

Using the Techumseh longitudinal data, Garn and colleagues (1981) corroborated this income to fatness notion. They followed up 564 girls and an almost equivalent number of boys for 18 years. Both sexes revealed a differential fatness change (skinfolds) that was related to income. Comparing gains in fatness over time, the authors found that the poorer put on more fat that did the richer. Thus, as adults, the poorer became the fatter; while as children, they had not been that way. Likewise, Huenemann's (1974a) results showed that the fat at six months of age were not necessarily economically disadvantaged.

Her study illuminates another population characteristic that seems to be connected with childhood obesity—race. More of the obese children in her study are Oriental as opposed to Caucasian or Black. According to Garn and colleagues (1975), Blacks seem to be fatter than Whites initially—in infancy—but not in childhood. Moreover, Blacks with higher incomes are fatter than are poorer Blacks, just as Whites from higher economic groupings are fatter than poorer Whites. Foster, Voors, Webber, Frerichs, & Berenson (1977) find in the Bogalusa Heart Study data on over 3500 juveniles ages 5 and up, that White children (about 2150) have thicker triceps skinfolds—2.5 mm thicker—than those of their Black counterparts (about 1350).

It is possible that these racial comparisons were affected by socioeconomic status. DuRant et al. (1980) indicated that more than 45 percent of the Black children in the Foster study were members of economically disadvantaged families—families having incomes below the poverty level. Only about 16 percent of the White youths, however, were that poor. Accordingly, perhaps the fatness differences in that study reflected to some extent the socioeconomic differences that existed. DuRant and associates, in their investigation of obesity among Whites and Blacks, attempted to avoid this potential bias; they sampled only from low-income families. Using the weight-for-length index (see Chapter 1) and establishing obesity, overweight, and thinness criteria based on this index, they measured 1830 youths, over 1600 Blacks and 220 Whites; some of the children were younger than one year of age and some were older than 17. The authors found that a lower percentage of Blacks compared with Whites were obese—Black males least, Black females next but differing less definitely from the two remaining groups. A different picture emerged for the overweight and thin categories and showed once again that category of excess in a study had influenced outcomes. Whereas higher percentages of Whites than Blacks fell into the obese grouping, lower percentages fell into the overweight one; and a greater percentage of Whites fell into the thin classification.

Also trying to remove the potential bias of income level on the race to fatness comparison, Garn and Clark (1976) showed in the TSNS data that, as stated above, Blacks were fatter than were Whites in infancy, and then they changed. Whites, as a group, became fatter. From ages 4 to 90, males stayed fatter, but not females. They switched again at about the end of adolescence—White women tended to become less corpulent than did Black women.

These economic and racial connections to fatness development and outright obesity in children are intriguing, to be sure. Equally fascinating are the familial connections. But, just as in studies on socioeconomic and racial involvements, studies on family-line connections are often perplexing. At times they are inconsistent. Sgaramella, Galante, Jayakar, and Pennetti (1980), investigating 2044 Northern Italian families, found that familial linkages with childhood obesity are weak (cf. Ravelli & Belmont, 1979). Likewise Keller, Colley, and Carpenter (1979), using the Colley (1974) data described earlier, report little similarity in degree of obesity between parents and children. As they note, however, obesity information on mothers and fathers (excessive weight for height) is questionnaire data; it may be inaccurate. Nevertheless, their study suggests that the parents of the heavy child may not, at the time they are measured anyway, be heavy too. Differently stated, but in keeping with the Keller and co-authors' results and commentary, overweight in mothers and fathers only weakly predicts excess weight and excess fat in children, although parents probably influence how fat their children are.

Mayer (1975) most likely would agree with the last part of this conclusion. He describes a strong influence. The probability of having a fat child rises with parental fatness from 7 percent if both parents are of normal weight, to 40 percent if one parent is obese, to 80 percent if two parents are obese (see also, Farrell, Layton, Ford, & Tervo, 1981 for handicapped children; Huenemann, 1974a; Kowalczyk, 1976; Simić 1980; Wilkinson et al., 1977b).

Garn and Clark (1976) corroborate the trend that Mayer proposes: The fat beget the fatter. TSNS data, nearly 21,000 parent–child pairs and nearly 30,000 sibling pairs, reveal familial connections. Lean parents tend to have leaner youngsters. Obese parents tend to have fatter ones. Even if only one parent is corpulent—it matters little which parent that is—the child's corpulence is significantly affected.

Moreover, obese children with brothers and sisters tend to have obese brothers and sisters (cf. Sgaramella et al., 1980). Garn and Clark (1976) write of families with three children, "There is an 80 percent chance that at least one of the two siblings of an obese child will also be obese" (pp. 452–453). The family environment is shared. Support for the concept that the obese are likely to share their environment with other obese family members comes from the Tecumseh project. Corroboration is based on the results obtained from more than 2900, four-member families—over 11,000 persons. Garn, Bailey, Solomon, & Hopkins (1981) note that, unlike the situation in which there are three nonobese members, the probability of finding an obese fourth is high if the other three are obese; the probability jumps from 13 percent to greater than 40%.

Thus far we found that class, racial, and family variables influence obesity in children; that connections exist is indisputable. But the prediction equations that unscramble the foregoing data—equations that enable us to forecast with accuracy which children from which families will be obese—are still unattainable. There are still unknowns (see Rona & Chinn, 1982). Disagreements still exist among the outcomes of the studies. Investigators still differ in how they define obesity and in how they measure many of the variables to which they believe it may be linked.

Prenatal Connections

Moving away from possible social, racial, and familial contributors, we may ask about the environment of the fetus and the ways that this environment connects with childhood obesity. We cannot, however, move too far afield of these other contributors, for they frequently influence what the expectant woman does during her pregnancy. Her actions during pregnancy may well affect the environment in which the fetus develops. The fashion-conscious pregnant woman, for instance, who starts her pregnancy slightly overweight, may restrict her calories in order to attenuate the level of gaining she expects and the post-pregnancy weight-loss difficulties she fears. By doing so she creates an abnormal environment for the fetus and possibly impairs its neurologic development as well as its intelligence (Berendez, 1975; Churchill & Berendez, 1969). Moreover, by doing so she possibly increases the risk of having a low birth weight infant, and that in turn would increase the risk of perinatal morbidity and mortality (Powers, 1980). The economically disadvantaged woman living in a developing country, forced by circumstance to consume carbohydrates excessively and protein deficiently, may dramatically elevate the chances of having an obese infant (DeSchampheleire, Parent, & Chatteur, 1980). Prenatal practices and the factors discussed in the previous section are related.

Remaining cognizant of this relationship, let us nevertheless limit inquiry here to two frequently studied variables affecting the environment of the fetus: mother's weight and her weight gain during pregnancy. The outcome that most of the studies are interested in when investigating them has to do with the infant's weight at birth.

Gross, Sokol, and King's (1980) investigation deals with the first variable—weight of the mother. In over 2000 pregnant women, more than 10 percent of whom weighed in excess of 90 kg, they studied labor complications and birth weights. Although problems during labor were fewer than those seen in past studies, the weight of mother to weight of the baby relationship was, as has often been found (Simić, 1980): Heavy women give birth to heavy babies (see also Whitelaw, 1976 on skinfolds). Furthermore in the Gross (1980) study, the likelihood of heavy women bearing infants who were large for gestational age was great; also great were the chances of these women delivering post-term. Further, almost 10 percent of the overweight mothers compared with just under 4 percent of the nonoverweight ones, a significant difference, gained below recommended levels during pregnancy. It is therefore remarkable, as the authors point out, that despite reasons militating against its happening (for example, gaining poorly) significantly more overweight mothers gave birth to heavier babies.

Repeating this finding, Harrison, Udall, and Morrow (1980) first enumerated 249 nonobese, 54 moderately obese, and 24 massively obese women. They applied percent overweight criteria to assess obesity; for example, they called those women who were 50 percent over standard weight massively obese. Their report on the 327 women they identified was based on data obtained over a two year period and combined the results of separate investigations. They found that of those women said to be massively obese who, in addition, gained inadequately during pregnancy, 75 percent in fact lost weight. Yet they also found that the risk of a massively obese woman bearing an infant whose weight at birth was elevated, an infant weighing over 4 kg, was more than 30 percent; this risk was significantly higher than that for women weighing appreciably less (see also Edwards, Dickes, Alton, & Hakanson, 1978). I have not said that heavy women give birth to obese infants, for neither heaviness nor largeness at birth unequivocally produces obesity at birth (Edwards, et al., 1978; Lloyd, 1977; Udall et al., 1978). But, as indicated, there is substantial evidence that pre-pregnancy weight of the mother and birth weight of the baby are correlated (see also Peckham & Christianson, 1971).

What role might weight gain during pregnancy have in this correlation? Apparently inadequate gaining, though undesirable in terms of fetal development (because it will possibly mar neurologic development) does not, if the gravida is extremely overweight, lead to low birth weight babies. Greater than adequate gaining—gains that markedly exceed the approximately 11 kg (Powers, 1980) that is expected—has other effects (Lloyd & Wolff, 1980; Niswander & Jackson, 1974; Simpson, Lawless, & Mitchell, 1975). To illustrate, Udall and co-workers (1978) scrutinized the weight-gaining histories of 109 mothers, 33 of whom, based on degree of overweight (20 percent overweight) before pregnancy, were labeled obese. Heavier mothers gave birth to infants categorized as large for gestational age. Lighter mothers had babies categorized as appropriate for gestational age. More important to the issue at hand, however, Udall and co-workers compared weight increases of the mother during pregnancy with skinfold thicknesses, in eight sites, of infants. The association was clear: Mothers gaining a great deal of weight, greater than 18 kg, were quite likely to have heavier babies who were also fatter than babies born of mothers gaining much less weight.

Does it matter when during pregnancy the gaining occurs? It occurs throughout, but customarily the 11 kg gain is divided unequally among the three trimesters: weight increases less during the first trimester—about 9 kg less—than during the two remaining (Powers, 1980). When this pattern of weight change is disrupted, consequences befall the fetus. Some of these may effect the development of obesity.

Ravelli, Stein, and Susser (1976) attempted to explain this phenomenon. They surveyed the medical records of hundreds of thousands of 19-year-old men undergoing induction into the Dutch military to ascertain how many of them were obese (20 percent overweight). They asked further how many of them were exposed to the Dutch Famine of 1944 to 1945 and, critically, when these men were exposed, in utero. It seems that period of exposure effected prevalence of obesity. Groups starved during the first two trimesters showed higher obesity rates after 19 years than did those starved during the third trimester and initial three to five months of infancy. Comparisons were made to unstarved controls, males conceived and born after the famine. To account for these results, Ravelli and associates, invoked the fat-cell proliferation theory (see below) and the notion that malnutrition caused disordered hypothalamic function. Admittedly speculating, they suggested that starvation during the last trimester and early infancy possibly caused restricted fat-cell development and by so doing led to lower obesity rates later on. Starvation before the last trimester, in contrast, caused developmental problems in centers regulating food intake and growth; as a result, once food became more plentiful, appetite and obesity problems arose (Hawk, 1977).

Whatever the mechanism, it appears that life in utero affects future weight status. Excepting Ravelli and colleagues' study, the period of concern in this section of the chapter has been infancy. Let us now look more closely at what has been implied by the investigations of the association between prenatal practices and birth weight to see whether high birth-weight babies really do run a grave risk of becoming obese children. Also, more generally, let us look at whether and when overweight (obesity) in childhood foretells subsequent overweight (obesity) in childhood.

Early Excess, Later Excess Connections

Not many reports can state reliably that fat babies are destined to become fat children. For not many researchers make birth to $time_2$ to $time_3$ to $time_n$ fatness comparisons that apply more than weight criteria to estimate corpulence. There are, however, studies indicating that heavy babies are, more than are light or average babies, candidates for the status of heavy children (Börjeson, 1962;

Illingsworth, Harvey, & Gin, 1949; Mossberg, 1948). There are other reports indicating that they are not candidates (Dorner, Grychtolik, & Julitz, 1977; Committee on Nutrition, 1978). In a phrase, disagreement exists.

Fisch and colleagues (1975) assessed overweight and overweight change, dividing weight by height, in a sample of 1786 babies. They labeled about 5.4 percent (96) of them as "very obese" because when born these infants exceeded the 95th percentile in weight for height. Longitudinally following these overweight babies, the authors determined relative weights at 4 and 7. Of those measured at age 4 (22 were not), 26 percent still were at or above the 90th percentile; more than twice that many were at or above the 70th percentile. Of those measured three years afterwards (all but one child), nearly 20 percent were above the 90th percentile and well over 55 percent were above the 70th percentile. Thus, some overweight newborns remain overweight; the number depends on the measures and criteria used. Clearly, though, many overweight newborns do not, by any standard measures and criteria, remain overweight. Moreover, as Fisch and co-workers noted, overweight in childhood does not necessarily reflect the presence of overweight at birth; more than a few of the overweight 4-year-olds in their study had no history of being overweight newborns. Categories of weight status shift over time.

Also illustrating this shift in weight category, Dine, Gartside, Glueck, Rheines, Greene, & Khoury (1979) further suggest that as the measurement interval increases, the proportion of children staying heavy decreases. Dine and co-workers followed 476 children from birth to age 5 and calculated weights, heights, and various relative weight indices incorporating these measures. They discovered, starting with the fifth year, a continuously decreasing percentage of heavy children, those at or above the 90th percentile; that is, 77 percent of the very heavy 5-year-olds were very heavy at age 4, but only 50 percent were that heavy at age 2, and even less, 19 percent at birth. Looking in the opposite direction—younger to older—Fisch and colleagues showed that overweight at age 4 had portended overweight at age 7 far better than had overweight at birth; more than 75 percent of the very heavy 4-year-olds had become very heavy 7-year-olds (see Wilkinson, et al., 1977b). Therefore, once again, it seems that predicting whether or not a child of a specific age will be overweight becomes more difficult as the time between data collections lengthens.

The first data collection may occur at a period later than immediately following birth. Using information from infant welfare centers in England, Asher (1966) compared the time$_1$ weights of 137 children (the six-month weights) with time$_2$ weights (3 to 5 years of age). Almost half of the overweight six-month-olds were overweight at the second assessment. In contrast, fewer than 7 percent of the 105 children not overweight at six months were overweight at the later measurement. Evaluating 269 other overweight youngsters—those in treatment for obesity—she found that 44 percent of them had been overweight infants. And, finally, comparing school children who had been above the 97th percentile between the ages of six months and one year with those not overweight at these times, she noted that significantly more of the overweight-as-infants group were heavier as children. Asher, therefore, sees heaviness early in life as presaging heaviness later in childhood. In her words, "Overweight children cannot be counted on to 'grow out of' their obesity" (p. 673). Similarly, Lloyd (1977) points out that even though most overweight infants do become normal-weight children, many, about 20 percent, do not (see also Brook, Lloyd, & Wolff, 1972; Court & Dunlop, 1975; Eid, 1970).

Is overweight during infancy a significant danger sign of childhood obesity? Clearly, not all researchers think that it is (Dine et al., 1979; Golden, 1979; Myres & Yeung, 1979; Neyzi, Saner, Binyildiz, Yazicioglu, Emre, & Gurson, 1976; Poskitt, 1977). Sveger (1978), studying Swedish children, found that only 13 percent of obese infants, obese on a weight-for-length measure, are obese at 4 years of age. Poskitt and Cole (1977), in an investigation of weight- and skinfold-change (four sites), show that the obese infant stands a greater chance of becoming overweight at age 5 than he does of becoming obese at that time. Their report, a follow-up of the 300 infants originally evaluated by Shukla, Forsyth, Anderson, and Marwah (1972) yields $time_1$ to $time_2$ body-type data on 68 percent of the original sample—$time_1$ is infancy, $time_2$ is about age 5. There is a 33.3 percent chance that an obese infant will become an overweight child, but only about an 11 percent chance that he or she will remain obese. Nonetheless, the tendency to stay overweight may, as the authors speculate, foreshadow subsequent obesity—the obese infant who becomes the overweight child may become obese in the future.

Rather than weight during infancy, perhaps rate of weight gain during this period is a main danger sign of childhood obesity (Dorner, et al., 1977). Eid (1970) says it is. He separated his sample of infants into rapid, average, and slow gainers by tabulating how much weight they put on during the first six weeks, three months, and six months following birth. He then examined these children when they reached 6 to 8 years of age, taking height, weight, and skinfold measurements on them (see Weil, 1977, p. 177 for a criticism). Eid concluded that the rapid gainers eventually became the heavier children; significantly more of the obese and the overweight 6- to 8-year-olds were traceable to this rapid-gainer group.

Mellbin and Vuille (1976) do not share the pessimism inherent in Eid's conclusion. They see no compelling reason for taking steps to prevent rapid weight gain during infancy if the objective is to prevent overweight in childhood. Their view emanates from an investigation of monthly weight-gain records of nearly 1000 infants. Data, taken for one year following birth, were compared with weight levels reached at 7 and 10 years of age. Rapid as opposed to normal gainers were those infants who exceeded the 90th percentile of gaining during the first year or those who exceeded the 97th percentile in any four-month interval; two other, intermediate criteria were applied as well. Seven-year-old boys, not girls, with a history of rapid gaining in infancy posted comparatively high relative risk scores; 10-year-olds evidenced a marked decline in risk. Therefore, overweight in childhood, as the authors indicate, even if predictable from rapid gaining in infancy, appears to be only temporary (see Vuille & Mellbin, 1979).

Other risk factors have been suggested. Kessen (1980), for instance, offers a composite picture involving familial, appetitive, and skinfold variables. He predicates his analysis on Milstein's (1978) dissertation which shows that thin infants have the least liking for sweet tastes. Kessen and Milstein speculate that the high-risk infant has "moderate to thick" skinfolds, overweight parents, and marked responsivity to food cues in general, sweetness in particular; Kessen acknowledges the need for research to support these speculations (see Grinker, 1981; Grinker, Price, and Greenwood, 1976).

The main question this section poses is prospective: Do early excesses promise later ones? Another query that some studies included here consider is retrospective in nature. That is, have later excesses, which are documented, arisen from earlier ones. This is equivalent to asking to what extent those overweight now are representative of a population having been overweight before. Fisch and coworkers (1975) ask and answer both questions. Not only, as indicated above, had 26 percent of the 74 previously overweight babies in that study retained their overweight at year 4, but also 18 percent of the overweight 4-year-olds had been overweight babies. The two kinds of inquiry often yield different answers, and the answers often vary depending on time elapsed between measurements, the measures being used, the criteria of overweight (obesity) being applied, as well as the authors being read (Dine, et al., 1979; Grinker, 1981; Lloyd, 1977; Weil, 1977).

Therefore, comparing studies is difficult and drawing conclusions is premature. Much work still needs to be done before we know when and why early-to later-excess connections arise, and when and why they do not. Possibly, a significant step forward will be taken once researchers identify the pertinent characteristics and backgrounds of obese children known to have been obese infants and monitor new samples of obese infants having these backgrounds and characteristics (or those likely to develop these characteristics). Perhaps by naming and tracking some combination of the variables and practices considered before and those to be considered next, researchers will be helped to take this step.

Connections with Feeding: Fat-cell Proliferation

Tightly connected to weight gain, fat gain, or gains in both during early life is feeding (see Jelliffe & Jelliffe, 1975). It would seem logical that some portion of the changes resulting in these body components and resistance to changes in them would be closely related to feeding. One theory says if feeding is excessive at critical stages of development (cf. Noppa, Bengtsson, Isaksson, & Smith, 1980), perhaps due to genetic susceptibility (Winick, 1978), the child will have a hard time maintaining a state of thinness as an adult. The notion, briefly, is that fat children who become fat adults may well be saddled with an unremitting condition traceable to the morphology of their adipose tissue.

As said in Chapter 1, surplus calories lead to an enlargement of adipose tissue through triglyceride storage in already existing fat cells (hypertrophy) or through the formation of new fat cells (hyperplasia). Many fat adults who became fat as children evidence fat-cell hyperplasia, whereas many fat adults who became fat as adults predominately show fat-cell hypertrophy (Salans, Cushman, & Weismann, 1973). There are, however, adult-onset obese individuals with excessive numbers of adipocytes, which indicates that the relationship between age of onset of obesity and fat-cell hyperplasia is inexact (Hirsch, 1975; Powers, 1980; Rodin, 1979b; Salans, 1981).

Notwithstanding this inexactitude, Knittle (1975) maintains that obese young-sters, in contrast to their slimmer peers, experience fat-cell proliferation earlier. He cites longitudinal data on obese and nonobese youths, some as young as 2 years, and he finds that fat youngsters have both larger and more numerous adipocytes (see also Brook, Lloyd, & Wolff, 1972; Knittle, Ginsberg-Fellner, & Brown, 1977; Knittle, Timmers, Ginsberg-Fellner, Brown, & Katz, 1979). According to Knittle (1975), adipose hypercellularity (exceeding adult levels) may occur in the 6-year-old; some of these hypercellular children show enlarged fat cells as well.

Central to the idea that intractable obesity is built early is the finding that weight loss among obese children and adults is accompanied by fat-cell shrinkage rather than fat-cell diminution (Ginsberg-Fellner & Knittle, 1981; Hirsch & Han, 1969; Salans, Horton, & Sims, 1971). Studies, however, are needed to see if hypercellu-lar obese patients who have maintained their weight losses for long periods demonstrate fat-cell number changes (Salans, 1974). Nevertheless, observations on the apparent stability of adipocyte number and the likely periods of adipocyte development—during the latter part of gestation (Powers, 1980; Ravelli, et al., 1976), during year one, and during the years between 9 and 13 (Salans et al., 1973)—leads Knittle as well as others (Ginsberg-Fellner, 1981) to warn: Treat the obese child early. Treat him before his hypercellularity reaches adult norms. Early treatment, it is contended, could slow the rate of fat-cell proliferation (see Hager, Sjöström, Arvidsson, Björntorp, & Smith, 1978).

The warning reflects the pessimism already articulated: Excessive numbers of adipocytes condemn the possessor to a lifetime of unremitting starvation (Grinker & Hirsh, 1972; Khan, 1981) in order to stay thinner and, because of this required starvation, the odds are poor for doing so. As Nisbett (1972, 1974) contends, the body defends against any penetration of its baseline stores of body fat—its set-point for body fat—and seeks to restore the equilibrium perturbed by a prolonged negative energy imbalance.

The argument is compelling; circumstantial evidence can be marshalled to support it; but as Nisbett appropriately cautions, logic and indirect evidence do not demonstrate that obesity in adulthood, if begun in childhood, is unmodifiable

(Simić, 1980); that proposition is unproven. Moreover, no one has as yet devised a valid way to define an individual's set-point (Rodin, 1975). Even more basic, no one has as yet isolated and examined the required signal from unfilled fat cells to the central nervous system that could sufficiently influence eating to return the individual to a fat state (Hirsch, 1975). Furthermore, criticisms of fat-cell counting methods exist (Gurr & Kirtland, 1978; Jung, Gurr, Robinson, & James, 1978; Roche, 1981); questions remain about the literature on animals on which much of the discussion about critical periods, severity of obesity, and adipocyte hyperplasia in humans is predicated (see Coates & Thoresen, 1980); and there are contradictory data and opinions (Ashwell, Priest, & Bondoux, 1975; Garn et al., 1975; Garrow, 1978a). Longitudinal study of adipose tissue cellularity is needed (Grinker, 1981; Sjöstrom & William-Olsson, 1981); so also is continued study of the ways and the effects of attenuating the proliferation of fat cells in the young.

Connections with Feeding: Early Practices

Disagreement exists not only about what fat-cell excesses in childhood do to initiate refractory obesity in adulthood, but also about what the behavioral progenitor, feeding, does to initiate and sustain obesity in children. That is, there is argument not about the logical notion that feeding affects weight and fat, but about presumed results: whether or not children are overfat because they overeat (Chapter 6) and, relatedly, whether or not infants who become overfat children do so because they are overfed (see Eid, 1970; Ferris, Laus, Hosmer, & Beal, 1980; Filer, 1978; Goldbloom, 1975; Poskitt & Cole, 1978; Sveger, 1978; Taitz, 1974). Two controversies pertaining to feeding in early infancy as the underpinning of obesity in later periods will be discussed in this chapter: breast-feeding versus bottle-feeding, and timing of solid-food introduction into the infant's diet (Kramer, 1981).

Soon after giving birth the mother has to determine how to feed her baby. Opinion differs on various facets of her predicament. Proponents of breast-feeding argue that breast milk is naturally superior to proprietary formula in meeting the infant's health and nutritional needs (Canadian Paediatric Society, 1978; Nutt, 1979; Powers, 1980; Taitz, 1974). More to the point of this section, they also argue that breast-feeding is less likely to be associated with infant obesity, with child obesity, or with both (Collipp, 1980b; Dorner, 1979; Neumann & Alpaugh, 1976; Ounsted & Sleigh, 1975; Taitz, 1971).

Thorogood, Clark, Harker, and Mann (1979), for example, report a 15 percent difference in prevalence of overweight that they feel is due to type of feeding; at the one-year checkup, more of the breast-fed babies compared with the bottle-fed babies were lighter for their size. Powers (1980), in her review, writes: "Breast-feeding for the first 4 to 6 months not only provides all the nutrients the baby needs, but also probably decreases the likelihood of later obesity " (p. 60).

One problem with nourishing with manufactured formula that she and other professionals identify has to do with feedback. When the infant is fed by bottle, the feedback is external not internal. Mother watches the bottle empty and by so doing judges whether her charge has eaten a sufficient amount; mother not baby, therefore, controls the magnitude of intake (Wright, 1981). This is one way that bottle-feeding (see Pollitt & Wirtz, 1981) does its damage, if, in fact, it does damage. Feeding by bottle deprives the infant of control over the amount consumed and thereby over the ability to regulate consumption. After studying 40 mother–infant pairs, 21 breast-fed infants and 19 bottle-fed infants, Crow, Fawcett, and Wright (1980) speculated that this feedback problem was central to obesity development. Even if their suspicion that overfeeding is more likely to result from bottle-feeding than from breast-feeding is correct, the evidence implicating overfeeding in infantile and childhood obesity is inconsistent. Moreover, there are those who disagree with the basic notion that breast-feeding, for whatever the reason, so definitely precludes obesity (Dine et al., 1979; Ferris et al., 1980; Golden, 1979; Huenemann, 1974a; Lloyd & Wolff, 1980; Wolman, 1980).

For example, Dubois, Hill, and Beaton (1979) found, in a retrospective inquiry using interviewing methods, no marked differences between the feeding practices of mothers with overweight infants versus mothers with nonoverweight infants. In their study, 47 heavy babies, those above the 90th percentile in weight for age, were compared with 42 normals, those between the 25th and 75th percentiles; the infants were 4- to 9-months old when the data were collected. Of the overweight group, 34 percent were never breast-fed. Similarly, of the nonoverweight group, 40 percent never were breast-fed. Also, proportionately fewer heavy infants were breast-fed for less than one month and more than three months. A comparison of even heavier infants, those above the 97th percentile in weight, again with normals, revealed parallel histories of being breast-fed.

Fomon (1980), like Yeung, Pennell, Leung, and Hall (1981), reported that type of feeding in infancy—breast versus bottle—did not predict childhood obesity. Fomon drew his conclusions from longitudinal data on more than 380 children, of whom 255 were bottle-fed during infancy and 131 were breast-fed; approximately 13 percent more of the formula-fed babies were boys, and approximately this percentage more of the breast-fed babies were girls. Measuring subscapular skinfold thickness and weight divided by height, he showed that obesity at near 4 months correlated significantly with obesity at age 8. It did not, at the eight-year assessment, correlate well with type of earliest feeding practice used.

Akin to disagreements about the outcomes of initial method of feeding are those about hazards, namely subsequent obesity, of introducing solid foods into the infants diet early, a practice no doubt encouraged by the baby-food industry (see Hancock, 1977; Powers, 1980). Some researchers and practitioners place a fair amount of blame on what they view as premature introduction (Eid, 1970; Khan, 1981; Laditan, 1981; Merritt & Batrus, 1980; Myres & Yeung, 1979, table 2;

Taitz, 1977b). Powers (1980) cautions waiting for more than four months (cf. Collipp, 1980b).

Others see time of first solids to be less of a basis of an obesity problem (Huenemann, 1974 a and b; Lloyd & Wolff, 1980; Weil, 1977; Yeung et al., 1981). Indeed, Dubois and colleagues (1979) detected later introduction of solids, and significantly later introduction of strained desserts, in their overweight group. On the whole, though, group differences were trivial. Likewise, Wolman (1980), in her study of 164 children infancy to age 4, found no relationship between time when solids were first presented and prevalence of subsequent obesity. As she reveals, however, approximately 90 percent of her sample were on solids before the third month, and that makes the early-to-late comparison a bit shaky. Moreover, as she also reveals, her five measures of obesity influenced the prevalence estimate. Further research is necessary, for, at present, indisputable evidence bearing on an association between time when solids are first given and later obesity is unavailable (Committee on Nutrition, 1981; Weil, 1977).

More generally, it remains to be seen exactly how feeding strategies during infancy affect infantile and childhood obesity (Morris, Farrier, Rogers, & Tapper, 1982). As Dubois and co-workers maintain, mothers who bottle-feed their babies and early on give them solids may not be guilty of fattening their children.

The Mother–Child Relationship and Other Post-natal Connections

During infancy, to a great extent much of the relationship between baby and mother does center around food (Lloyd & Wolff, 1980). The child cries and the mother, interpreting the cry as a call to be fed, gives food. The results for both mother and child of doing so increase the probability of future actions being similar. The child learns that crying is an instrument for obtaining food, and the mother learns that feeding is an instrument for ending loud crying; moreover, the mother may come to believe that her actions, by stopping crying and bringing on other signs of satisfaction, mean that she has done the right thing, that she is a good mother.

Bruch (1969, 1970, 1973, 1981) has been foremost in articulating far-reaching consequences that the mother–child relationship has on childhood obesity (see also Birch, Marlin, Kramer, & Peyer, 1981; Weil, 1975). Bruch maintains that plying the infant with food at his every cry and continuing to use food as the pacifier during his development may well breed a youngster who confuses his internal states. For Bruch, awareness of hunger and satiety contain learned elements, as do frustration, anxiety, and tension. As a result of confusion, the child may grow obese and stay that way (In Bruch's thinking, therefore, overfeeding teaches faulty linkages between internal states and eating; overfeeding early in life sets the stage for overeating later on)(see Chapter 6 for further discussion). The contradictory messages that many obese children hear, those that tell them to eat, to enjoy, and to suffer the outcomes, may add to this misguidance.

Among the other post-natal factors potentially affecting the ontogeny of childhood obesity are inactivity (Ross, Daniels, & Douglas, 1980; Chapter 6); illness, infection, surgery (Powers, 1980; Schwartz, van Gilst, & Rexwinkel, 1978; Weil, 1975) and, apropos of the mother–child relationship, separation. Kahn (1970), for example, surveyed the medical records of over 140 children under 12 years of age. Half, referrals to an obesity treatment center, were overweight; the others (less five), matched for age and sex with the overweight group, were not. Nearly four times more of the overweight children (a significant amount) had been placed under the care of a mother surrogate (that is, a friend or relative), and often the biological mother had never visited during the time of separation. For approximately 78 percent of the overweight children who had been separated from their mothers and for whom ages of overweight-onset had been discerned, gaining started almost coincidentally with the separation.

Genetic Connections

If the fat do indeed beget the fatter, as the TSNS data previously reviewed suggest, is this phenomenon due to environmental influences or is it the result of heredity? Poskitt and Cole (1978) suggest that it is due to heredity. Investigating the dietaries of the children they followed up in their 1977 study (see above), they found that calorie intake was an undiscriminating variable; the overweight and nonoverweight ate alike; that is, amount of energy consumed was similar. Significant, however, was that mothers and children resembled one another in excess weight: More overweight youngsters had overweight mothers than did nonoverweight youngsters.

Therefore, Poskitt and Cole conclude genetic variables more than dietary ones may have played a greater part in deciding who would be overweight at age 5 (see also Apfelbaum, Fumeron, Dunica, Magnet, Brigant, Boulange, & Hors, 1980; Koh, 1981). Genetic variables may also underlie the transmission of body type: Fathers contribute mesomorphy (muscularity); mothers, endomorphy (roundness) (Withers, 1964). Family-line effects, as indicated above, are evident.

But why? Years ago Gurney (1936) could show, as Garn and Clark (1976) and Mayer (1975) have been able to do subsequently, that when both parents are obese the progeny are more likely to be obese than when one or neither parent is obese. Nonetheless, it is still unclear whether corpulent youngsters inherit this excess or whether they acquire it from the worlds their parents, grandparents, aunts, uncles, teachers, and peers create for them. It is also unclear whether having obese brothers and sisters reflects a common heredity or a common environment.

Nature versus nature arguments about the causes of childhood obesity have been with us for quite awhile. Studies on twins have tried to settle these arguments.

Also concerned with family-line effects, these studies have investigated the genetic connection by exploring variance in common between relatives.

The contribution of genetics to this variation is called heritability (cf. Committee on Nutrition, 1978); heritability ranges between zero (no genetic effect) and one (total genetic dominance). Because estimating heritability is sounder if such extraneous variables as age and sex on adiposity are removed (Hawk, 1977), studying same sex twins is reasonable. Monozygotic twins are genetically identical and therefore should show a correlation of one in regard to any characteristic that is completely genetically determined. Dizygotic twins, because half their genes are shared, should show a correlation of .5 in regard to any characteristic that is completely genetically determined. If the correlations obtained veer from these expectancies, variables other than genetic ones are responsible; heritability estimates decrease from 100 percent as these other variables exert control.

Applying this logic, Börjeson (1976) calculated heritability from a ratio of intrapair skinfold (triceps, abdomen, subscapular) differences; he computed the ratio for samples of dizygotic and monozygotic twins. Differences between twins at the measured site should be less for the monozygotic pairs since, as said, they have all their genes in common. This essentially is what Börjeson found after comparing 61 pairs of dizygotic twins with 40 pairs of monozygotic twins living in Sweden; the criterion for obesity was that one or both twins have subscapular skinfolds exceeding the 90th percentile on the Tanner and Whitehouse (1962) standards. The mean difference between dizygotic pairs of twins was more than three times greater than that between monozygotic pairs at the triceps and subscapular sites and nearly three times greater at the abdominal site. Assuming each set of twins, be they identical or not, live in a similar environment, overall differences between the monozygotic and dizygotic twins reflect heredity (Hawk, 1977). Börjeson concluded that there is a major genetic contribution to childhood obesity (see also Brook, Huntley, & Slack, 1975).

The extent of the contribution, however, is still far from clear (See Rony, 1940; VonVerscheuer, 1927). For example, Newmann, Freeman, and Holzinger (1937) find greater weight differences among pairs of monozygous twins raised apart compared with the weight differences of those growing up together (cf. Shields, 1962). In addition, difficulties and potential sources of error, in drawing conclusions from twin studies, per se, do exist—zygosity determinations may be incorrect, and prenatal environments of monozygotic twins may be dissimilar, prejudicing judgements about post-natal effects on fatness (Powers, 1980).

Another strategy for investigating the heredity–environment issue in childhood obesity is to study parent–child similarities when parents are biologically related to the child and when they are not (see, for example, Withers, 1964). Shenker, Fisichelli, and Lang (1974) studied the latter category. They learned that male infants raised by overweight foster mothers were significantly heavier at several measurement times (for example, 6 months, 7 months) than were those raised by nonoverweight foster mothers; trends were similar for the female infants. The most parsimonious explanation for these results is that overweight foster mothers created different environments for their babies (fed them more, perhaps) than did the lighter foster mothers. Certainly, biological linkages between mother and child were nonextant. (See also Mason's 1970 finding for obese pets of obese pet owners.) Comparing both categories listed above—biological versus nonbiological—Garn, Cole, and Bailey (1977) reported fatness increases for both natural and adopted children that varied with parental fatness combinations (that is, one obese parent, two obese parents); it would be difficult to apply a genetic explanation to these results (cf. Biron, Mongeau, & Bertrand, 1977; Garn & Bailey, 1976; Mayer, 1975).

At present, the view concerning nature versus nurture in childhood obesity is that both genetic and environmental forces are involved (Börjeson, 1980; Brownell, 1981; Grinker, 1981). Understanding how each contributes, especially how and when environmental control is able to attenuate or overcome the effects of genetic predispositions (Bray, 1976), is a current challenge.

Rarer Forms of Obesity in Childhood

Varieties of obesity exist in which afflicted children are generally short and fat because of such endocrinologic and other endogenous circumstances, as decreased thyroid function (Collipp, 1980b), excessive cortisol (Douglass, 1980), or tumors (Golden, 1979). Among the rare forms that may be transmitted genetically are the Laurence-Moon-Bardet-Biedl Syndrome (LMBB) in which the obese child with hypogenatilism is retarded, often has decreased visual acuity that disintegrates into blindness in adulthood, and has webbed (syndactyly) or extra (polydactyly) fingers or toes. Also, in the Alstrom-Hallgren Syndrome diabetes and nerve deafness are added to obesity and childhood blindness. Furthermore, infants with the Prader-Willi Syndrome (HHHO) show marked hypotonia (poor muscle tone). As the infants grow, classic symptoms are hypotonia as well as hypogenitalism, hypomentia (retardation), and obesity (see Holm & Pipes, 1976; Orenstein, Boat, Owens, Horowitz, Primiano, Germann, & Doershuk 1980); according to Bray (1976), the genetic basis of the Prader-Willi Syndrome, however, is still uncertain. Those with the syndrome frequently demonstrate a voracious appetite that interferes with treatment. Detailed discussions of this affliction and the others mentioned, as well as the Summit Syndrome and triglyceride storage disease, are available (Bray, 1976; Collipp, 1980a; Douglass, 1980; Goldstein, & Failkow, 1973; Sells, Hanson, & Hall, 1979). There have been many and varied therapeutic attempts: dietary (Coplin, Hine, & Gormican, 1976; Pipes & Holm, 1973), surgical (Anderson, Soper, & Scott, 1980; Chapter 1), and behavioral (Altman, Bondy, & Hirsch, 1978; Heiman, 1978; Marshall, Elder, O'Basky, Wallace, & Liberman, 1979; Thompson, Kodluboy, & Heston, 1980; Chapter 5).

It is apparent that the epidemiology and natural history of childhood obesity, as discussed thus far in this chapter, are unsettled, complex topics. They evince intricacies, some of which may be traceable to interdependencies among elements. I have, for the most part, surveyed these elements as if they were independent contributors, occasionally suggesting possible interrelationships.

Interconnections may, however, be the rule. For instance, there may be a complex interplay among overnutrition during pregnancy, fat-cell development in utero, weight at birth, overfeeding in infancy, and overweight as well as overfatness at that time, that will become manifest in childhood, adolescence, and adulthood; and the results of this interaction of contributors may be affected by gender and socioeconomic variables. Furthermore, there may be a relationship between timing of overfeeding in childhood and genetic predispositions to obesity. Possibly, the capacity to be overfed, the capacity to acquire a protracted surplus of calories, may be most visible during later childhood (Brook, Lloyd, & Wolff 1972); if so, early treatment may be easier than later treatment (Powers, 1980). The proof of such a speculation, and more generally the recording of all the interconnections among the potential contributors to childhood obesity awaits further research—a familiar and necessary refrain in the literature on the prevalence and beginnings of childhood obesity and in the discussions of this volume.

Concomitants

Here the discussion shifts from possible connections to possible physical, psychological, and social problems facing the child who becomes obese. Before commencing, four points need to be made. First, concomitants may become contributors; the child who is teased because of the shape of his body may isolate himself, abuse food and television-watching, and therefore grow even more obese. Second, the data in this section, as in the previous one, are correlational, not causal. For every anomaly mentioned it is unknown to what extent obesity brings that anomaly on, or to what extent other variables coincidental with childhood obesity cause it. Third, the strategy of much of the research documented here is to appraise, cross-sectionally, groups of overweight boys and girls and to tabulate what has happened to them. Longitudinal inquiries that follow developing children to identify the onset and course of physical, psychological, and social difficulties are decidedly rare. Fourth, only some of the children who become obese will be discussed here. Many remain unscathed. Why they remain so and why numbers of their brethren do not is unclear. It is to the unlucky ones, however, that much of the literature on concomitants and the ensuing discussion is directed.

Injuries, Discomforts, and Diseases

Surveying medical records in a retrospective inquiry, Willmore and Pruitt (1972) reported that significant numbers (20 percent) of overweight boys between the ages of 2 and 13 were accidentally burned; the survey covered six years and included 108 boys. Additionally, the records of an almost equal number of girls, age range the same as in the male sample, were inspected; overweight, however, did not prove to be a significant discriminator. As the authors suggest, possibly some overweight boys receiving burns were just too slow to escape the consequences of their mischief. In other words, perhaps their burns could have been avoided had they been more agile. The same could be said for the 86 nonoverweight boys (80 percent) who also were burned; it also could be said for the four overweight and 95 average-weight girls in the study.

Commenting on the physical discomfort that assails some obese children, Stimbert and Coffey (1972) identify musculoskeletal problems in the lower extremities (for example, knock-knees); they note that such difficulties, when seen, are more common among obese children who have been obese for a long time. Mobbs (1970) discovered the presence of physical defects (flat feet for example) in each of the six childhood obesity case histories he reviewed; some of the children depicted had, in addition, difficulty exerting themselves. Davies, Godfrey, Light, Sargeant, and Zeidifard (1975) also observed this exertion problem in their study of 17 obese females, of whom six were under 13 years of age. Obesity, as measured by weight and skinfold, seemed to reduce performance when actions required maximal or close to maximal effort; at lower levels of exertion the conspicuous performance drops were absent.

Disease-Related Risk Factors. Rarely, except when children are extremely obese (as with some Prader-Willi children) do clinicians worry about their perishing from being fat. There is concern, however, that obesity and overweight are bedfellows with a host of physical difficulties, such as fatty liver, respiratory tract infections, carbohydrate intolerance, diabetes mellitus, hyperinsulinemia, depressed growth hormone release, susceptibility to disease (Brook, 1980; Chiumello, Guercio, Carnelutti, & Bidone, 1969; Deschamps, Desjeux, Machinot, Rolland, & Lestradet, 1978; Hager & Thorell, 1979; Kappy & Plotnick, 1980; Lasarev, 1978; Martin & Martin, 1973; Murata, Fujita, Yamazaki, Hoshina, & Imai, 1978; Petrash, 1977; Weil, 1975).

One untoward condition currently receiving much attention for its potential relationship to overweight and obesity in children is cardiovascular disease (Levine, Hennekens, Rosner, Gourley, Gelband, & Jesse, 1981). Risk factors of elevated blood lipid levels and elevated blood pressure have been identified in heavy and fat youngsters. The concern is whether the chances of future cardiovascular mishaps are greater among those manifesting these risk factors. Early intervention for those in whom the seeds of cardiovascular problems are planted early might attenuate later morbidity and mortality (see Kannel & Dawber, 1972; Lauer & Shekelle, 1980; VanBiervliet & deWijn, 1978). There is also some evidence that overweight and obese children do indeed display higher concentrations of serum cholesterol and triglycerides, but the positive correlations are small. Frerichs, Webber, Srinivasan, and Berenson (1978), using Bogalusa Heart Study data, report that little of the total variability in lipid levels is attributable to obesity and overweight (see also Berenson, 1977; Berenson, Foster, Frank, Frerichs, Srinivasan, Voors, & Webber, 1978).

Similarly, Lauer et al. (1975), after studying more than 4800 school children in Muscatine, Iowa, found that the correlations of weight and triceps skinfold with cholesterol and triglyceride levels are weak. At the extremes of the variables, however, stronger relationships appear. Of the 493 heaviest children falling within the upper decile of relative weight, nearly 18 percent have cholesterol levels at or over the 90th percentile; even more, nearly 25 percent, have triglyceride levels that are likewise exaggerated. Similarly, of the 555 fattest children, skinfold thicknesses greater than the 90th percentile, the number showing elevated cholesterol, is almost 18 percent; and the number showing elevated triglyceride concentrations is almost 24 percent. Perhaps even stronger relationships between these anthropometric measures and blood lipid profiles will emerge as more epidemiologists study the lipoprotein carriers of serum cholesterol instead of just total cholesterol (see Coates & Thoresen, 1980; Frerichs et al., 1978; Garrison, Wilson, Castelli, Fenleib, Kannel, & McNamara, 1980; Chapter 1).

More striking than the aforenamed relationships are those of overweight and obesity with elevated blood pressure (see Ellison, Newburger, & Gross, 1982). Thus, Berenson (1977), summarizing Bogalusa study findings, reports that anthropometric measures account for more of the variability of blood pressure data than that of blood lipid observations (cf. Frerichs et al., 1978; Siervogel, Frey, Kezdi, Roche, & Stanley, 1980; Voors, Sklov, Wolf, Hunter, & Berenson 1980). Voors, Webber, Frerichs, and Berenson (1977) show for 5- to 14-year-olds that ponderosity (weight/height^3) correlates positively with systolic blood pressure in particular (cf. deCastro, Christianson, & Lollar, 1976b; Voors, Foster, Frerichs, Webber, & Berenson, 1976). According to Voors, Webber, and Berenson (1978) size of the body (for example, arm circumference, height) correlates with systolic and diastolic blood pressure even in 2.5- to 5.5-year-old children (cf, Berenson et al., 1978).

From the Muscatine study, Lauer and co-workers (1975) obtained positive correlations between skinfold thickness and diastolic ($r = .36$) as well as between skinfolds and systolic ($r = .39$) readings. Again evaluating extreme scores, they showed blood pressure data for the fattest and for the heaviest youngsters. Almost 30 percent of the most corpulent evinced systolic blood pressures at or greater than the 90th percentile, and nearly that many (27.7 percent) have equivalently marked diastolic readings. Percentages of children demonstrating elevated weights and blood pressures agreed with these values—approximately 29 percent for systolic and about the same for diastolic terms.

Lynds, Seyler, and Morgan (1980) also documented this elevated blood pressure–overweight relationship. They did so using a sample of 1692 Black school children, ages 5 to 11; roughly 11.5 percent of these youngsters had high systolic pressures and slightly more than that had high diastolic pressures. Lynds and colleagues assigned all the children to one of five weight categories and then compared how many of those with elevated blood pressures, systolic and diastolic, were in each category. Chances were great, as the authors noted, for the children with elevated blood pressure to be heavy, above the 90th percentile in weight-for-height; indeed, chances were far greater for them to be obese by this weight-for-height criterion than to be below the 10th percentile in weight-for-height. On the whole, therefore, overweight and other measures of obesity appear to be associated with the higher levels of blood pressure (Berchtold, Jorgens, Finke, & Berger, 1981).

In fact, significant hypertension among obese and overweight youths has been seen (New & Rauh, 1980). Court, Hill, Dunlap, and Boulton (1974), assessing 209 juveniles ranging in age from just over one year to almost 18 (mean age 10.5 years), reported high positive correlations between percent body weight as fat and both diastolic ($r = .70$) and systolic ($r = .81$) blood pressures; subscapular skinfold thickness also correlate significantly with these pressure readings. Subjects varied from 3 to 113 percent overweight; more than 114 of them (over half the sample), having blood pressures at or above 90mm Hg diastolic or at or above 135mm Hg systolic, were hypertensive. Of these youths, 21 (mean age 10 years) were even more definitely hypertensive, diastolic blood pressure greater than 95mm Hg. Similarly, Londe, Bourgoignie, Robson, and Goldring (1971) found a significant difference between numbers of overweight youths, ages 4 to 18 years, but most under 13, who were hypertensive versus normotensive. In excess of 50 percent of the hypertensive subjects, compared with 14 percent of the normotensive ones, weighed above the 90th percentile.

Hence it appears that some overweight and overfat youths are at a greater risk than are their lighter and thinner contemporaries for discomfort and disease. Yet the lower limits of high-risk overweight and obesity are unknown. More than overweight and obesity must be considered in predicting who these unfortunate youths will likely be. For as Court and associates report, serious blood pressure elevations are absent in most of their sample; some of the heaviest and fatest were normotensive. Therefore, again, not all overweight or obese children will suffer from adverse physical conditions happening sometime in childhood, adolescence, or adulthood. Nor are all destined to suffer from the event discussed below.

Despair

Too often society condemns the obese person. Unlike the diseased or the deformed, the fat may be seen as having a weak character. A boy with excessive breast development and visible rolls of fat around his middle is at odds with the value of thinness so entrenched in our culture, and we usually let him know it. Perhaps his parents and peers tell him that he has failed to do what he is supposed to do to avoid fatness or that he has done something to bring it on. Perhaps by their words and deeds they tell him that he is the architect of his plight (Maddox, Back, & Leiderman, 1968) and that he therefore deserves harassment; he may agree (Allon, 1980; Cahnman, 1968; DeJong, 1980). As Cahnman writes, he may be ill-treated, thought of as, and come to believe he is responsible for his condition, and he may be led to accept his mistreatment as fitting. LeBow (1981a) cites a thin adult, once a very fat child, who recalls:

My first grade teacher opened up my eyes, making me realize that what my parents called my healthiness and my robustness might be something more. She engineered my being elected that year's Santa Claus. Her reasoning was simple. As she put it to the class, "He (meaning me) has more meat on his bones!" I liked the idea of being Santa because everyone else wanted to be it. The joys were passing out gifts, wearing a special costume, and receiving lots of attention. But there were drawbacks, too. Indeed, something felt wrong with the whole thing. I felt uneasy. I sensed that my parents were not overjoyed either when I explained why I was chosen, namely that the meat on my bones (which they knew they helped put there) won me the honor.

In time my position in grade school and everywhere else, for that matter, became sharper. I was the fat one or, more accurately, one of the fatties. I didn't really like the other blimps because they looked funny, especially when they played football and baseball. And, most of all, nobody who was anybody liked them.

My friends called me names, too. I was inured to their epithets, however, and at least until the fourth grade took my greater size to mean greater strength. But in the sixth grade I learned something new: fatness definitely was not toughness. All the thin kids who fought me, beat me!

The kings were the guys with the V-shapes. Stan, to name one of them, had noticeable muscular contours. Four of these royal ones allowed me to enter their kingdom, primarily as court jester—if I could get them to laugh I could get them to accept me, or so I thought.

But they teased quite a bit and played pranks. One time they told me to go home and get my swimming trunks, and we would all go to the pool; yet when I returned to the meeting place, everyone had gone. Eventually, I forgave them for disliking me, because at that time in my life it was simpler to forgive such conduct.

My first job was delivering papers. It was boring but at least you could hide your front and back sides with the paper sack. Selling papers on the street corner was more lucrative, yet more visible and hence more painful. You couldn't snack on the corner because people looked at you as if to say fat boys should never eat. Once I was a busboy at a fancy department store restaurant. The worst thing about the job was having to wear the white uniform. For some reason, the establishment thought boys should have waist sizes no bigger than 30 inches and that hips should be possessed only by girls. The uniform chaffed, and I looked strange waddling around in it. I quit the job within two weeks.

Society told me I should not be fat. Failing to live up to the standards set before me meant rejection. I still frequently hear the "be's": be thin, be coordinated, be strong—and the important "have"—have willpower. But very little was within reach that told me how to be thin, coordinated, and strong, or where to find willpower and how to give it a boost. The rebukes cried out more loudly than did the remedies.

I still feel distance from others as if I walk around them not towards them. The fringes of the world in which I live are my world. My fear and my pleasure look alike, for I hate being noticed while I long to be accepted—both mean attention. But the eyes that watch me sting. From the many whom I touched, I learned that I was grotesque, actually burlesque. My body was ludicrous. Yet, unlike the bent limb, the scarred face or the twisted frame, my affliction was a crime and I was a criminal. I was weak, too. I was responsible for my curse, and because I was guilty of making myself funny-looking, I legitimized the abuse I endured.*

Some Studies of Stigmatizers. Peers of the obese child mete out this second-class treatment. When given choices about who they prefer as friends, about who they care to resemble, and about who they describe as possessing positive or negative attributes, many of the peers of the obese child, some obese themselves, downgrade the corpulent (see Edelman, 1982).

Lerner and Gellert (1969) surveyed 45 kindergarteners who exhibited this disaffection. These children looked at photographs of lean, average, and portly 5- and 6-year-olds. Significant numbers expressed negative attitudes toward the fat children in the pictures, wanting not to look like them (see Lerner & Korn, 1972; Lerner & Pool, 1972). Over 20 years ago Richardson, Goodman, Hastorf, and Dornbusch (1961) witnessed a similar phenomenon in 640 10- and 11-year-olds. These children differed from one another in socioeconomic status, religion, race, sex, residence (rural versus urban), and whether or not they were handicapped. The task they were given was to rank six drawings of youngsters according to whom they liked the most, the next most, and so on; as choices were made, drawings were removed until every drawing was rated. The pictures were alike in all but two respects—sex of the child depicted and type of impairment presented (being in a wheelchair, on crutches, disfigured head or face, obese); one drawing was of a child without any handicap whatsoever. To control for sex of the child pictured biasing the choice, Goodman and colleagues showed the girls, girls and the boys, boys. Regardless of their own background, race, and physical disability, the tested children ranked the totally unimpaired child the highest and the obese child the lowest.

Sampling from a younger population, using other methods, Staffieri (1967) demonstrated essentially the same phenomenon—looks affected likes. Stimuli were silhouettes of children differing in body builds. Staffieri tested 90 males, ages 6 to 10 years mainly, and assigned them to one of three groups based on how the youngsters themselves were shaped—thin, muscular, or fat; one triad at each of the ages was represented. Boys were interviewed about peers who either resembled them in body contour or who were different from them. They were shown silhouettes that were identical to each other except in the body shape each portrayed—thin, muscular, or fat. The boys were then asked to evaluate these drawings using 39 adjectives (for example, strong, weak, stupid, smart, naughty, healthy, etc.).

Whether or not the rater was himself fat, muscular, or thin, endomorphs were negatively viewed. Whereas 58 of the respondents saw the fat silhouette as stupid, only eight saw the muscular form that way. Endomorphs were described as cheats, lazy, or mean far more than were the mesomorphs: These muscular fellows were characterized as having lots of friends, being clean, smart, neat, brave, good-looking. Paralleling these ratings were sociometric ones of current friends; they showed unmistakably that fat children were derogated (see Lerner, 1969a; Lerner & Schroeder, 1971; Staffieri, 1968).

Evaluating the responses of 60 7- to 11-year-old females to silhouettes similar to those just mentioned, Staffieri (1972) again revealed that ill-feeling was directed against the endomorph more than it was against other body-builds. Unfavorable adjectives (stupid and ugly, for example) were disproportionately applied to the endomorph, and "best friend" judgements were quite low—3.3 percent. Likewise, Dyrenforth, Freeman, and Wooley (cited in Wooley, Wooley, & Dyrenforth, 1979) disclosed that even in preschoolers, negative feelings toward fatness existed (cf., Horan, 1982). About 95 percent of their sample preferred a thin to a fat rag doll; obese children preferred it too, despite 60 percent of those studied (three) identifying more in appearance with the fat doll.

I am reminded of my own 4-year-old's description of two birds he viewed one day from our living room window. "The thin one," he said, "is strong; the fat one stuffed himself." He may have been echoing what his friends and parents say and feel. I would hate to admit complicity in this stereotyping, yet I know full well that much of it starts in the home. Elders disparage many things, and children imitate what they say and do.

Ridiculing fatness is no exception. Many adults denigrate the obese (Lerner, 1969b), and some adults, when the obese person happens to be a child, will alter overt mistreatment but not negative feelings (Morgavan, 1976). To show that adults may hold derisive attitudes toward obese youngsters, Goodman, Richardson, Dornbusch and Hastorf (1963) replicated and extended their earlier work (see Richardson et al., 1961 discussed above). The methodology was the same; they presented drawings of children with and without handicaps and had respondents rank them. None of the subjects in the Goodman study, however, were handicapped; moreover, 72 of them were adults who dealt in some capacity with handicapped children. As before, results showed children ranking the drawing of the obese child last. Further, they showed adults doing the same. Similarly, Maddox and colleagues (1968) noted that adults find it harder to like the obese child than to like other children. These investigators applied the Richardson and co-workers' drawing technique to Whites and Blacks from varying backgrounds; males and females were in both racial groupings. In addition, the authors attempted to uncover the reasons behind the rankings, finding that pity as a frame of reference led the adults to downgrade the drawing of the overweight child; the fat child was, in other words, less pitied than was his peer with a noticeable deformity.

There is every reason to believe that today, as in the past, the stigma of obesity confronts the young. Television frequently portrays fat persons, real and animated alike, as clumsy. Comic strips picture them as laughable. Joke books, gum wrappers, movies, and nursery rhymes do the same. Stigmatizers are abundant; they forcibly carry their messages. Now more than ever before it is unfashionable to view the fat infant as the healthy infant. From such sources, which not only directly influence obese youths but also color their interactions with family and friends, children learn about themselves. Being fat is, for some, traumatic; it shapes the self-definitions that underlie any psychological (Bruch, 1975; Turner, 1980), self-concept (Sallade, 1973; but see Day, 1982) and body-image distortions (Nathan, 1976; Stunkard & Burt, 1967; see also, Leon, Bemis, Meland, & Nussbaum, 1978) they happen to manifest.

What has essentially been said is that many obese youngsters, but by no means all (Coates & Thoresen, 1980), face turmoil resulting from a negative social impact that is traceable to their body shapes. Further research is needed to corroborate this view (see Dyrenforth, Wooley, & Wooley, 1980 for an update) and to discover which obese children are candidates. Nonetheless, clinical experience does suggest that many of those rebuked by parents and agemates for looking fat are currently, or soon to be, locked in a vicious circle of rejection, isolation, and further rejection. They are at risk of entrapment by a system that punishes them for obesity and that, by so doing, augments the probability of maintaining obesity. They may hear several contradictory messages (see Appendix G) that are at the heart of this paradox—messages given at home and at play that act to close the vicious circle. I often observe them in my own work with obese juveniles.

Double Messages

Finish Your Dinner if You Want Dessert, But Stop Eating So Many Sweets So You Won't Be Fat.   Those 12 and under hear this message. It has several supports in parents' belief structures, the group who so frequently state it. To waste not is to want not; to leave food on your plate is to mock your good fortune; to eat all that is before you is to nourish yourself well; to eat dessert is to be rewarded; to be a fat child is to be an overeater of sweets. Take, for instance, what may happen to an overweight 10-year-old boy. He is served an enormous, in his eyes anyway, well-balanced meal, comprised of salad, meat, potatoes, corn, peas, and milk. For dessert there is apple pie and ice cream. If he balks at downing the entree, he is told about the many starving children in the world that he is somehow demeaning; he is ungratefully refusing what they would joyously welcome. Or he is told that wasting food is expensive because today's food is costly. Or he is told both. Whatever message is given, when his parents find these ploys to be no longer effective, they will pose a more drastic, immediately compelling threat: no dessert if food from dinner remains on the plate. This scare often does the job. A few hours later or the next day the contradiction arises. While dressing the boy finds that his pants are tight; he complains. His mother and father, in response, admonish him for eating too many pies and cookies; these, they say, are making him chubby. By so answering, the parents denigrate stimuli they have only a short time ago designated as fitting rewards. This is a rapid and perplexing switch.

One objective in therapy is to convince parents that desserts are allowable positive reinforcers, if planned for that day or evening, and that they are legitimate consequences of half-eaten meals—better these than levers to increase eating. The responsibility for wasting belongs to the server of the food as much as to the eater. The obese child should not be forced to compound the error of having too much food served by having to consume it all in order to receive even more food; dessert need not be the reinforcer of massive consumption. Parents should be taught also that eating less, as a behavioral objective, is facilitated by giving less food, a practice that accomplishes the reduction of waste as well.

Food Is Splendor, But Fat Is Ugly.   The contradiction here is not a two-sided verbalization; it is a discordance between what is done in the home and what is said there. Illustrating it are families displaying copious amounts of rich and tasty food and housing fat models who eat and love it while they condemn fatness. Obese children of all ages may enjoy and suffer from a family who say that less than plenty is insufficient, even sinful, and that obesity is sometimes a punishable offense.

Recalling this inconsistency, the formerly fat child quoted in LeBow (1981a) above writes further:

> Eating was the most fun on Sunday. Brunch could be lox and bagels, salami and eggs, kippers, bacon, ham, and toast with butter . . . all washed down with skim milk. (The nonfat milk was a half-hearted bid for lower calories; at least we felt as though we had something low-calorie and were better for doing so.) Our home was a lot like our food—kept perfect in every way. I used to peel my fat legs off the plastic covers on the living room sofa in order to get up after the television program had ended.
>
> Dinners during the work week never equalled the mid-Sunday grandeur, but I have since learned that they also verged on the superior—meat (brisket), never less than two cooked vegetables (cooked with lots of butter and love), some raw carrots and celery (but who wants them?), potatoes fried crisply, sometimes rice, sometimes both. Pie, for afterwards, never sat naked on the plate but was dressed in ice cream (ice milk once in awhile because it sounded low-cal). The food parade never ended!
>
> Even television and its companion the TV tray could not interrupt it. We usually sat down at six o'clock and began eating when we saw our filled plates. I always ate all the reasons that were visible on my plate to continue eating—when the food was gone, I stopped to refill, or just stopped. Rarely was I only satisfied. And never, perish the thought was I left hungry. For me, to be full was to be bloated.
>
> Indeed, during my childhood food was love, and eating was ecstasy. Food,

concern, and affection played on the same stage before the same audience of six who applauded and gave every indication that repeat performances would be highly approved of. Food was the great performer, who even could boast a special holiday show.

Friends and relatives also at times put on food-extravaganzas and rewarded you for feats of consumption that were beyond the call of duty. For instance, I once went with my family to a large party where fried chicken lay beside an array of side-dishes and desserts and after-dessert nourishments . . . all on a table inviting you to gorge; the more I did so, the more the "healthiness" of my appetite drew attention. I performed well. And I was applauded.

Yet eating had its drawbacks, too. My family touted anti-fat propaganda as much as anyone else. My grandparents and parents were fatness-defilers who warned that corpulence, ugliness, and weakness shared the same seat at the dinner table. My older sister was often punished for hiding cookies though she always claimed her innocence— loudly.

But at the same time, we could unite in our common affliction. I was a lot like my father. On those glorious Sundays I frequently tried on his pants and came downstairs for approving laughter, which I learned to love. At thirteen I was nearly his height, but he was king in the waistline. I kept getting closer, however, to dethroning him.*

Eat To Be Friendly, But Best Friends Are Not Fat.   This is a contradiction that older obese children and adolescents hear. It is a paradox of social eating and remaining thin. Obese youths who, in order to socialize, frequent restaurants reknown for their fatty and carbohydrate-rich cuisine, may fall victim to it. Consider, for example, an overweight 12-year-old girl trying to diet, who after school follows her friends to a local coffee shop or fast-food restaurant. While there she must decide whether or not to eat. If she chooses to do as her peers, she conforms to the first part of the message: She eats to be a friend. But by doing so she helps bring about a violation of the second part of it and, relatedly, risks being teased for being an eater who is fat. If she chooses not to eat anything she confirms that something is wrong with her. She totally violates the first part of the message and, in addition, admits to being fat, calling into question her status as friend. Adding insult to injury, she again risks being teased, this time for being a rigid dieter. She could avoid the entire situation, but by doing so she risks exclusion from many social plans. In reality, therefore, she is damned no matter what she does, punished every way she turns.

Play With Us To Be One Of Us, But We Don't Like Fatsos Who Aren't Good Athletes.   Children and adolescents learn many age-appropriate actions by forming alliances with peers on the playing field. When prevented from these sports, or when relegated to an inferior place on the field, a child is denied opportunities for social as well as physical development. Too often it is the obese youngster who is

*Michael D. LeBow, *Weight Control: The Behavioural Strategies* (Chichester: John Wiley & Sons, Ltd., 1981; pp. 227–228). Copyright © 1981 by John Wiley & Sons, Ltd. Reprinted by permission of the publisher.

so denied. The reason is largely that a winning-at-all-costs mood pervades both organized and unsupervised sports, and thus directs coaches and team captains to search for the best athletes. Fat children may be excluded because they are seen as lacking such prowess; they do frequently lack it. Although many coaches appear to forget, they are, however, teachable. Even if placed on a team, chances are the obese youth will be assigned a shock-absorber or battering-ram position. As a poor player, he will come to feel awkward, burdensome, and least desirable as a teammate. Ridicule on the field, matched by ridicule off of it, may well lead to withdrawal from future contests (for example, seeking medical excuses from physical education classes); this avoidance diminishes the chances of ever acquiring the athletic skills needed to become valuable in the eyes of significant others. In brief, exile soon helps fulfill the prophecy of being too uncoordinated to play.

The fellow quoted in LeBow (1981a) explains:

> I liked sports in my junior high school years, but I never could make the first team. In school, the coach, who was also my math teacher, was a V-shape who wore his shirt two buttons open at the top, when the weather permitted. He didn't like fat kids, I was certain of that. Being a no-nonsense guy about athletics, his formula was simple: If you are not good enough, you are no good.
>
> I felt badly about being second rate in his eyes and just accepted his denigration of me. He represented the epitome, the model man, who continually tried to prove that fatness was ugliness caused by weakness. And he represented the leader of the best I so longed to be one of. Organized sports eventually became punishing, so I stopped trying out for the teams. Even after-school sports became unpleasant, for often I was the one who went on the side that had exhausted its choices but needed one more player.
>
> High school, likewise, was an athletic nightmare. One day during swimming the coach yelled, "Everybody out of the pool," and like regimented troops all the V-shapes pulled up with great ease. I couldn't get out. The laughter was deafening. I laughed as loudly as everyone else—what else do you do?
>
> For some strange reason I had a mandatory wrestling class in the tenth grade. The coach was more of an inverted V-shape like me but, in contrast, was strong and sturdy. He adored his mightiness and with equal gusto hated my weakness. So, he was fond of demonstrating various holds on me. I weighed over 200 pounds at that time and was 5 feet 6 inches tall—a perfect specimen for him. My doctor, appreciating my dilemma, wrote me an excuse that let me out of gym entirely; aperiodic asthma saved me. I never returned and in so doing cut off one source of the fitness that I so desperately needed.
>
> I stayed home my fifteenth summer finding relief in TV and food. The outside was still anti-fat with a vengeance, and I was still fat with a great visibility. Teachers and peers loathed my shape. I continued to accept their views as the only ones possible. Yet, by now, my proximity to my own fatness at least made me a little more tolerant of it.*

*Michael D. LeBow, *Weight Control: The Behavioural Strategies* (Chichester: John Wiley & Sons, Ltd., 1981; pp. 233–234). Copyright © 1981 by John Wiley & Sons, Ltd. Reprinted by permission of the publisher.

In sum, I have recounted four contradictory messages that obese youths may hear (Rallo, 1982); no doubt there are others. At the very least, these messages confuse. Moreover, they may interfere with therapy by intensifying the problems obese children have in following the prescriptions designed to make them thinner.

Should Therapy be Offered?

Answering this question requires answering two of its components: Is it needed? And does it work? Those who argue against treatment for obesity in children (see, for example, Rappoport, 1974) often respond no to both of these queries. Opposers say that therapy is unlikely to be successful because many youngsters lack the motivation necessary for it to work (see Chapter 6); failing to make it work increases the chances of youngsters defining themselves as failures. Also, opposers say that weight and fatness problems in childhood, unless extreme, are unlikely to be permanent; they say that at best, evidence that the fat stay fat is equivocal (see Committee on Nutrition, 1978; Grinker, 1980; Hawk & Brook, 1979).

In contrast, proponents of early intervention answer yes, in particular to the question about need. They argue that development often fails to erase the problem; they argue that fat children become fat adults (Brownell & Stunkard, 1980a; Court, 1979; Israel & Stolmaker, 1980; Lloyd & Wolff, 1980; Nutt, 1979; Simić, 1980; above for shorter $time_1$ to $time_2$ comparisons). They can offer some evidence. For example, Abraham and Nordsieck (1960), from a 20-year follow-up on 50 overweight and 50 nonoverweight boys (the Hagerstown study), report substantial differences between these groups. Over twice as many of the overweight boys (86 percent) become overweight adults. Even more dramatic is the difference between the two groups of females at follow-up. Approximately 60 percent more of the 50 overweight versus the 50 nonoverweight girls become overweight women.

Considering boys and girls together, Abraham and Nordsieck found that overweight children are far more likely than are nonoverweight children to become overweight adults. Only 30 percent of the lighter-for-height youngsters become heavy adults; 70 percent do not. But 83 percent of the heavy-for-height youngsters become heavy adults; 17 percent do not. As Stunkard and Burt (1967) illuminated, the chances against an overweight child growing up to be a nonoverweight adult, outgrowing excessive heaviness, are therefore greater than 4 to 1 if reduction has not occurred during childhood; it is decidedly worse if it has not happened by the end of adolescence.

Similarly, Abraham, Collins, and Nordsieck (1971), after a 35 to 40 year follow-up, discovered that markedly overweight youths failed to drop beneath average weight in adulthood; in fact, 63 percent were markedly overweight adults (see Stark, Atkins, Wolff, & Douglas, 1981). Furthermore, Rimm and Rimm (1976) suggested, in a retrospective account, that obesity in childhood relates strongly to obesity in adulthood. From surveying more than 73,000 women who belonged to a popular self-help weight-loss group, they found that the most overweight were the most likely to have been fat youngsters; those adults having the greatest weight problems in comparison with those having the least weight problems were two to three times more likely to relate childhood histories of these difficulties (cf. Rimm, Rimm, & Hartz, 1976; Ullman, 1976). The age of onset in childhood that might best predict adult problems was, however, unstated.

Charney, Goodman, McBride, Lyon, & Pratt (1976), like several others mentioned previously in this chapter (for example, Knittle, 1975; Ginsberg-Fellner, 1981; Salans et al., 1973), suspect that obesity may be determined quite early in life; they do so after collecting weight measurements at two times on the same sample of individuals. First, they scrutinized thousands of pediatric records in order to obtain a sample of persons who, as infants, were at the 90th percentile in weight at six weeks, three months, or six months, those who were between the 25th and 75th percentiles at each of these times, or those who were below the 10th percentile during one of them. Approximately 400 persons met criteria. They then sent these individuals, already adults by the time of the study (20- to 30-years-old), a current weight-status questionnaire; to correct for reporting errors, that is, to develop a correction factor, they assessed a few in person. Analyzing the data, 366 returns, Charney and colleagues discovered that overweight infants risked becoming overweight adults. Compared with infants who failed to exceed or reach the 90th percentile in weight a minimum of one time during their first six months, those who did were 2.6 times more likely to be overweight adults (cf. Weil, 1977), 36 percent compared with 14 percent.

Accordingly, a relationship between excesses in childhood and adulthood appears for numerous individuals. Yet data are far from consistent. Here, as with studies depicting intervals shorter than childhood to adulthood (see above), the research strategies differ (for example, prospective versus retrospective); the obesity criteria differ; and the samples of children and adults tested differ in socioeconomic status, background, and so forth. Based on this relationship when it is found and on studies showing parent–child correspondences in obesity, it appears possible that not only do many obese, overweight adults pass these problems along to their progeny but also their progeny grow to pass it along to their own children. For numbers of obese children, consequently, there is a need for treatment. Identifying these children, however, is an undeveloped science.

Regarding treatment effectiveness (the second query), there is evidence that weight-control measures exacted in childhood do reduce the disease-related risk factors (Coates & Thoresen, 1980; Widhalm & Schernthaner, 1979; Chapter 1). There is less documentation that they improve a child's social relationships; nevertheless, many practitioners would undoubtedly attest, from clinical experience, that they do.

When treatment is offered, the therapist should be watchful, lest parents and caretakers force it on unwilling youths. Battlelines should not be drawn, for when they are, treatment is often doomed from the outset, bickering is often fostered (Chapter 6), and the child's negative view of himself and his body is often increased.

With young or institutionalized children (the retarded, for example), caretakers may be supervised in making such small, undramatic changes as reducing the availability of high-calorie treats and augmenting play opportunities. These could have profound results, not the least of which could be improving the child's chances of avoiding marked obesity. Older children could also prosper from such alterations, but these youths are usually drawn into the formal therapy process itself (cf. Aragona, Cassady, & Drabman, 1975).

Therapy will work well for some children, but not for all. Researchers and practitioners still do not know enough about its far-reaching effects (its effects on the child's self-perceptions and feelings of self-worth, and its durability), or about who needs which methods. Examples of how to design a therapy predicated on the child's uniqueness—particular skills, needs, environment—are rare. Indeed, there is a dearth of proven health-care strategies to offer (see Chapter 1). Subsequent chapters examine the behavior therapist's contribution to eliminating this deficit, a contribution that is now only in its earliest stage.

CHAPTER 3

Behavioral Treatment: Part I

Therapy is behavioral because it attempts, through the application of principles of learning that have their origins in scientific research, to help individuals to alter unwanted actions (Wilson & O'Leary, 1980). Characteristic of behavior therapy or, as it sometimes is termed in this book, behavior modification, is the process by which it is carried out. That process, parts of which will be illustrated in this and subsequent chapters, is comprised of three interrelated stages: assessment of behavior and its environmental concomitants; intervention to change behavior; evaluation to monitor the current effects of intervention, to understand the behavior changing role of intervention, to determine the long-range results of intervention, and to decipher the clinical impact of intervention in the patient's social milieu. As will be evident presently, this process may take several forms in the behavioral control of obesity and often, unfortunately, is markedly abridged.

Chapters 3, 4, and 5 examine what aids exist in the camp of the behavior therapist for the overweight youngster; principles and methods are discussed and practices exemplifying their application are shown. Behavioral technology currently being offered to overweight youngsters is addressed. Also addressed, however, are behavioral tactics of the adult weight-control literature that are not as yet prominent in child treatment; some may soon be. For the behavioral strategies used in treating overweight adults are the seeds from which a major part of the behavioral care of the overweight child, as a research and treatment area, will grow.

Behaviors and Methods of Acceleration

The technology of operant conditioning (see, for example, Skinner, 1953) underlies much of what is directed toward helping the obese child reduce. This technology concerns itself with antecedents, behaviors, and consequences. Behaviors and consequences will be discussed in this chapter.

Operant conditioning focuses on behaviors called operants that are to be distinguished from respondents. Respondents are elicited behaviors that are seemingly involuntary, in the sense that when stimuli for them are presented they, with apparent automaticity, follow. For example, provided that no physical reasons arise to prevent it, when a bright light is focused into the eye, the pupil constricts; pupil constriction thus is a respondent. Respondent conditioning is possible, as Pavlov (1927) demonstrated at the turn of this century; respondents can be attached to previously neutral stimuli. A defining characteristic of the respondent, be it attached to other stimuli or not, is that it is controlled by its antecedents. The operant, in contrast, is controlled by its consequences, by events following it.

Operants, such as running, walking, tying a shoelace, turning a doorknob, occur everyday; they happen most often in sequences aimed toward some ultimate end. Those operants plaguing an overweight child could be snacking between meals, watching television six hours daily, being chauffered about, and more. Such actions are modifiable. They may be made less likely, less probable, as other more desirable behaviors are made more likely, more probable. This change in probability is most clearly expressed as a change in frequency or a change in rate (that is, frequency in a specified period). Accelerating behavior, therefore, means making it more frequent, more probable, or making it occur at a higher rate. Decelerating behavior means the opposite; that is, making it less frequent, less probable, or making it occur at a lower rate. A child may, after treatment, go to the corner candy store three times per week instead of six. If so, the rate of his visits has been decelerated. He goes half as often, a reduction of three in frequency.

Is this change beneficial? The answer, in part, depends on whether or not there has been a corresponding reduction in calorie intake and weight. To know, the therapist must tabulate both the quantity of food the child buys at the store and eats soon afterwards as well as the child's weight before and after the deceleration in behavior takes place. Perhaps the child keeps his weight stable by increasing his purchases and consumption as he reduces his visits. The point, albeit obvious, reflects the importance of considering the interrelationships of behavior change, body change, and energy change when judging the worth of a behavioral intervention; usually the point is overlooked.

Negative Reinforcement

To accelerate an operant behavior beyond its customary level of occurrence—its baseline or pretreatment level—one must change its consequences. There are two ways to do so: positive reinforcement and negative reinforcement. Negative reinforcement should not be confused with punishment, a technique for decelerating behavior; negative reinforcement is for accelerating behavior. With negative reinforcement, an individual learns to behave in ways that help to avoid or remove events that, colloquially, are unpleasant; actions that avoid or remove such events become probable when the events are likely. Sometimes unadaptive, illicit eating is maintained in just that way. For example, the obese preadolescent girl who joins her peers after school at a nearby restaurant (see Chapter 2) eats a slice of apple pie not because she is hungry but because she wants to avoid being teased about dieting. Teasing is the consequence that the peer group issues for violating the norm: "Eat to be one of us." Between-meal eating, therefore, is negatively reinforced.

The girl has a conflict. She can eat and not be teased, or she can diet and not gain weight. Negative reinforcement is involved in both possibilities. If she chooses to diet in the face of peer ridicule, her punishment is immediate. If she chooses instead to eat, her punishment—gaining weight—is delayed. Her decision is affected by the immediacy of the consequence; remote consequences have a weaker hold (see Ferster, Nurnberger, & Levitt, 1962). Indeed, for many obese children, adolescents, and adults, dieting becomes a private action because when obvious it draws unwanted attention, attention to their being different; the discomfort of immediate recognition outweighs the pain—the more remote pain—of gaining weight and girth.

Making food substitutions describes an adaptive role for negative reinforcement. An obese child, told by his therapist to snack on carrots rather than on potato chips, asks his parents to buy vegetables to avoid having calorie-rich snacks available in the home; by so doing he avoids the temptation of chips. Teaching children to make these substitutions may, however, be tremendously frustrating. Having parents try to teach their children to do so may be equally frustrating. Negative reinforcement has some value in changing parental actions in this regard. Kirscht, Becker, Haefner, and Maiman (1978), for example, suggest that threatening communications about the dangers of being fat are helpful in increasing parental compliance with weight-control prescriptions and attendance at weight-control sessions.

Negative reinforcement has been applied in behavioral control programs for overweight adults. Ferster and colleagues (1962) recommend it for bringing the ultimate consequences of being obese closer to the act of illicit eating, for solving the immediacy–delay problem just addressed. They taught their patients to say personally meaningful and punishing things to themselves when compelled to eat unplanned-for food. The idea was to associate the nasty statements with the acts of between-meal eating so that the act of eating, or rather approaches to eating, became aversive. Once starting to engage in these acts becomes unpleasant, efforts to escape should become strong.

Penick, Filion, Fox, and Stunkard (1971) also used the negative reinforcement procedure to bring about weight loss; unlike Ferster and co-workers, however, they did not focus directly on eating. They told their patients to devise plastic "fat bags" to store suet. The bags, containing ounce-size portions of the animal fat, were kept in the refrigerator. When a patient reduced a pound, she threw away an ounce of suet from the fat bag. Presumably, behaviors culminating in weight loss were reinforced by the removal of suet. There have been other attempts to negatively reinforce in order to treat obese adults, but these attempts are infrequent when compared to those relying on the acceleration technique described below.

Positive Reinforcement

Suppose a behavior therapist seeing the conflicted preadolescent as described above, wished to strengthen her dieting behaviors without applying negative reinforcement. To do so, he or she would first have to separate dieting into its components. If one were to order low-calorie snacks—snacks under 200 calories—when in the company of friends who are eating, for example, a list of foods and drinks conforming to this criterion would have to be generated. It could not include items that, if ordered, would engender ridicule; also, ideally the list should be comprised of foods and drinks on the menu of the most-frequented restaurant; the therapist and the patient could construct the list together, while both visit the designated place.

Having identified the dieting components, the therapist would next have to develop a recording strategy and a method of strengthening the desired changes. The patient could possibly be directed to mentally note whether she orders a low-calorie snack, a high-calorie one, or none at all when in a restaurant with friends. She could actually record her behavior later, at home. Self-reports of compliance with the recommenation could then be praised during the next treatment session or before, by telephone.

There are various consequences the therapist may employ in addition to approval. Regardless of what these consequences are, if they follow an action that increases in frequency and becomes more probable in similar situations, then the operation of giving them is called positive reinforcement. If something is said to the patient after she reports ordering low-calorie snacks and her reports of compliance increase, positive reinforcement has occurred; however, the accuracy of the reports is in question unless there are other sources of information (for example, peer reports) to corroborate it.

Positive reinforcement is a procedure in which behavior accelerates because of the consequences of that behavior; these consequences are called positive reinforcers if the behavior leading to their presentation increases. Both positive and negative reinforcement accelerate behavior. With negative reinforcement certain consequences are avoided or escaped. With positive reinforcement certain consequences are received.

As a therapy, positive reinforcement is deceptively simple: Give something to the patient that he likes for doing something good and he will get better. It is not that easy, however. Helping an obese child to safely change the shape of his body is a complex and delicate matter. In addition to the problems of selecting targets (that is, behaviors to change) and of retrieving data (glossed over above, to be further addressed) are two problems basic to applying the positive reinforcement procedure: finding and giving positive reinforcers.

What Levers Do Therapists Have?

Sometimes a specific consequence, an event or commodity, that seems like it should be a positive reinforcer is not for a specific child, in a specific setting, trying to alter a specific behavior. Determining which levers exist can never be done independently of the patient, setting, and behavior; however, leads as to what might function as positive reinforcers may come from knowing their classes.

One class, primary reinforcers, will accelerate behavior that produces them for everyone deprived of them. They are from birth capable of affecting what we do. Air, water, food, and rest are examples of these primary reinforcers. The necessity of depriving an individual before these events become behavior strengtheners makes some of them impractical. They lose their potency rapidly—as soon as they are used—because the deprivation originally responsible for their potency disappears. What's more, their routine and continued use is unethical; depriving persons of basic necessities is not justifiable.

Acquired reinforcers, another class, are not inborn rectifiers of need states; rather, they are learned consequences that are potent without creating specific deprivations. They become positive reinforcers during development through association with already powerful consequences. Acquired reinforcers vary in the degree to which they are central to one's obtaining many other reinforcers. If they are very central—that is, if having them makes possible having many other reinforcers—they are called generalized (generalized–acquired) reinforcers. Unlike primary reinforcers, generalized reinforcers do not quickly lose their power to reinforce behavior. Relatedly, they do not require that specific deprivations be created in order for them to become powerful. Their function is not to eliminate physiologic needs. Money, for instance, is a generalized reinforcer because it literally buys many primary and other reinforcers. Individuals do many different things to obtain money, even if they already are rich. Equally powerful, for some persons even more powerful, are attention and approval. We do various things to get these social consequences because having them increases the chances that our other actions will be reinforced. As Ferster and Perrott (1968) write about approval: "We ask a favor from someone who is smiling more readily than from someone who is frowning because of the greater likelihood of the favor being granted" (p. 191).

Various consequences have been used in behavioral programs.

Food and Drink.   In our society of plenty, numerous consumables continue to function as positive reinforcers even when hunger is absent; an ice cream cone will reinforce behavior even after a heavy dinner, as will such treats as soda pop, candy, and doughnuts. These edibles are ubiquitous and powerful.

Because they are potent and available in developed countries, can they be used in childhood obesity control programs? Some behavior therapists have tried (see, for example, Wheeler & Hess, 1976, Application 3). A very real concern in using them, however, is that they not become counterproductive, that they not spoil the behaver's efforts. A trip to the doughnut shop on the weekend may reinforce low calorie snacking during the week; desirable food substitutions occur daily. But if the intake of doughnuts on Saturday and Sunday results in a calorie surplus, (calories available from the weekend exceed the reduction achieved from food substitutions during the week), the positive reinforcement procedure will not contribute to weight or fat loss. Perhaps though, at the beginning of treatment, changes in behavior (snacking-control) are seen as vital, even if calorie overages on the weekend are needed to bring them about. Nevertheless, in the long run procedures causing calorie excesses, despite countable improvements in desired behaviors, are, as suggested before, self-defeating.

Another problem with edible reinforcers is that they may convey the wrong information to the overweight child. The boy or girl with a history of eating when angry, happy, sad, bored, or anxious (see Bruch, 1973, Chapter 2) might be better served by a positive reinforcement procedure that does not say "good" actions are paths to tasty foods.

Points, Trinkets, Money, and Praise. Less problematic than food and drink as reinforcers are the tangible, economic, and social consequences of points (tokens), toys, money, and praise. They may be used in various ways to increase the desirable behaviors of obese children; illustrations in the ensuing pages are a sample of some of the possibilities. Praise is valuable for all children, regardless of age. The other consequences, however, are more dependent on the child's age and maturity.

LeBow, Buser, Coles, Hanel, and Vallentyne (1979), for example, used pictures of animals to reinforce young children for adhering to activity regimens, whereas older youngsters simply graphed their progress (feedback). All the children (ages 7 to 12 years) also received points for increasing activity (for example, for walking to school instead of being driven). For the younger children the points were backed up by toys and fun activities; for the older children, points were exchanged for other items as well as for trips. The backup consequences made getting points worthwhile; exchanges of points for backup reinforcers took place every four weeks. The program lasted for approximately four months and served 18 obese children. At its conclusion, eight of the youngsters had lost weight, but five had gained. Nevertheless, all had reduced their waist sizes by 2.5 cm to over 20 cm. Also, skinfolds taken at the triceps had decreased, and the children had grown taller.

Applying a generalized reinforcer, one of several methods to treat an obese 11-year-old boy, Kaoukis (1980) employed the visual display pictured in Figure 3.1; he called it the two-bucket system. Each bucket had six levels, the objective for the boy was to fill both of them, one with fat, weight, and calories, the other with money. For every half-pound loss, the boy made an insert into the fat bucket and the therapist put 15¢ into the money bucket; a five pound reduction equalled $1.50. The boy could withdraw the money when he reached a new level of weight loss, but he was only allowed to advance to a new level if he had not relapsed or, if

Figure 3.1
Two-bucket System

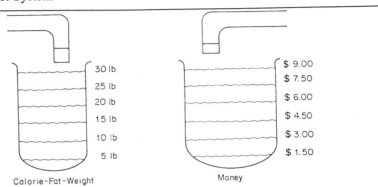

The bucket system is a tool in a comprehensive weight reduction program. The child is told that losing weight can be profitable. At this point, the youngster is shown the two buckets. He is told that as the fat bucket is filled with excess pounds, calories, and fat, the money bucket is being filled with money. The objective is to fill both buckets to the top.

The rules of the system are as follows:
a. For each half pound lost, a "glob" will be placed in the fat bucket and a coin will be put into the money bucket.
b. When 5 lbs have been lost, ten "globs" will be present in the fat bucket and 10 coins will have been placed in the money bucket. The 5 lb mark in the fat bucket and the $1.50 mark in the money bucket are the first levels or goals of the bucket system.
c. The child will not be paid until he reaches a bucket level.
d. If the child does not maintain his reduced weight he does not receive any further remuneration.
e. It is explained that he will receive money for losing weight only if it advances him to a higher level in the buckets.
f. The child is also told that he must lose weight according to the rules of the weight reduction program in order to be remunerated.

Text and figure adapted from Kaoukis (1980).

he had, that he lost the regained weight in addition to the stipulated five pounds; thus, hovering about the same weight was not reinforced. Kaoukis' system could be modified to suit younger patients if gradations in the weight bucket were reduced, perhaps to one pound, and if money in the second bucket was replaced by points or toys.

Activities. Opportunities to participate in certain activities may be used to accelerate desired activities. For instance, running and screaming are, for nursery schoolers, activity reinforcers that have been used to strengthen their being quiet (see, for example, Homme, deBaca, Devine, Steinhorst, & Rickert, 1963). Having time to do as you please has been used as an activity reinforcer for older children who are deaf (Osborne, 1969). Exploring a one-way mirror, operating a dictaphone, and running a videotape machine have been used in the treatment of a 10-year-old obese child (see Application 1, Chapter 5). Answering the telephone, turning on the faucet in the kitchen sink, sitting down in a special chair are reinforcers that have been used for overweight adults (Horan & Johnson, 1971; Tyler & Straughan, 1970). Employing activities to reinforce activities is a seminal idea. Premack (1965) laid down the principles for doing so; these were later extended for use in applied settings (Ayllon & Azrin, 1968; Homme et al., 1963; Homme, 1965), though not without criticism (see Danaher, 1974). The basic idea, the Premack Principle, is that behavior that is very probable in a given situation may be used as an activity reinforcer for behavior that is less probable in that situation. After naming behaviors to change and identifying potential activity reinforcers—going to a movie, watching television, playing tag, checkers, or chess—the therapist's task is to juxtapose the two actions. One technical difficulty is that many patients require immediate reinforcement in order for effectiveness; often, however, it is impossible to give an activity reinforcer right away; reinforcement is delayed. A movie after a week of good behavior is a distant outcome and, therefore, may be too remote to be effective. One solution is to combine acquired and activity reinforcers. Thus, as illustrated in the LeBow and co-workers' (1979) report, a child may earn points that he saves toward the purchase of some activity reinforcer by complying with treatment prescriptions; points can be delivered immediately. Beck and colleagues (1980) studied 43 overweight youngsters between the ages of 8 and 12 years. Those who were taught routine daily exercises outperformed, in weight losses and body-mass index changes measured at follow-up, those who were taught the more prolonged activities—daily sports and recreations (see also, Dickson, Szparaga, Epstein, Wing, Koeske, & Zidansek, 1981; Epstein, Nuss, Wing, Koeske, Zidansek, & Dickson, 1981; Epstein, Wing, Koeske, Ossip, & Beck, 1982). To reinforce exercising, Beck and colleagues gave the children points contingent on the expenditure of calories; the points bought such reinforcers as family outings.

Feedback. As suggested, a change in an action often generates its own positively reinforcing consequence, and that perpetuates action. In other words, by realizing progress from our past actions we increase their future likelihood. Seen, progress is a reinforcer. Behavior therapists were not the first to learn this, for since the dawn of history those involved in sustained effort have evaluated their achievements, and many people have persevered from the experience of doing so; others have been punished by seeing the results of their labors, and have quit in the face of failure; still others, unhappy with what they have produced, have modified their efforts and tried again.

Dieters fit into each of the three categories: There are those who have seen their dieting efforts pay off; there are those who, seeing them defeated, stop forever; and there are those, the most numerous class, who, having failed, are still game for every new diet that comes along. Feedback from what we do affects what we continue to do.

Among the sources of feedback for dieters are records of calorie intake and calorie outgo, records of adherence to treatment directives, and graphs of weight loss. Fisher, Green, Friedling, Levenkron, & Porter (1976) used weight graphing to generate therapeutic feedback (see also Loro, Fisher, & Levenkron, 1979). Patients weighed themselves daily and evaluated whether they were above or below a designated goal. They plotted weight-expected against time-dieting to construct their personal graphs. On these graphs patients drew diagonal lines from their initial weights plus almost 1 kg at the top of the ordinate to the last days on the program; these days were depicted at the point to the right of the abcissa. The lines were the critical weight lines that were not to be crossed. The program worked. After a mean of less than 40 days, 11 patients lost roughly 4.3 kg.

Fisher and co-workers' simple graphing tactic permitted daily feedback, but unless patients kept mental or written notes of what they did to reduce, they could not see how they went about it. Since they were not taught the how-to information, it is unlikely that they made behavioral records and related weight-loss successes to behavior-change efforts. Had they attempted to see these relationships, they would have been quite fortunate in realizing progress so rapidly. Daily weight losses are atypical, and fat losses take still longer to become evident. Tying body modifications to behavior modifications is difficult for the patient; feedback in the form of body changes is often delayed. One sees neither a difference in a bathroom scale reading nor a difference in the way clothes fit from each refusal to snack. Both changes, particularly the ones in fatness, usually arise long after many similar refusals. Thus, because transformations in targeted actions only poorly reflect body alterations, they may have to be specifically highlighted and specifically reinforced, especially in working with children, in order to bridge the gap between behavior change and its ultimate result. The clearest effects of the attempts to modify behavior are the modifications in behavior that result; if they are important in losing weight and fat, they must be repeated over and over again. It is necessary to explicitly reinforce them until the child comes into contact with the fruits of his labors that will then sustain him in continuing to behave adaptively.

Summary of Available Levers

In sum, various classes of reinforcers exist, and there are numbers of reinforcers within each class. Determining what they are for a particular child is an empirical problem. Suggestions about what to try, however, are available. Phillips, Fischer, and Singh (1977), for example, list possible activity reinforcers, among which are riding in a car, hunting for frogs and snakes, watching television, hiking, fishing, pool. They also list toys (for example, matchbox cars, dolls, electric trains, bicycles), crafts, food, learning, items for personal appearance, and more. Patterned after Cautela and Kastenbaum's (1967) survey of reinforcers for adults, the Phillips and colleagues' schedule reports a test–retest reliability of .598 over one week. Ease of administration is a strength. Additional ways for finding a youngster's reinforcers are interviewing the child and his parents and (most time consuming) directly observing him. Combining survey, interview, and empirical observation methods may prove to be useful. The objective is to create an array of reinforcers—a reinforcer menu (Addison & Homme, 1966)—that allows the therapist to switch reinforcers as necessary. The data gathered as the child progresses in treatment dictate when to switch.

Having discussed the levers therapists can use, we can turn to the second problem they face when using the positive-reinforcement procedure.

How Are Reinforcers Best Administered?

There are six rules. Exceptions to following them exist, successes occurring despite violations; but following the rules maximizes efficient use of the positive-reinforcement procedure.

Administer Reinforcers Contingent on Behavior. There should be an explicit relationship between the outcome of a designated action and the action itself, and the child should know about it; he should be clear as to what is desired and what comes from behaving as desired. Contingencies, relationships between behaviors and consequences, are to be specified at the start of intervention. Accordingly, if a child is to substitute fruit for cookies at the Monday, Wednesday, and Friday after-school snacks, the therapist must state exactly what appropriate substitutions are and what compliance each day will bring (for example, an hour of "extra" television at night).

Administer Reinforcers Soon After Behavior. How prompt the reinforcer–administrator (therapist, parent) needs to be varies, depending on the child being treated and the complexity of the behavior being accelerated. Very young children and the developmentally impaired profit from immediate reinforcement. Thus, allowing a retarded child an outing at night for eating only the meals served him during day and evening will likely be less productive than giving him hourly points toward the outing if he lives up to the contingency.

Similarly, praising an 8-year-old obese girl for making low-fat and low-sugar food choices as soon as she makes them at lunch in a cafeteria (see, for example, Application 7, Chapter 5) has a better chance of working than does praising her recollections of doing so three hours later. The girl recalls accurately and responds well to delayed reinforcement, but selecting criterion foods may be a complex undertaking for her; if so, immediate praise will be more informative and corrective than will delayed praise. In this vein, approving of her weight losses at the end of the week, if that is all or most of what is done, does not optimize the value of praise, for it is doubtful that the consequence will have a major impact if the actions the child takes to achieve the loss remain unclear to her.

Administer Enough Reinforcers that are Powerful.   Enough and powerful are inexact words. How much reinforcement is enough and which consequences are powerful (such as praise, movies, money) depend on the patient and the behavior asked of him. Ten cents for bed-making may do much to ensure that a 7-year-old keeps his room tidy but nothing toward getting him to eat more salads and fewer sweets. There is even less that a modern 12-year-old living in an affluent society would do to earn a dime, but he may do much for approval; 4-year-olds care nothing about money, but they respond well to toys and praise. Therefore, the criteria of enough and powerful, as with the initial selection of reinforcers, are affected by the patient's age and maturity and the task in question.

Applying too much and too little reinforcement and employing weak consequences have the same result: Behavior changes little, if at all. Excessive reinforcement bankrupts the reinforcer–administrator or allows the child riches that obviate continued compliance. Likewise, too little reinforcement and weak reinforcers lead to quitting—the payoff is not worth the effort. Even if powerful at the outset, the potency of the consequence dwindles as the event that obtains it becomes more difficult to complete. Losing weight, for instance, becomes harder as time passes, and so monetary incentives for reducing (the kinds of consequences often used) should be augmented to offset the increasing difficulty; a dollar per week at the start of treatment for losing a ½ kg could be raised to $2 by the 50th week for the same amount of weight loss. Similarly, if a patient tires of keeping food records, the payoffs contingent on compliance could be enlarged. Efforts to keep reinforcers powerful may be necessary.

Patients in weight-control programs frequently receive payments for progressing; they are paid from funds they deposit with the therapist just before the start of treatment. To exemplify, Mann (1972) asked his adult patients to surrender items they valued—jewelry, medals, clothes, and trophies; he promised to return them contingent on weight loss. How valuable these items remained to the adults surrendering them was probably critical to Mann's findings.

Jeffery, Thompson, and Wing (1978), though not specifically testing the amount or power variable, did find that large returns produced dramatic results. Thirty-one adults received 10 weeks of behaviorally based instruction on how to reduce. The patients, all quite overweight at the start, were placed in one of four groups—three financial incentive conditions and a control. The reinforcement was earning back portions of a $200 deposit, $20.00 weekly for losing about 1 kg (weight group), keeping to a certain calorie intake level (calorie group), or attending sessions (attendance group). By tying large reinforcers either to weight reduction or calorie intake reduction, Jeffery and associates produced good effects; reinforcing attendance was less productive, however (cf., Wing, Epstein, Marcus, & Shapira, 1981). Patients in this study, as noted, did not appear to take drastic measures to retrieve funds. Mann (1972), in contrast, found that some of his patients did; they took diuretics and laxatives to promote reinforceable weight losses. Evidently, powerful reinforcers had a negative byproduct. If large returns are attendant upon continued reduction, and if continuing to reduce is difficult, the reinforcers may be ultimately damaging. The more powerful the reinforcers are, the more important it is to monitor the steps patients take to acquire them. Certainly, using powerful reinforcers is not bad practice, but in doing so researchers and practitioners should look not only at the measurable changes in the body that result but also at how these changes are obtained.

Administer Reinforcers Sincerely. A powerful reinforcer, such as praise, will lose its potency if given halfheartedly or overzealously. Sincere delivery is mandatory. Perhaps insincerity in the reinforcer–administration accounts for some of the variability in patient response to behavioral treatment. One way of being insincere in a behavioral weight control program is to request that patients keep food records, to accept them graciously at the end of a week, and then, in front of the patient who has labored over them, to file these records without reading them. Therapists guilty of this neglect are not backing up praise with actions that confirm the importance of these inventories. In effect, patients are told that they need not bother complying. Time spent scrutinizing records in the patient's presence is well worth it, both to strengthen adherence to a valuable prescription and perhaps to weaken the chances of attrition (Stuart, 1978).

Administer Reinforcers Consistently. This dictum concerns scheduling reinforcer delivery. The way to most efficiently strengthen behavior is to reinforce it every time it happens. Consistency of this sort, however, demands either continuous observation or permanent products; suppose food-intake charting is to be strengthened; the chart is then a permanent record generated by the behavior of recording consumption. The overweight child asked to record could be reinforced for doing so after each meal. To run the program, parents and school personnel would have to monitor him carefully, surveying his charts every few hours. This nearly continuous watching would be time consuming. Less costly would be surveying a week of food records gathered daily. Rather than meal-by-meal monitoring, the unit of behavior observed before reinforcement is administered is larger, and fewer people are needed to run the program. But there is a price for making the job easier. Precision in strengthening a behavior is often sacrificed when units are large because even though the food-intake recordings are permanent products, errors in their constuction may be present; and these mistakes are more easily buried in a seven day tactic as opposed to one done meal by meal. Whatever way you tackle strengthening record keeping (meal by meal, day by day, or week by week) avoid the hit-and-miss system of reinforcement. Administer reinforcers consistently.

Once the behavior to be accelerated is strong, however, reinforcers may be delivered intermittently. Theoretically, it would be possible to strengthen an obese child's compliance with treatment prescriptions by consistently administering reinforcers contingent on his acting as desired and then making the desired actions endure by tapering off reinforcement—switching to an intermittent schedule (see, for example, Ferster & Skinner, 1957; Ferster, Culbertson, & Boren, 1975).

Practically, on the other hand, the task of switching would be difficult. The amount of control over the patient's reinforcers needed to change from consistent to intermittent rarely exists in the obese child's environment; the topic has, therefore, received little attention. Recently, however, DeLuca (1982) did investigate the effects of intermittent schedules of reinforcement on exercising in obese and nonobese youngsters. She recruited several fifth-grade boys, obese and nonobese, for her intensive study. The job for each child was to pedal a stationary bicycle (programmed to simultaneously ring a bell and flash a red light) five times weekly for one-half hour a day. The bell and light signals followed either a minute of pedalling (an interval schedule) or a designated number of bicycle-wheel revolutions (a ratio schedule); the behavioral requirement of the ratio schedule, wheel revolutions, equalled the average number of revolutions of the interval schedule. The children earned points backed up by previously selected items from a reinforcer survey for turning on the bell and light. Looking at rate of pedalling, DeLuca found increases for all children on the interval schedule and for all but one (a nonobese child) on the ratio schedule. She also reported fitness improvements and body-fat decreases attributable to her program. The clinical value of such methods for obese children (for example, hooking up a stationary bicycle to the TV at home so that the children's pedalling will bring in a clearer picture) awaits further demonstration; so also does the entire topic of making consistent reinforcement for healthful actions intermittent.

Producing Behavior

The behaviorist believes that the obese child will profit from increases in the frequency of specific behaviors. Negative and positive reinforcement are two procedures for helping the child to accomplish this; positive reinforcement, understandably, is the more popular of the two. Unwanted side effects are less likely when applying positive reinforcement, and ordinarily it is easier to engineer. For use, the behavior to be strengthened must already occur at some level. If it does not, it must first be produced.

How difficult it is to produce a behavior depends on what the action is and, relatedly, on the skills of the patient being treated. Usually the simplest method is tried initially: that is, instruction. When the information on how to reduce is available, patients frequently are simply told what it is. To be maximally effective, these instructions should be exact. They should explicitly specify what behaviors are prescribed. Simple tasks may be stated in their entirety, while those more complex should be broken down into their parts and arranged sequentially; each step should be instructed and performing it reinforced; advancing to a new step should occur after the patient masters preceding ones.

Another tactic for producing behavior, less often used in obesity programs, is modeling (see Janzen & Doleys, 1981; also see Application 4, Chapter 5). By observing the therapist clearly demonstrate an activity and by being reinforced for correctly imitating it, a patient can learn a new behavior or can increase the complexity of some other one that he already is able to perform. If the activity to be produced and then to be accelerated is complex, the following steps are valuable:

1. Specify the behavior, and sequentially arrange the parts that comprise it, from first to last
2. Demonstrate each part clearly
3. Reinforce the patient's correct imitation of each element shown
4. Advance from one step to the next only when the patient masters the previous ones.

When all the parts can be performed correctly, they should be linked together to form the whole behavior that is then demonstrated in its entirety. Imitation of the total behavior eventually becomes the requirement for reinforcement (LeBow, 1973).

Instructions may be used with the demonstration–imitation tactic. Gradualness in overcoming hurdles and practice in performing new behaviors are essential. For example, initiating ½ hour of jogging in an otherwise healthy but out of shape overweight 12-year-old sixth-grade girl requires that the patient assemble the correct equipment, set proper objectives, select a course, and begin a walk-jog-walk sequence (see, for example, Bowerman, Harris, & Shea, 1978). She should practice the sequence three to four times weekly, gradually lessening the walking components as the jogging is increased. How fast she accelerates will depend on how she feels when exercising. She should not demand too much of herself too quickly or become sluggish and fail to try harder. She might develop a self-rating form of perceived effort and apply this to pace changes in the program. Reinforcers for progressing could be praise from the therapist and feedback from self-observed accomplishments in behavior and body change.

Acquiring and strengthening new eating and activity habits are not the only ways in which the overweight prosper from behavioral technology. Strategies for decreasing the frequency of problematic actions, actions that cause weight gain or that interfere with weight loss, can also be applied.

Behaviors and Methods of Deceleration

Five operant conditioning-based deceleration tactics are identified here. Each plays a role in the behavioral control of obesity.

Aversive Stimulation

Operationally, behaviors that decrease—that is, those that become less probable in the future—after producing identifiable consequences may be said to be punished. When a child touches a hot stove, he quickly withdraws his hand. The behavior of touching stoves that appear to be hot is less likely to occur in the future. For the child, the results of the action are crying (respondent behavior) from pain and surprise as well as becoming less likely to touch stoves in the future.

Aversive stimulation is effective, but there are potential problems with it, unwanted side effects (Bandura, 1969). The punished individual may take steps to avoid those who punish; behaviors successful in avoiding or escaping from aversive stimuli are likely to become strong through the process of negative reinforcement.

In a therapy relying on aversive stimulation, avoidance has been found to interfere; Meyer and Crisp (1964) illustrate. They attempted to treat two overweight, hospitalized women by shocking them with an 80 to 90 volt electric shock when the women approached tempting food. One woman did well under this punishment procedure, receiving 10 shocks in all and losing 9 kg during the first six weeks; she lost over 23 kg more during the next 20 months. The other patient fared worse. She lost next to nothing. After one practice shock, she managed to avoid ever being shocked again by not touching the tempting food placed before her. She apparently eliminated the opportunity to be treated by never coming into contact with the aversive stimulus.

Measuring both the palatability and the consumption of tempting food, Abramson and Jones (1981) found the aversive stimulation procedure more effective than one devoid of pain. Their subjects were told to follow junk-food cravings and choices by snapping themselves with a rubber band worn on the wrist. Like Meyer and Crisp, Abramson and Jones used overt procedures. Cautela (1966, 1967, 1972) applied covert ones, the most prominent in the literature on weight control being covert sensitization. He discussed its theoretical rationale in operant-conditioning terms and saw it as the covert analogue of what I have called aversive stimluation (see Cautela & Baron, 1977). Covert sensitization, therefore, is a deceleration method. It relies upon imaginal representations of both the behavior to be decreased and the aversive consequences to be attendant on failing to decrease it. Patients imagine eating a proscribed food and then vomiting it; they must practice the technique in front of the therapist and at home. In rehearsals, they are to try to imagine the sensations of being where troublesome eating occurs, giving in to temptation, and then the horrid consequence of relenting to the temptation.

Studies investigating this method's value for the obese adult are contradictory; some find it to be potent, others do not (Diament & Wilson, 1975; Harris, 1969; Janda & Rimm, 1972). The conditioning principles underlying the method also have been challenged (Diament & Wilson, 1975; Foreyt & Hagen, 1973). The view that today prevails among many obesity therapists is that covert sensitization's major service is adjunctive, not primary (see, for example, Stuart, 1967). Whether the technique has use in treating overweight juveniles is unknown; it may yet prove to be of some value to obese adolescents who have unremitting food cravings.

Removing Positive Reinforcers

An alternative to presenting aversive, unpleasant consequences in order to decelerate overt or covert behavior is to remove something pleasant when the behaver acts in a proscribed way. The main result of doing so is the same: the proscribed act decelerates, becomes less likely to occur in the future. Parents, teachers, and therapists have tried controlling children in this way, sometimes succeeding, sometimes not.

Time out is one of the two variations of the basic operation. Time out means that the individual is forced to spend time away from something he enjoys because he has done something condemnable. For instance, a 6-year-old who leaps out of his chair at school, runs around the classroom, and shouts may be pulled out of the classroom and made to stand in the hall for 10 minutes. If being in class is desirable in his view, then being removed from it contingent on jumping up, and so on, should decrease the bothersome conduct. Ayllon (1963) applied this reasoning to stop an almost 114 kg hospitalized psychiatric patient from pilfering food; she stole when in the hospital's dining area. Time out for stealing—she was removed from the dining room—appeared to work. She stopped her thievery, and because her food supply was as a result less, the reduced nearly 32 kg. Had the eating place been an unpleasant setting, or had the attention from the staff that occurred when she took extra food been sought, she would have probably gotten worse instead of better. The method would have boomeranged. Likewise, if the 6-year-old had hated the schoolroom, or if he had liked being where passersby recognized him, he would have probably become a greater behavior problem for his teacher. In effect, for both the child and Ayllon's patient, time out would have amounted to removal from a negative setting (negative reinforcement) and admission to a positive one (the chance for positive consequences). Application errors do occur. Monitoring the individual's response to treatment methods will help correct them.

Use of time out is not at all that frequent in the behavioral control of obesity. More often the second variation of removing positive reinforcers is found (see Application 5, Chapter 5; Coates, Jeffery, Slinkard, Killen, & Danaher, 1982). This technique makes forbidden actions expensive and is called response-cost; the expense is a loss of money, prizes, or other valuables. In other words, when patients behave undesirably, they forfeit positive reinforcers.

As stated, Jefferey, Thompson, and Wing (1978) kept portions of patients' two-hundred-dollar deposits for failing to meet calorie-intake quotas, for failing to attend sessions, and for failing to reduce. In brief, patients lost money when they ate too much, missed sessions, stayed the same weight, or gained. Although the program worked, the authors indicate a potential problem with it: When response-cost is applied to the events of failing to reduce or to gaining, it is possible to accidentally punish appropriate eating and actions related to it because weight may fluctuate regardless of behavior change.

Reinforcing Other Behavior

The rationale of this method is that of the positive reinforcement procedure. Reinforcing other behavior is a deceleration method, however, because the behavior accelerated by reinforcement competes with the proscribed action; the behavior strengthened is incompatible or interfering. There are basically two ways to apply this deceleration method: First, identify a behavior incompatible with the behavior to be decreased, and then positively reinforce the incompatible action until it is strong enough to compete with the undesirable one. For instance, instead of using time out to decrease jumping, running, and shouting, the teacher discussed in the above section on time out could have reinforced the child's remaining seated and quiet; being seated and quiet competes with jumping, running, and shouting.

Behaviorists trying to teach the overweight to alter their environments often have asked them to find incompatible behaviors that can be substituted for between-meal eating (see, for example, Stuart, 1967). Ferster and associates (1962) refer to these incompatible actions as a pre-potent repertoire; the repertoire replaces unwanted behaviors. A woman who complains of uncontrollable urges to snack at 3:00 p.m. could be told to go for a walk at that time, provided that walking is pleasurable to her. Or, she could be told to call a friend, read, or write a letter when the disposition to eat arises. Ferster and co-workers advise patients to reserve such pleasant activities for hours when illicit eating is probable so that the chances of using them when they are needed is high.

The second way to apply the positive reinforcement procedure as a deceleration method is to deliver reinforcers following an interval during which the patient behaves adaptively . . . no matter what the actions are, so long as they are not those proscribed. The obese Prader-Willi child who is described in Application 2, Chapter 5, was awarded stars for periods of *not* stealing food.

Applying positive reinforcement, an acceleration method, to diminish the probability of unhealthy actions among obese children is a wise strategy. More use should be made of it. It is often a reasonable alternative to punitive methods. Also, it may be associated with coming to see the therapist as a giver rather than as a taker and by so doing encourages the obese youngster to remain active in therapy longer instead of searching for ways to end it.

Extinction

Extinction is the act of discontinuing reinforcement; it is a way to decrease the frequency of positively and negatively reinforced behavior. A child who tantrums may do so because the tantrums bring attention. If attention is the culprit that positively reinforces tantrumming, extinction would be ignoring tantrums; as a result of applying this method, the tantrums should diminish.

The 6-year-old who nags his mother for candy at the supermarket often receives the candy on an intermittent schedule and attention from mother on a continuous one; stern "no's" follow loud requests until a number of the requests have been made or until they become intense, whereupon the candy is given. Consequently, nagging remains strong. To apply extinction and reduce pestering at the market, mother would have to stop answering the demands—an admittedly difficult feat, especially in public. Also, mother would have to stop giving candy at the store. She can expect nagging to get worse for awhile but eventually to abate. She could help herself triumph by giving the child treats at home, perhaps after meals or at scheduled snack times. Of course, for extinction to benefit the child's weight, he must consume less candy at home than he would have at the market. But even if he replaces what he no longer has at the store, he still may be helped behaviorally; the setting change delimits the cues to junk-food eating, cues that could bother him in future years.

Satiation

Satiation works, quite possibly, by reducing the potency of a positive reinforcer until the reinforcer no longer is reinforcing at all. Operationally, satiation involves giving the patient an overabundance of positive reinforcers; how much is too much is measurable by monitoring behavioral effects.

Ayllon (1963), in a much quoted study, treated hoarding with satiation. He oversupplied the hoarder with the hoarded commodity. The patient, the food stealer discussed above, also collected towels and by so doing disrupted the ward routine. Consequently, her nurses tried to stop her by applying the satiation procedure. They gave her towels by the dozens until her customary level of 19 to 29 jumped to 625. Following that, after several weeks of satiation, she began to rid herself of towels, and thereby ended the procedure. The woman's hoarding decreased not only by treatment's end but also during the ensuing year. Perhaps the towels, previously effective as positive reinforcers, became aversive. That this may have happened is suggested by her exclamation, "Get these dirty towels out of here" (p. 57).

As a behavioral procedure for reducing unwanted eating, satiation could amount to using the act of eating to control long-term overeating. That is, by consuming a favorite food to excess one could make the food unpleasant and as a result the probability for consuming it in the future less. Hagen (1976) did so on purpose. Many do so by accident. Binge eaters, however, appear to be resistent to this kind of satiation, for numbers of them eat to discomfort, even illness, only to return to binging on the same foods a few days or weeks later. The clinical value of applying satiation in a comprehensive behavioral weight-loss program and for whom it is most suitable are issues needing further study.

CHAPTER 4

Behavioral Treatment: Part II

This chapter continues the presentation of methods found in the behavioral control of obesity; the emphasis is on multi-element tactics.

Contracting

Contracting with adults, adolescents, and children, in addition to being a key part of many a multi-element weight-loss program, is a way to supply patients with the multiple treatments. It consists of developing a clear, written agreement that parties to it believe will help the patient to become thinner; the agreement designed is a behavioral contract. It details a *quid pro quo* arrangement between those signing it, and it lists consequences for doing and not doing the agreed to things. These consequences, the fuel of the contract, may be various items of value that are administered for living up to the contract or withdrawn for failure to do so.

Examples of Contracting

Several years ago I treated a 32-year-old, 109 kg woman for 47 weeks using a system of renewable five-week contracts. She loathed the idea of embarking on a long-term commitment to reduce but felt more sanguine about tying herself to consecutive short-term agreements. She recognized this as a ploy; nevertheless, by breaking down the task into small units, she entered into the agreement more comfortably and more full of hope.

To start, she surrendered $20.00 to me; she did this at the beginning of each contract. I returned money to her at scheduled sessions contingent on her losing weight (about 1 kg weekly), keeping food records, restricting calories to a prescribed level, and exercising. I kept money if she failed to meet objectives and if she neglected to notify me that she could not attend sessions. Forfeited money was sent in her name, with her approval, to an organization she abhorred.

In all, she signed seven of these contracts. For the first three of them, she reached or exceeded her objectives, losing almost 17 kg over the course of a few months. After the third contract, however, difficulties arose. For contract four, she decided against weekly sessions, preferring to meet bi-weekly instead. I modified the document accordingly, but she managed to reduce only about 1.4 kg all told. Several weeks later, after returning from a vacation, she began contract five. To her own great pleasure, she lost enough weight on her trip to start this new agreement at the level she previously had bargained to reach.

So, with renewed confidence in her efforts and pride in her accomplishments (by now she had lost nearly 21 kg) she set to work on the next commitment. Unfortunately, she also had to go to court to obtain more child-support payments from her ex-husband. This battle resulted in a great deal of stress for her and led to a weight gain, the first one since the start of the program, of about .5 kg; a long-standing pattern of hers was to use food to alleviate distress, but the relapse was slight and was, therefore, an indication of control. As I look back, however, it may have been less painful for her had I stopped the contract when she went to court. The advantage of doing so, in addition to subtracting from her woes, would have been not pitting the regimen against forces that could have compromised it and brought on premature termination.

Luckily this patient did not drop out in the face of adversity. Instead, she prevented herself from a marked relapse. She signed the sixth document but lost only half the stipulated amount of weight. Several weeks afterwards, an interval during which she shed the remainder, she negotiated contract seven; again, however, she reduced only a portion of the agreed upon amount. Then, treatment ended because she moved. I do not know if she maintained her losses. Overall, she reduced 24 kg, which is 22 percent of her pretreatment weight; her reduction rate was approximately .5 kg weekly.

These contracts, as most in the weight-control area, were time limited. They lasted for designated periods, the durations of which were agreed to in advance of the signing. Some contracts, however, are event limited, in that specific events must happen (for example, 4 kg must be lost) before termination. Actually, the above contracts were both time and event limited; they specified five-week operating intervals and 4.5 kg losses. Terminations occurred when either circumstance occurred, no matter which happened first. The task for the patient was to lose the weight before the time elapsed, but not too fast; by not being paid for losses in excess of .5 kg above the weekly criterion (cf. Martin & Sachs, 1973), she was discouraged from reducing more than 1.4 kg a week.

Behavioral researchers and practitioners design weight-control contracts to run for weeks, months, and sometimes more than a year. Table 4.1 (LeBow, 1976) is a sample 53-week agreement, strictly time limited, having five phases; two therapists and one patient signed it.

Seven requirements are specified in Phase A, weeks 1 to 13. Weight loss of a pound a week below basal weight results in one dollar, record-keeping yields fifty cents, and so forth. The number of treatment sessions each week is two, but money is paid out once every seven days; for requirements 6 and 7, however, money is given only near the end of the first 10-week period.

The patient is paid for the tasks he accomplishes. If he gains during the week, he not only remains broke but also loses ground, that is, he makes it tougher on himself to

Table 4.1
A Sample 53-Week Contract

PATIENT

I realize that this is a contract for losing weight and that my signing it signifies my complete understanding of its contents. There will be five phases to this fat-control program wherein I will have the opportunity to earn back monies constituting some portion of my fees.

Weeks 1 to 13 (two sessions per week, ten money-exchange days). During this time period, I will have 10 opportunities to receive payment for my fat-control efforts. During each of these 10 opportunities, I will be paid the following amounts for the following events:

1. One dollar for each pound lost below my basal level of weight. The basal weight is the lowest amount of weight I have reduced to as determined on any one of the money-transaction days. My beginning weight will be determined at the first group meeting. My basal weight can never increase from this amount or any reduction that I achieve as measured during a money-transaction day.

2. Fifty cents for one week's accurate collection of food-related data.

3. Fifty cents for one week's accurate collection of exercise-related data that indicate the achievement of a pre-set exercise goal.

4. Fifty cents for making an innovative diet or exercise change. (This will be determined by Drs. LeBow and Skopec.)

5. Fifty cents for making the most constructive suggestion(s) to a fellow group member concerning his exercise, eating, or nutrition. (This will be determined by a group vote.)

6. One dollar and fifty cents for each inch lost from waist from basal waist measurement. Waist size will be determined before the group begins and measured once again for money return on the tenth-point transaction day.

7. One dollar for passing a quiz concerning knowledge of the behavioral control of fatness. (This quiz will be given near the end of the tenth week of treatment. Its contents will be material that has been discussed during each group session. To pass the test, one must achieve a score of 70 percent or better.)

Therapists reserve the right to make changes in the contract as seem necessary to them during this phase.

Weeks 14 to 18 (one session per week, five money transactions).

1. One dollar and fifty cents per pound lost from basal weight.

2. Fifty cents for one week's accurate collection of food-related data.

3. Fifty cents for one week's accurate collection of exercise-related data that indicate the achievement of a pre-set exercise goal.

4. Fifty cents for making an innovative diet or exercise change. (This will be determined by Drs. LeBow and Skopec who also shared in the project employing this contract.)

5. Fifty cents for making the most constructive suggestion to a fellow group member concerning exercise, eating, nutrition.

6. One dollar and fifty cents for each inch lost from waist from basal waist measurement. (Measured on fifth money-transaction day of this phase.)

Therapists reserve the right to make any changes in this contract as seem necessary to them during this phase.

Weeks 19 to 24 (one session every two weeks, three-money transaction days).

1. Two dollars per pound lost below basal weight.

2. Fifty cents per each week's accurate collection of food-related data.

3. Fifty cents per each week's accurate collection of exercise-related data that indicate the achievement of pre-set exercise goal.

4. One dollar and fifty cents for each inch lost from waist from basal waist measurement. (Measured on third money-transaction day of this phase.)

Therapists reserve the right to make any changes in this contract as seem necessary to them during this phase.

Weeks 25 to 33 (one session every three weeks, three money-transaction days).

1. Two dollars per pound lost below the basal weight.

2. One dollar per each week's accurate collection of food-related data.

3. One dollar per each week's accurate collection of exercise-related data that indicate the achievement of pre-set exercise goal.

4. Two dollars for each inch lost from waist from basal waist measurement. (Measured on third money-transaction day of this phase.)

Therapists reserve the right to make any changes in this contract as seem necessary to them during this phase.

Weeks 34 to 53 (one session every four weeks, five money-transaction days).

1. Two dollars per pound lost below basal level weight.

2. One dollar per each week's accurate collection of food-related data.

3. One dollar per each week's accurate collection of exercise-related data that indicate the achievement of a pre-set exercise goal.

4. Two dollars for each inch lost from waist from basal waist measurement. (Measured on the last money-transaction day of this program.)

Therapists reserve the right to make any changes in this contract as seem necessary to them during this phase.

BONUSES

Records will be kept of all money earned. Bonuses of five dollars given to:

a. The person earning the most money.
b. The person losing the most weight.
c. The person losing the most inches.
d. Each person who reaches a weight that is set as the goal and which falls within the desirable weight category for that person as derived from the appropriate statistical tables.

PENALTY

The full session fee will be deducted from anyone who misses a scheduled therapy session unless appropriate reasons are given in advance. In addition, the equivalent of five dollars will be subtracted from the "a" under "Bonuses" making the earning of this extra income less likely for the person missing an appointment.

THERAPISTS

We, the therapists, agree to do everything in our power to help the undersigned lose weight.

We, the therapists, will provide the undersigned with what we believe to be a workable and medically safe approach to weight and fat control.

_____

Patient's Signature

_____

Therapist's Signature

_____

Therapist's Signature

SCHEDULE OF SESSIONS AND PAYMENTS

Phases	Sessions	Payments	Weeks in Progress
A	Twice each week	10 (once a week)	13
B	Once each week	5 (once a week)	5
C	Once every two weeks	3 (once every two weeks)	6
D	Once every three weeks	3 (once every three weeks)	9
E	Once every four weeks	5 (once every four weeks)	20

From Michael D. LeBow, *Approaches to Modifying Patient Behavior* (New York: Appleton-Century-Crofts, 1976, pp. 57-59). Copyright ©1976 by Appleton-Century-Crofts. Reprinted by permission of the publisher.

recapture funds the next week—he must reduce the amount of weight gained, plus at least an additional pound, before he will fall below his basal weight. But even though he has temporarily put on pounds, if he has been a diligent recorder and good advice-giver (stipulations 2, 3, 5), he will be paid.

The amount of money available for desired outcomes grows in the later phases of the contract—as time advances, so do the payoffs. Thus, a weight loss yielding one dollar during Phase A, yields twice that during Phase E. Likewise, exercise and food data double in value. Some requirements are removed. As the contract ensues, sessions are reduced in number from twice per week in A to once every four weeks in E, and the allotted money-transaction days are lessened from once a week in A to once every four weeks in E. The number of treatment sessions, payment days, and weeks involved in each phase is summarized in the last part of the table.[*]

The increasing payments accompanied by decreasing treatment sessions reflects a declining contact feature that is built into each contract. In a phrase, therapists gradually see the patient less but progressively pay him more for his weight-control triumphs. Bonuses are an added feature for noteworthy progress. Penalties as well are possible. Thus, if the patient misses a treatment session without giving notice, he is fined. Also a clause is added to each phase stating that therapists reserve the right to change the contract as they deem appropriate. After carefully reading the document, the patient signs it and then begins treatment. During this time he is paid in cash by the therapists who obtain funds from the monthly charges for therapy. The patient can earn back almost half the funds he contributes, if he complies with his end of the bargain.[**]

Contracts vary not only in objectives and lengths but also in frequency of reinforcement (and reinforcers used). Coates, Jeffery, Slinkard, Killen, & Danaher (1982), for example, daily reimbursed adolescents for weight loss; daily contact

[*]For evaluative purposes (Part E) the contract is abandoned for three weeks during Phase A.

[**]From Michael D. LeBow, *Approaches to Modifying Patient Behavior* (New York: Appleton-Century-Crofts, 1976, p. 60). Copyright © 1976 by Appleton-Century-Crofts. Reprinted by permission of the publisher.

Table 4.2
Weight Loss Contract for the Retarded

THE CONTRACT

This contract is entered into signed in good faith by:

Parents: _____

Student: _____

School: _____

per _____

(Principal)

and

_____

(Teacher)

Consultants:

_____

_____

This is a short term contract, to be renegotiated for each phase.

This contract is good from

_____ to _____

The parent agrees to:

1. Count and record portions of each food group whenever eaten.
2. Send signed food and points record to school daily.
3. Praise student each day for sticking to diet.
4. Award "cooperation points" on this basis.
   a. Good cooperation — 2 points
   b. A little nagging — 1 point
   c. Poor sportsmanship — 0 points
      (do this 4 times per day — after each meal and once in the evening for between-meal cooperation)
5. Provide chances for the student to spend his points, according to the agreed upon list.

6. Note on food and points record the times of day praise is given.
7. Indicate on food record in comments column whether the student spends extra points.
8. Indicate type of extra exercise and duration.

The student agrees to:

1. Eat only the foods on the diet.
2. Take the signed record to school each day.
3. Not complain about the diet.
4. Try to get more exercise.

The school agrees to:

1. Weigh the students on Mondays, Wednesdays, and Fridays, and keep a careful record of these weights.
2. Send home a note on the last day of the school week showing:
   a. The student's weight that day
   b. The net weight loss for the week
   c. The points earned for weight loss (1/4 kilogram = 10 points), points earned for bringing sheets in daily, plus any extra points earned for exercise (to be negotiated on an individual basis)
   d. The total points earned during the week
   e. The number of points the student has spent at school, his request for spending points at home, and the number he has banked for spending during the week.

From Michael D. LeBow, *Weight Control: The Behavioral Strategies* (Chichester: John Wiley & Sons, Ltd., 1981, p. 76). Copyright ©1981 by John Wiley & Sons, Ltd. Reprinted by permission of the publisher.

was significantly effective. Table 4.2 (LeBow, 1981a) shows a contract requiring even more frequent checkups and reinforcement.

This device was used in the treatment of obese, retarded young adults. As evident, several opportunities existed daily for reinforcement by praise and points redeemed by commodities and activities. Parents and teachers in a day-care center were monitors and deliverers of positive consequences. Students were the receivers; they were charged with the task of eating designated foods—a diet of 1200 calories accompanied the contract—and with cooperating. Consultants were the overseers of the contract, handling, or at least trying to handle, disputes among the students, parents, and teachers.

Many disputes arose. Most did after the first few months when it became obvious that although the agreement was acceptable to students and teachers, parents were becoming progressively more dissatisfied with it. Their main complaint was the work. For many of the mothers and fathers, all of whom had the best of intentions at the outset, continuous monitoring proved to be formidable; they felt overburdened by it and underrewarded from doing it; reinforcers were not powerful enough.

Perhaps money from treatment deposits, had they been required, would have helped these parents to follow the strictures of the program (see, for example, Application 5, Chapter 5); seeing their children lose weight was insufficiently rewarding. It was too late, however, to redesign the contract and build in immediate reinforcers for parents. In other contracting schemes troubles may surface earlier, allowing therapists to change agreements with the signatories' consent. Suppose, for instance, an 11-year-old obese boy contracts to complete food records, to forsake second helpings at dinner, and to hold television down to 90 minutes daily; his mother agrees to cook his favorite meals at least three days a week, to quit nagging him to lose weight, and to take him swimming on the weekends. Also let's say the mother assumes the job of giving her son points, eventually redeemable for an array of backups. The child takes on the role of evaluating his mother's performances. The therapist reviews records, cashes in the child's points, and agrees to return portions of a monetary deposit to mother contingent on the mother's compliance and the son's progress.

Such a trade-off between mother and child could benefit the youngster. Trouble could arise, however, if mother, so pleased to see her boy succeed, decides to reinforce extra; say she decides to give him rich, unplanned-for treats. This inadvertent sabotage, defeating to both child and parent, would call for either directing the mother to desist or, if the pattern were too ingrained, redesigning the contract.

Contracting and Trapping

The contracts in Tables 4.1 and 4.2 above provide consequences for cooperation, sportsmanship, food recordkeeping, exercise recordkeeping, constructive suggestions, size losses, and more. As noted, contracts also may be designed for attending therapy (Jeffery, Thompson, & Wing, 1978)—daily, weekly, monthly, or even more intermittently—and for weight loss. Recall Mann's (1972) study in which he recruited seven females and one male in order to investigate the effects of contracting for weight loss; all of his patients signed weight-change agreements. They gave Mann personal treasures that he gave back when they became lighter or that he kept when they failed to do so; actually, he donated forfeited treasures to charities. Each contract specified three weight-based arrangements: just under a 1 kg loss was to be positively reinforced, whereas just under a 1 kg gain resulted in loss of treasures; two-week reductions, a pre-set amount, were to be positively reinforced, whereas failure to reduce resulted in a loss of valuables; reaching goal weight was to be positively reinforced from a special list of treasures, whereas dropping out resulted in forfeiture.

Mann's contracts were powerful. The weekly rate of loss averaged approximately 1 kg during the first phase of treatment, which occurred after the initial baseline, and over .5 kg during the second phase of treatment, which followed the reversal. But why were the contracts so potent? Mann answered this question by likening his documents to behavioral traps (Baer & Wolff, 1967). When individuals wanting to reduce give the therapist valuables to return if they do reduce they entrap themselves. After signing the contract, they must either comply with the weight-loss imperative or lose their treasures. And if the treasures are indeed treasurable, the trap is strong. In brief, Mann's system may have trapped his patients and forced them to lose weight.

The notion of trapping seems well-suited to the task of designing comprehensive programs for obese children, for trapping also entails searching for behavior changes that allow the child entry into more natural behavior-changing environments, environments that support and extend the progress only begun in therapy (Baer & Wolff, 1967). Once penetrated, these new environments are not easily left (see Stokes & Baer, 1977).

The therapist's task is to find these environments and to initiate changes that will allow the child to enter them. Thus, treatment goals may be fostering weight loss as well as teaching athletic and social skills. Once a few of these skills are mastered, the child becomes more acceptable to his peers, and thus joins their games and sports. By playing more with his agemates he will become even less isolative and perhaps thinner. Trapping the child into his peer group and letting this group continue and extend the modifications started in therapy helps to break the vicious circle of rejection, isolation, loss of social and athletic skills, weight-gain, and further rejection (see Chapter 2). In brief, trapping may prove an effective way to bring about enduring and extensive change (Stokes & Baer, 1977).

But trapping a child into his peer group is beneficial only if the peer group teaches him adaptive behaviors that do not ultimately cause him harm. The long-term outcomes, however, of many seemingly appropriate changes are unknown (see, for example, Steele, 1980). That is, where the peer group will lead the child in five or ten years is impossible to say. Judgments about the value of trapping into the peer group therefore rest on what the immediate value of joining appears to be—that is, reduction of isolation, social acceptability, weight loss, and so on.

Likewise, trapping an individual into losing weight by using a strong contract is beneficial only if the contract does not ultimately cause him harm. Still, it is easier to recognize the untoward results of contracting than the problems set in motion by the peer group because the abuses of contracting are more immediately apparent. The question to ask is what steps do patients take to fulfill the contract. The danger to be wary of is that they may try to wriggle free of a trap by behaving unhealthily; they may try to do so because it is difficult to lose weight steadily, week after week. As noted, some of Mann's patients took laxatives and diuretics to meet the weight loss requirements (cf., Jeffery, Thompson, & Wing, 1978). Not only are such methods unwholesome, but when relied on they preclude learning adaptive strategies that are needed to maintain and continue the losses; in short, the wrong tactics are acquired.

With strong contracts that encourage behavior change as well as body change as opposed to agreements that dwell soley on body change, patients need not demonstrate weight reduction to regain valuables. Instead, they need only comply with prescriptions—or at least say they comply; notably, Jeffery and colleagues' patients did lose weight commensurate with adherence to behavioral directives and by so doing indicated honest reporting.

Contracting and Behavior Therapy Techniques

Contracting and the techniques discussed in Chapter 3, some of which form the very contracts designed, may be combined. Obese adults most often receive behavior-therapy packages. So also do obese children. Packagers hope that their treatments will sufficiently change the patient's world in order to change his shape. The methods discussed thus far that compose the packages, however, are not the mainstay of researchers and practitioners seeking this alteration in the environment. Other methods, to be discussed next, have been more prominent (see Ferster et al., 1962; Stuart, 1967, 1971; Stuart & Davis, 1972). These other procedures have been used to teach patients self-control skills, skills it is believed that will enable them to continue prospering independently of professional involvement. The assumption is that individuals taught the principles of self-control, that is how to manipulate their own behavior in their food and activity worlds, will remain better after formal intervention. Unfortunately as yet, there is far too little proof that they will.

Self-monitoring

Self-monitoring is self-observing. You look at what you do or intend to do. The self-monitor may observe and record the types, quantities, and preparations of the foods eaten at each meal, or the calories per meal, or both. Or, he may observe and record the number of mouthfuls taken during the day (Fowler, Fordyce, Boyd, & Masock, 1972), or the urges he has to eat (Stuart, 1978). Furthermore, the self-monitor may observe and record the situational accompaniments of each eating episode, daily activities, and recreations. Stuart (1967), for instance, had his patients watch what, when, and how much they ate each day as well as how they prepared their foods; moreover he had them note feelings and activities associated with eating, and he had them record their weights four times daily. Various aspects of obesity can thus be observed by obese persons watching themselves. Which aspect is best to observe, however, is still open to question (see Romanczyk, Tracey, Wilson, & Thorpe, 1973).

Why ask patients to observe themselves in the first place? There are two reasons: First, the data are useful in formulating a treatment because they suggest problem areas or because they provide baselines against which to evaluate treatment effects, or because of both; second, the data, as they are obtained, may cause patients to alter their behaviors. In regard to the modification possibility, self-observation enables patients to evaluate their actions against what they view to be appropriate behaviors and then to chastise themselves for violating these standards (see Kanfer, 1970, 1977; McFall, 1977).

The two purposes of self-monitoring, therefore, are assessment and treatment. But these two purposes sometimes conflict because the potential reactivity of self-monitoring—that monitoring can change behavior—limits its accuracy as an assessment tool. A patient who loses 1 kg during the first week of baseline is perhaps demonstrating the reactive effect of self-monitoring, and undoubtedly he will be glad about this effect. Yet he is likely to soon find out that the reactivity of self-monitoring dissipates, and thus its potential as a treatment in its own right is limited (see, Joachim, 1977; Mahoney, 1974; Stollack, 1967). After several weeks of having the patient monitor his behavior, the therapist will probably get more accurate disclosure about what customarily goes on.

Monitoring Eating

To assess eating behavior before intervention, patients may observe and record consumption after the fact—immediately after. Forms for doing so abound; a typical one is shown in Table 4.3 (see Jeffrey & Katz, 1977; Jordan, Levitz, & Kimbrell, 1976b; Stuart & Davis, 1972). With it, patients record time of meal, feelings before eating, and food consumed. BLDS stands for breakfast, lunch, dinner, snack. Patients also note quantity of food eaten and activities occurring before, during, and following the meal. Calorie data usually are supplied by therapists after the records are turned in. In the sample entry, Donald Boudreau ate a quarter pounder, fries, and milkshake, which he purchased at McDonalds. He downed the meal at 1:15 p.m., feeling upset about his car bill. Prior to lunch, he had retrieved his automobile from the mechanic; while eating he did nothing else, and afterwards he returned to the office.

During intervention, patients may observe and record what they have eaten or what they intend to eat either a day or so before the meal or perhaps immediately before it. Noting intentions long ahead of the act, planning intake, or noting them just as the act is about to happen may both be especially helpful as therapies. They are likely to influence and are useful in attempting to influence food choices.

The youngster who received the two-bucket system was also asked to plan his intake, with his mother's help, to a level not exceeding 2000 calories per day. Table 4.4 presents the planning form he used. As soon as he finished a meal, planned or otherwise, he completed the food record form depicted in Table 4.5. The letters BLDS at the top of the box, one box per meal, mean the same as indicated above. In the first column, the youngster wrote what he ate; in the second column, he wrote the quantity of every food; in the third, the calories; in the fourth, the preparation. Below the box he totaled calories for the meal and then deter-

Table 4.3
Food Chart

FILL OUT IMMEDIATELY AFTER EATING EACH MEAL

Name: _Donald Boudreau_

Date: _Nov. 12_

Unless instructed otherwise, do
not record calorie information.

Time	Feeling	Food (BLDS)	Qn.	Cals.	Before	During	After
						Activities	
1:15pm	Upset	Quarter Pound-er (from McDonalds)	1/4	518	Picked up car	ate alone. no reading, ch.	back to work
		Fries (	Sml	211			
		Vanilla Shake	Reg	323			

From Michael D. LeBow, *Weight Control: The Behavioural Strategies* (Chichester: John Wiley & Sons, Ltd., 1981, p. 39). Copyright © 1981 by John Wiley & Sons, Ltd. Reprinted by permission of the publisher.

Table 4.4
Sample Meal Plan

| Day & Date Planned For | *Tuesday March 6* |
| Daily Calorie Intake Goal | *2000* |

Morning Meal

Food	Quantity	Calories	Preparation
white bread	2 sl	130	toasted
butter	1/2 t	50	—
banana	1 (140 g)	85	fresh
milk	1 glass	160	whole

Afternoon Meal

Food	Quantity	Calories	Preparation
white bread	2 sl	130	reg.
salami	84 g	260	from pkg.
mustard	1 tsp.	8	from jar
apple	1 (144 g)	82	fresh
milk	1 glass	160	whole

Evening Meal

Food	Quantity	Calories	Preparation
spaghetti with meat sauce	abt. 350 g.	475	boiled spag., browned meat, simmered
carrot	1 (50 g)	22	fresh
milk	1 glass	160	whole
animal crackers	16 g (8 cookies)	70	in box

Snacks During the Day

Food	Quantity	Calories	Preparation
Calorie slush fund		200	

Total: _____ *1992* _____

Deficit from Goal: _____ *– 8* _____

Free Foods Not Counted

83

Table 4.5
Food Record Form

WEEK 1   DAY Wednesday   DATE March 7

MEAL   B (L) D S   Meal # Today ___2___

	Type	Quantity	Calories	Preparation
Food 1	white bread	2 sl	130	regular
Food 2	salami	84g	260	packaged
Food 3	mustard	1 tsp.	8	from jar
Food 4	apple	1 (144g)	82	fresh
Food 5	milk	1 glass	160	whole
Food 6				
Food 7				
Food 8				

Total Calories for Meal: _____640_____

Time Begin Eating: _____12:15_____

Feeling: _____Hungry_____

Remarks: _____

TOTAL CALORIES THUS FAR TODAY: _____1065_____

mined, in last line on the box, his calorie intake up to that point. The final line on the final box showed him his total calories for the day. Also, he recorded times, feelings, and any observations he had. Thus, the planning form pictured intentions, whereas the food-record form pictured performances. By completing both, the youngster was able to compare them and find exactly where they did not match. These disagreements, violations in plans, were then investigated thoroughly to determine what contributed to them (for example, seeing food, watching others eat); afterwards, behavioral strategies were invoked to thwart their reoccurrences. Chapter 5, Application 9, lists common sources of disagreements, other details of this program, and results for this boy.

Many children, however, find such devices far too complex. They require simpler instruments if they are to monitor themselves without maximum parental assistance; happily, several uncomplex strategies are available. Table 4.6 portrays a simple tactic, an exchange-diet card system that one of my graduate students is currently using to gather the self-monitored consumption data of the 132 cm, 45.4 kg girl of 8 years that he is seeing. The child fills out the card, which holds a week's worth of data; she requires very little help from her mother. On it she writes down the number of food exchanges eaten each day (for example, see Sunday's entry), but she monitors meal by meal. The exchanges, taken from Stuart and Davis (1972), are listed across the top of the card and days are listed down its side; the child places a tick when she consumes an exchange, and on the reverse side she writes why she veered from her allotment, if she happens to do so.

Six food groups comprise the Stuart and Davis plan, as indicated in the table. The diet allows for variety and flexibility in selections because the foods within each of the categories are interchangeable. Thus, the child can substitute asparagus for celery in the vegetable group and peanut butter for sausage in the meat group, provided that amounts are watched. The youngster's mother is given primary responsibility for weighing and preparing foods, although the child helps. Results thus far are encouraging. The girl has steadily and slowly lost weight—3.2 kg in 10 sessions over 14 weeks; furthermore, during this period, she has lost 5.1 cm from her waist. Moreover, she has successfully completed several behavioral programs enabling her to reduce plan violations most of which are overages in the miscellaneous category; her junk-food benefactors are parents and grandparents.

Foreyt and Parks (1975), also employing the Stuart and Davis exchange-diet, illustrated another easy way to self-monitor intake. They used their system to treat retarded adults, but it is applicable to normally intelligent youngsters as well. They had tokens, differing in color, to represent food categories—six colors for six categories; red signified meat, yellow meant cereal, white was milk, green vegetables, orange fruit, brown miscellaneous. Each patient, three women, was given a day's supply of tokens and a plastic box with two compartments. To monitor ingestion, each had to transfer tokens from one compartment to the next as she ate throughout the day, the right color for the specific food.

Table 4.6
Self-Monitoring For Obese Children On An Exchange Diet

	Meat	Cereal	Milk*	Vegetable	Fruit	Misc.**
Allotted Daily Exchanges	8	6	3	3	5	4
Monday						
Tuesday						
Wednesday						
Thursday						
Friday						
Saturday						
Sunday	xxxxx	xxxxxx	xx	xxx	xxxxx	xx

This diet is taken in modified form from the Stuart and Davis (1972) 1700 calorie regimen.

*This is a minimum recommendation for a child.

**Fats, Sweets, Candy, Syrup, Sugar, Carbonated Drinks.

Foreyt and Parks noted that this monitoring system eliminated the need to calorie count, enabled caretakers to encourage patients to eat balanced diets, and helped staff at the training center where these women passed the day to communicate with parents about total consumption. The authors reported no difficulties having the patients transport the token boxes between home and the center; in fact, "The subjects seemed proud to carry the boxes with them" (p. 28).

The ways in which the monitoring system helped them learn adaptive food-selection practices was unsaid. There were low-calorie choices in the presence of high-calorie foods and there were refusals to snack, but the impact of monitoring on these decisions was unclear. The program was comprised of several tactics, in addition to the colored-token system, including positive reinforcement for weight reduction; component effects were not analyzed. The package, however, worked, or so it seemed. After 11 weeks of treatment, weight losses ranged from more than 2 kg to almost 5 kg; the lightest patient lost the least. Reductions continued over the 29 week follow-up, growing to 2.6 kg for the lightest woman and to 9.8 kg for the heaviest.

Epstein, Masek, and Marshall (1978) also color-coded foods. Their purpose, however, was not developing a monitoring method, although the possibility exists (see Epstein et al., 1981), but improving the selections of obese youngsters confronted by various kinds of foods at meals (see Stark, Collins, & Stokes, 1981; Application 8, Chapter 5). After separating foods into three categories, they gave each grouping a color—distinctions were based on nutritional and caloric densities—and instructed the children about eating: green foods (for example, milk, fish, green peas) were to be eaten in their entirety; yellow foods (potatoes, bologna, sausage) were to be eaten sparingly; red foods (candy, cakes) were to be avoided.

Monitoring Activity

As with self-observation of eating behavior, activity may be planned, or it may be recorded after it occurs, or both. A patient may monitor brief, daily routines, such as taking the elevator, taking the stairs, dressing, watching television, and sleeping; and he may monitor prolonged activities, such as playing tennis, swimming, dancing, chopping wood, and jogging. Furthermore, he may estimate the time and effort he expends in doing these things. Thus, the patient could list the minute he began an activity, what the activity was, and when he ended it, and then he could rate how hard he worked at it—mildly effortful to strenuous (LeBow, 1981a). The data could be subsequently translated into calories burned. Tables exist for doing so; they report calorie data that vary with type and time of activity as well as with weight of performer. During baseline, the therapist would make the calorie translation. During intervention, the patient would do so. Consider Table 4.7 for example. It is a form used to plan and record data on both brief and prolonged activities (LeBow & Perry, 1977). The 11-year-old boy mentioned earlier who planned his intake also forecasted his activities, one week in advance

Table 4.7
Activity Change Plan and Requirement Chart

Week of _May 28_
Program Week _13_

CHANGES

	Monday	Tuesday	Wednesday	Thursday
BRIEF (Activities)	walk to School ✓	walk to School ✓	walk to School ✓	walk to School ✓
PROLONGED	CE goal 135 Plans bike 30min ✓	CE goal 135 Plans bike 30min	CE goal 135 Plans bike 30min ✓	CE goal 135 Plans bike 30min ✓

	Friday	Saturday	Sunday
BRIEF (Activities)	walk to School ✓		
PROLONGED	CE goal Plans	CE goal 252 Plans swim 60mins ✓	CE goal Plans

PAST WEEK'S ACCOMPLISHMENTS ARE
THIS WEEK'S REQUIREMENTS

	Monday	Tuesday	Wednesday	Thursday
BRIEF (Activities)	take out garbage ✓		take out garbage ✓	
PROLONGED	CE goal Suggestions	CE goal Suggestions	CE goal Suggestions	CE goal Suggestions

	Friday	Saturday	Sunday
BRIEF (Activities)			
PROLONGED	CE goal 135 Suggestions Bike 30min ✓	CE goal Suggestions	CE goal 135 Suggestions Bike 30min ✓

for eight consecutive weeks; he recorded daily whether or not he lived up to his plans. On the left-hand portion of the diagram, Changes, he could propose, during the second week of activity planning, to walk to school for five days (Monday through Friday); also he could propose to bike for 30 minutes after school Monday through Thursday and to swim for an hour on Saturday; then he would translate these prolonged activities into calorie-expenditure goals (CE goal). Immediately following the completion of an activity or during the evening thereafter he would check the box where it was written, or, if failing to complete it, he would mark a "D" in the box.

He was required to take similar steps when trying to make his past successes, his changes, cumulative. That is, on the right hand part of the form, Past Weeks . . . , he listed his accomplishments for the previous week of the program, in this case what he managed to live up to during his first attempt to plan. His intention for week two was to complete all the activities designated on both halves of the chart—previous triumphs and new hurdles. He was allowed to vary his proposals somewhat, as he felt necessary, but he was strongly encouraged to meet all the calorie-expenditure goals. His activity program began soon after he had finished the food-planning segment (see above). It started near his baseline, obtained by using the baseline activity monitoring tactic mentioned, and increased to a level he felt to be tolerable. During treatment, compliance was variable and violations between plans and performances were handled behaviorally.

Monitoring Inactivity

Self-monitoring may be tedious and boring. This is a problem if it leads patients to fail to complete records or to distort information (Bellack & Schwartz, 1976). It also is a problem if it leads patients to drop out of treatment; aversive tasks are avoided when possible (negative reinforcement). But it is not necessarily a problem if it leads patients away from the specific act that is supposed to be observed and recorded. When, because self-monitoring is unpleasant, a patient refuses a snack so that he does not have to bother getting out his data sheets and writing out his behavior, the avoidance is working for him. It is working against him, however, when the behavior avoided is being more active, for it is contratherapeutic not to exercise so as not to have to record. What is needed is an alternative to charting activity when doing so amounts to punishing desirable behavior. One option is to monitor inactivity. Instead of placing aversive consequences after desired actions, they can be placed after undesirable actions, namely being sedentary. Jordan, Levitz, and Kimbrell's (1976a) activity clock seen in Figure 4.1 accomplishes this task. As the instructions read, patients mark a box when they are inactive for 10 or more minutes of a 15-minute period. There are 96 of these boxes for each day of the four days shown—48 on the a.m. clock and the same number on the p.m. one. Research on the applicability of this device and other tactics that monitor inactivity is needed for adults, adolescents, and children.

Regardless of the self-monitoring system developed, be it for collecting eating

Figure 4.1
Activity Clock
From Jordan, Levitz, and Kimbrell (1976a).

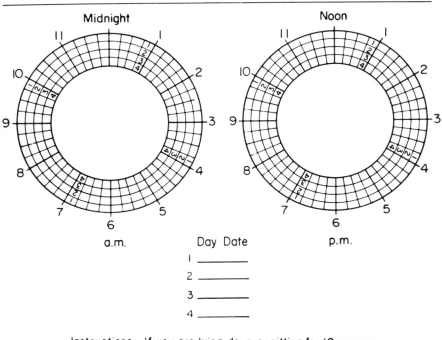

Instructions : If you are lying down or sitting for 10 or more
of any 15-minute period, fill in the space.

or activity data or both, its value as an assessment or treatment tool partly rests on how well the patient is taught to use it. Techniques for teaching are the techniques for initiating and strengthening any new behavior: for example, instruction, modeling, practice, feedback. Self-monitoring is best taught at a speed that accords with the patient's progress at mastering it; therefore, surveillance of monitoring practices is required. Noncompliance is too often found among adults, and although still undocumented sufficiently, is probably rife among children, too.

Stimulus Control

An obese 10-year-old girl comes home following a hard day at school and immediately after greeting her mother, sometimes before, dips her hand into a prominently displayed, well-stocked candy dish in the living room. Then she heads for the kitchen and enjoys a snack of cookies and grape juice. Finishing, she returns to the living room, turns on the television and, while watching her regular program, dips into the candy dish again. Monday through Friday this sequence of behavior unfolds . . . automatically.

This pattern exists among both nonobese and obese children. It illustrates connections between the environment, eating, and inactivity that are thought to be problems if the child grows fat or stays fat because of them. Therapists treating obese youngsters usually think such connections are damaging, but data on their actual effects are unreported. Routines, such as those set in motion by visible candy dishes and cookie jars, exemplify how operant behavior is controlled by its antecedents; in the parlance of behaviorists, antecedent control is stimulus control.

I discussed consequence control in Chapter 3 by examining such techniques as positive and negative reinforcement, aversive stimulation, response-cost, and so on. As described, changing a behavior's frequency is possible by manipulating its outcomes. Actually, antecedent control is not independent of consequence control, as will be shown, but it is often thought of as a separate avenue in the quest to make the obese person thinner. Moreover, it is not a new addition to the obesity therapies. In 1962, Ferster and colleagues postulated that overweight adults are controlled by too few of the right kinds of antecedents and too many of the wrong kinds; many precursors to unadaptive eating exist. Schachter (1971), also promoted the more general notion, which has been challenged (Rodin, 1977, 1979b, 1980, 1981; Wooley & Wooley, 1975), that the obese are externally impelled to eat; external control of the obese has been contrasted with internal control of their nonobese peers. One cue of interest to both groups of researchers has been time of day. Ferster and co-workers advised patients to eat at specified hours to delimit antecedent control. Schachter and colleagues investigated how powerful the temporal cue was, before any treatment, in determining eating above and beyond perceived hunger. Thus, neither group would be surprised by the daily, afterschool snacking practices of the aforementioned 10-year-old.

How might time of day control her snacking? One way might be by setting the occasion for it. Because a specific time of day regularly precedes snacking, a behavior strongly reinforced by carbohydrate-laden foodstuffs, time becomes a cue for the act. Notably, hunger may or may not play a part, and time alone may or may not be a sufficient cue; the child may have to be in her own home after the school day before she will seek food in the manner described above. Stimuli preceding behavior control its occurrence by indicating when, where, and under what conditions it will be reinforced.

Times, sights, and places are powerful determiners of our actions because they signal consequences to us. Thus, we greet those who have returned our greetings in the past. If a person ignores your hello on Monday, the chance of your greeting him when you see him on Tuesday is less than it would have been had he responded pleasantly the day before; the taciturn evoke a different response than do the loquacious, and we quickly learn to discriminate the two. Indeed, the discriminations we acquire throughout development are often quite subtle. Tones of voice and expression of face, for instance, cue pronounced variations in action. Different individuals with different learning histories respond differently to the same stimuli, as illustrated by the story of the little boy who was content only when in the presence of the disfigured. Hence, the reasons that we behave as we do are partially the result of the sorts of cues our environment provides.

Obesity researchers and therapists capitalize on this fact, for we are all affected by times, sights, places, and situations. But the concern is not so much how this antecedent control arises for each obese person. The concern is, rather, that antecedent control exists and that it is modifiable. Accordingly, the overweight are exhorted to eliminate control that is troublesome and to instill control that is helpful. They are told to rid their cupboards of snack foods because seeing these delectables sets them up to consume them, and they are told to pick a specific place to eat so that only one place cues eating. Unfortunately, when making these and similar demands, behaviorists are generally less moved by differences their patients bring to therapy than by suspected similarities; the variations on the stimulus control theme that are offered have not usually been borne from individual baseline data (LeBow, 1981).

Tactics

Today, stimulus control dwells on some aspect of eating; stimulus control of exercise behavior is rare. The focus is on consuming, serving, storing, buying, or cleaning up food, or on all of these facets (McReynolds, Lutz, Paulsen, & Kohrs, 1975). Stuart (1971), for example, advises his patients to eat without doing anything else while eating; to shop from a shopping list; to eat in a specific spot. McReynolds and colleagues instruct their patients to serve themselves last, to avoid making their table a training table, to stay away from areas of the house where eating is likely, unless one is going to eat, and to scrape leftovers into the garbage can rather than into the mouth. Stunkard and Mahoney (1976) warn their patients about leftovers, too, and counsel them to use shallow bowls and plates. Like Stuart, they also warn patients not to eat with such behavioral accompaniments as reading or watching television during dinner. Jordan and Berland (1981) caution their readers to store food away from sight, to buy small packages of edibles rather than large ones, and to prepare food only when it is needed, not too far in advance. The lists go on and on. Commonly used directives designed to narrow and augment antecedent control can be seen in Table 4.8 (LeBow, 1981a, p. 143).

The assumptions are that if patients follow the rules they will improve their chances to reduce and, if they do reduce, to stay lighter; evidence, however, is contradictory (Carroll, Yates, & Gray, 1980; Miller & Sims, 1981). Moreover, there is disagreement about the best way to apply the rules: Logic and some data indicate that simply telling the obese to alter their lifestyles, prescribing and

proscribing by instruction alone, is insufficient; perhaps, there need to be consequences for complying (Mahoney, 1974; Mahoney, Moura, & Wade, 1973); other
data suggest otherwise—that instruction is enough (Abrahms & Allen, 1974;
Jongmans, 1969). Both topics, the expected effects of stimulus-control treatment
and the most efficient way to apply it, are still questions in childhood obesity
therapy.

Slowing Eating Speed

Just prior to the beginning of this century, Horace Fletcher, a self-made mil-
lionaire, who happened also to be obese, laid down a principle for eating, much
like obese patients of today hear. He was a functionalist who believed that our
having 32 teeth meant we should chew each bite of food 32 times. "Nature will
castigate those who don't masticate," warned Fletcher (Carroll, Miller, & Nash,
1976, p. 375). He lost weight, but there is no evidence that his law helped him to
do so. Behaviorists still advise obese patients to slow down, although not by
chewing mouthfuls of food 32 times. The history of the behaviorists' wisdom is
more recent.

It was Ferster and colleagues (1962) who enjoined the overweight to be less
quick with fork and spoon. Using the ideas of antecedent and consequent control
derived from operant-conditioning reasoning, Ferster and associates conceptualized eating as a chain of behaviors leading ultimately to the ingestion of food.
Circumstances set the occasion for an eating-related action that is then reinforced.
The reinforcer not only strengthens the action preceding it but also precedes the
next eating-related action. For example, chewing food is a behavior resulting after
new food is placed in the mouth. Unchewed food in the mouth is the antecedent of
chewing. The outcome of masticating is having the feeling of chewed food; this
consequence, the reinforcer of chewing, also is the antecedent of the next link in
the chain, swallowing. Feeling chewed food in the mouth sets the occasion for
swallowing, and that produces another consequence, the completion of swallowing. If the eater refills the fork after swallowing, eating is probably not too speedy.
If, however, the eater allows the feeling of chewed food in the mouth to cue not
only swallowing but also utensil-refilling, then eating is likely, according to the
Ferster group, to be fast. Relatedly, if the overweight person chews incompletely
(as Fletcher warned against) and swallows early, eating will be rapid.

Whatever the specific problem, Ferster and co-workers and numerous other
behaviorists instructed the overweight to be slower eaters. Typical prescriptions
(Bellack, 1975; Stuart, 1978; Stuart & Davis, 1972; Stunkard & Mahoney, 1976)
follow:

1. Reduce the amount of food you put on your eating utensil. (Cut food into
   smaller pieces.)
2. Chew the food in your mouth more.

Table 4.8
Typical Stimulus Control Directives

Objectives		Instructions*
Breaking problematic connections between the environment and eventual eating	1.	If you are the chief cook, then prepare the next meal after finishing the previous one. That is, make dinner following lunch. This schedule will help reduce sampling.
	2.	Snack foods should be eliminated from the cupboard or be earmarked for others. Have those with whom you live keep their "junk food" in their own containers, and have them write their names on these containers, too.
	3.	Take food out of every room but the kitchen.
	4.	The majority of foods that you have on hand should require preparation before they are eaten.
	5.	Stop eating when you are doing something else that is pleasurable, such as reading. If you are going to eat, then eat, but that is all you should do.
	6.	When dining out ask the waiter not to serve bread before the meal.
Creating new connections between the environment and eventual eating.	7.	Develop an eating place in the home that is to be used only for that purpose, and only eat there when at home.
	8.	Use the same eating utensils and place mat. Also use the same specific dish and cup. This special plate and glass should be smaller than usual, though not too small.
	9.	Fill plates from the kitchen counter, not from the kitchen or dining room table. Second helpings should be harder to acquire.
	10.	Let the urge to eat at an unplanned time (i.e., between meals) signal an exercise break, telephone call, bath, or whatever is desirable at the moment, so long as it does not involve food.

Objectives	Instructions*
	11. Stock up on favorite activities by saving them for times when the urge to eat strikes. For example, do not read the paper until you feel like having a snack.
	12. Eat at designated times.
	13. Buy food when you are least disposed to eat (e.g., after a meal), and let a shopping list determine your purchases more than the sight of food on the shelves.
	14. After the meal is over, put leftovers away in opaque containers.
	15. If leftovers on the plate are too few to store, then immediately put them into the garbage or delegate a child, spouse, or friend to do so.
	16. Before you leave for a restaurant, consider the possible things you will allow yourself to eat there.

From Michael D. LeBow, *Weight Control: The Behavioural Strategies* (Chichester: John Wiley & Sons, Ltd., 1981, p. 143). Copyright ©1981 by John Wiley & Sons, Ltd. Reprinted by permission of the publisher.

*When listing stimulus-control directives several researcher-practitioners also include eating-pace tactics. For more suggestions, consult Bellack (1975); McReynolds et al. (1975); Stuart (1971); Stuart and Davis (1972); Stunkard and Mahoney (1976).

3. Swallow the food in your mouth before taking another bite. (Lay down your eating utensils after taking the bite.)
4. Interrupt your meals. (Talk more to your meal partners in order to delay the meal more.)
5. Use eating utensils for finger-foods (hamburgers).

Do the Overweight Really Eat Too Fast?

Some attempts to answer are conducted in the laboratory under controlled conditions (Adams, Ferguson, Stunkard, & Agras, 1978; Hill & McCutcheon, 1975; Kaplan, 1977; Mahoney, 1975b; Rosenthal & Marx, 1978; Warner & Balagura, 1975). Other attempts are orchestrated in the field setting, where there is less control but the situation is more natural (Dodd, Birky, & Stalling, 1976; Gaul, Craighead, & Mahoney, 1975; LeBow, Goldberg, & Collins, 1977; Mahoney, 1975b; Shisslack, 1977; Warner & Balagura, 1975). Generally, studies in both settings look at an array of rate variables, such as meal duration, bites per minute, and calories per minute. These studies require that observers learn to differentiate subjects into two or more weight categories and to learn to agree on the eating-rate measures they tabulate.

Training observers to do both is mandatory. Before investigating plate cleaning as a function of weight, sex, and social setting, LeBow, Chipperfield, and Magnusson (1982) took several weeks just rating the heaviness of university students. Observers, two at a time, watched students in a cafeteria checkout line, and applied Wing, Epstein, Ossip, and LaPorte's (1979) five weight classifications: "very lean person (like Twiggy), somewhat lean person (Farrah Fawcett), average person (Johnny Carson), somewhat overweight person (Archie Bunker), very overweight person (Santa Claus)" (p. 135). To bring reliability (degree of agreement) to 80 percent, we joined together the two lean groupings as well as the two overweight ones and by so doing formed three classifications—lean, average, and fat; the study required only these categories.

Training observers to gather reliable consumption data is more difficult. To accomplish this, LeBow and co-workers (1977) used videotapes of volunteers consuming hamburgers, french fries, and drinks—the meals eventually to be observed in a study of eating speed. A code was developed, also to be employed in the study, whereby biting into a hamburger sandwich was translated into a stopwatch click sounded into a tape recorder microphone. Similarly, eating french fries became scratching noises; chewing became taps; drinking, rubs. Observers practiced coding until they agreed on 90 percent of the observations made on each variable. During the study itself, conducted in a fast-food establishment, 34 overweight and 37 nonoverweight adults were observed eating. There were six reliability checks done; two observers, stationed in different parts of the dining area, made recordings on the same subject. Reliabilities ranged from .63 to .88. It was found that the overweight ate their meals faster than did the nonoverweight— chewing less, taking fewer bites, and pausing less between bites. However, other researchers have reached opposite conclusions (Mahoney, 1975b; Shisslack, 1978; Warner & Balagura, 1975). Methodological differences cloud the eating-speed studies, so making comparisons is difficult and the discovery of contradictions is not surprising. Therefore, in response to the question of eating speed among the overweight, we do not know if they eat too fast, for the tactic of attempting to find out, comparing overweight with nonoverweight adults, has disclosed numerous inconsistencies.

Far fewer studies have been done with children and, because of this, far fewer inconsistencies are apparent. In both laboratory (Keane, Geller, & Scheirer, 1981) and field settings (Drabman, Cordua, Hammer, Jarvie, & Horton, 1979; Drabman, Hammer, & Jarvie, 1977a, b; Geller, Keane, & Scheirer, 1981; Marston, London, & Cooper, 1976; Waxman & Stunkard, 1980) overweight youngsters, some as young as 1.5 years, appear to be the speedier eaters (but see Epstein, Parker, McCoy, & McGee, 1976).

Is Slowing Down Therapeutic?

The critical question arising from the data on children and adults is whether having an overweight person reduce his eating speed can benefit him. It can if he experiences a modicum of self-control (see Stuart, 1967) from having successfully done so; the experience can increase his motivation to persevere in treatment, whether or not he was a speedy eater at the beginning of treatment. The effects of continuing to follow the pacing directives, however, would have to be monitored to find out when the patient no longer deems the prescriptions to be valuable.

Slowing down also can be therapeutic if it reduces food consumption. Does slowing down result in eating less? It may not, according to Booth (1978, 1980). Reducing consumption speed may create cravings and retard feelings of fullness. He states, " . . . a meal could be slowed so much that the stomach never becomes full enough to pump energy into the duodenum fast enough to reach the absorption rates that induce satiety" (1980, p. 130). He goes on to caution that there is even a chance that reduced eating speed, keeping the quantity of food constant, produces greater amounts of fat in the body.

Does eating fast result in eating more? Some data on adults suggest that, no matter what the patient weighs, speediness increases the consumption of both liquid and solid food meals (Kaplan, 1977; see also Jordan & Spiegel, 1977; Jordan, Stellar, & Duggan, 1968; Spiegel & Jordan, 1978; Walike, Jordan, & Stellar, 1969). Further, some data suggest that ratings for foods already eaten (Kaplan, 1977) and appetite for foods to be served later (Wooley, Wooley, & Turner, 1975) also increase after speedy ingestion.

The questions about eating speed affecting food quantity and body weight are almost untested in children. Epstein and co-workers (1976) did find that when elementary school children laid down silverware between bites in order to reduce eating speed, changes in amount eaten resulted. These authors investigated the effects of bite-rate modification in six children, 7 years of age, three of whom were overweight and three of whom were not. The experiment lasted for six months and sessions occurred twice weekly at the school's dining facility. All children learned to take fewer bites and to eat less at the test meals, but weight losses were not remarkable. Epstein and co-workers told their subjects how to eat more slowly. Had more meals been slowed, perhaps weights would have declined more.

Be that as it may, the study demonstrates that eating rate is modifiable by instruction. Sash (1975) also appears to show that eating behaviors can be placed under instructional control and in addition suggests that the instructions can produce weight losses. In his clinical demonstration he told six obese boys, students at a boarding school who were ill-treated by peers for being fat, to take twice as long to eat their six daily meals, 1200 kcal. To help them do so, Sash had the boys cut food into small bites, chew each mouthful 10 to 15 times, refill the utensil after swallowing, not before, replace silverware on the table while chewing, drink water following every third mouthful, and talk during meals. Eighteen other boys, three groups, received portions of the treatment package, which included diet, exercise, and eating-pacing. Findings, untested statistically, indicated that giving more treatment components yielded better losses. Boys receiving pacing directives (this group also received the diet and exercise procedures) posted the best results; moreover, they took fewer mouthfuls per minute than did the other obese boys—approximately half as many.

Like Epstein and colleagues, Sash thus illustrated the plasticity of eating behavior. Perry, LeBow, and Buser (1979) also illustrated it and further suggested that the modifying procedures they applied differentially affected the eating style differences that emerged. In this experiment, however, modeling procedures, not instructions, were used to reduce consumption speed. From newspaper advertisements and a radio talk-show, 10 boys and 8 girls, ages 7 to 12 years, were recruited, of whom all were at least 20 percent overweight, weighing between 33.6 kg and 72.6 kg. Heights ranged from 120 cm to 155 cm; triceps skinfolds, from 21 mm to 34 mm; and ages of obesity onset, from 1 to 7 years. Each child consented to participate, had no chronic illness, and had a physician's permission to join. After several sessions of acclimating to the experimental set-up, he or she began baseline, the objective of which was to construct an eating profile; hamburgers were consumed while each youngster was videotaped.

Following baseline, the modeling conditions were implemented and effects were evaluated against a no-treatment control. One group of children watched a videotape of themselves eating at half-speed. The tape was constructed by having them eat while they listened to a small electronic device (12.7 cm × 7.6 cm × 5 cm) that could deliver clicks from 1 to 99 seconds apart. Knowing each child's baseline interbite interval—the time to the nearest tenth of a second between bites—the machine was set to twice the average interbite interval. Thus, if baseline showed a three-second average, the machine was set to six seconds; the pacer signaled when to take a bite of food. The other group of children watched a videotape of an adult eating half as fast as each of them had. During the test phase, youngsters in both groups and in the control returned once weekly, four times. They were told to avoid solid food after the midday meal on an experiment day, so that they would be hungry when served supper. They ate it after viewing the videotapes of themselves or adults eating slowly or after (controls only) viewing baseline tapes.

Unlike controls, experimentals changed in the way they ate, but they changed in different ways, depending on whom they watched eat. Children in the adult-modeling condition seemed to adopt a well-paced eating style, chewing more and longer than they had during baseline. In contrast, their peers in the self-modeling condition appeared to bolt food, chewing less for less time and pausing longer between bites than they had before. Why the different procedures produced these style differences is unknown. Total amount consumed was unaffected by either.

Perhaps amount consumed would have been affected had the method thatproduced well-paced eating been repeated in the home. That is, had well-paced eating been modeled in the setting in which most of the meals were taken, to the extent that the children would have adopted this style of eating for an extended period, amount ingested might have changed and weight losses might have resulted. A more comprehensive investigation of eating speed might shed light on what value slowing down has on total consumption and on body weight. Rallo (1982) is currently addressing this topic by videotaping meals in the homes of obese and nonobese children, observing parent–child eating speed correspondences, and teaching the adults to eat more slowly while their children watch; he intends to document pace of eating changes, food intake reductions, and weight differences, if any of these take place.

Conclusion

Eating speed is just one component of eating behavior, and tactics for modifying consumption pace are just one class of technique for directly altering the act of eating. For instance, bite counting is as yet untried with obese children (see, for example, Fowler et al., 1972). When bite counting, patients total their daily mouthfuls of food and try to reduce the total; automatic counting devices are available (WaterPik, 1977). Eventually, the strategy may prove useful in a comprehensive attack on a youngster's eating habits, perhaps as an initiation to self-monitoring.

Whatever is tried, it is imperative to avoid the error of attributing value to methods whose effects have not been measured directly. The attempts to modify pace of eating rest on the premise that the obese eat faster than do the nonobese, a questionable premise as we have seen, and on the premise that if fast, fat eaters can learn to eat like their thinner peers, the fat will come to resemble the thin in weight (cf., Mahoney, 1975a). This last assumption gains status as truth so long as researchers and practitioners continue not to gather information on the impact of rate-change strategies (Mahoney, 1975 a, b). Weight losses alone, subsequent to eating-rate modifications, are insufficient proof of the clinical utility of pacing techniques, or of any other behavioral procedures for that matter. As Mahoney (1975 a, b) implies, the behavioral control of adult obesity is riddled with fallacious reasoning of this sort. The domain of child obesity need not perpetuate the tradition.

Goal-setting

As part of the weight-control therapy, patients often agree to try to achieve explicit objectives. They might promise to reduce specific amounts of weight within specific periods, to eat specific foods each day, to not exceed certain calorie levels, to perform stipulated exercises, to attend all or most treatment sessions, and so on. Having patients set goals may be therapeutic (Stunkard & Mahoney, 1976), but why this may be so is unclear.

Perhaps it is the feedback that becomes possible only if reasonable goals are fixed in advance that makes setting goals therapeutic (e.g., Fisher et al., 1976). There is evidence on adults that techniques maximizing the likelihood of receiving information about progress are the most influential. Thus, setting proximal food-intake goals appears to be superior to setting more distant ones (Bandura & Simon, 1977), and setting smaller (more reachable) weight-loss objectives is better than setting larger ones (Jackson & Ormiston, 1977; LeBow & Skopec, 1973). With obese children, even less is known about goal-setting. Thus, information is lacking as to which areas are best set as objectives—calories per day, weight losses per week, fat losses per month, snacking frequency in the evening, television watching after school. Moreover, too little is known about how much change in any of these areas to encourage.

Support from Others

It has long been recognized that the social milieu of patients influences their behaviors, desirable and undesirable alike. Trapping someone into joining an existing community of reinforcement (see above) capitalizes on this fact. As fruitful as trapping is in mustering positive environmental forces, even more fruitful, perhaps, is directly teaching others to help the patient, enlisting helpers in therapy (Brownell, Heckerman, Westlake, Hayes, & Monti, 1978; Heckerman & Zitter, 1979; Israel & Saccone, 1979; Matson, 1977; Murphy, Williamson, Buxton, Moody, Absher, & Warner, 1980; O'Neil, Currey, Hirsch, Riddle, Taylor, Malcolm, & Sexauer, 1979; Pearce, LeBow, & Orchard, 1981; Rosenthal, Allen, & Winter, 1980; Saccone & Israel, 1978).

The outcome of doing so, at least the outcome hoped for, is maintaining and extending the progress the patient realizes from treatment. To date, results of this practice have varied (Brownell et al., 1978; Brownell & Stunkard, 1981a; Christensen & Barrios, 1975; Pleas, 1977; Wilson & Brownell, 1978); so also have the choices of helpers (spouses, friends external to the family), and the effects of enlisting the different kinds of helpers (Perri, Twentyman, Stalonas, Toro, & Zastowny, 1980). Varying as well are the roles helpers are assigned (for example, reinforcing weight loss, monitoring record keeping) and the intensity and method of instruction.

One way to possibly augment the value of the helper tactic is to teach the patient how to become the teacher of his own helpers, that is how to initiate and sustain their support (Mahoney & Mahoney, 1976a, b; Miller & Sims, 1981). As for overweight children, can they become teachers of their parents, grandparents, and peers and by doing so make these behavior modifiers more helpful (see Chapter 6)?

Cognitive Restructuring

Few of us would take sledgehammers to our cars when they break down. But many hapless dieters go on guilt-induced binges when they even slightly violate their diets, when they break restraint; they punish themselves instead of recouping from the slips. It may be that what they say to themselves at these times and before affects what they ultimately do. Mahoney and Mahoney (1976a) reason that covert messages, occurring during and after a weight-control program, influence the patient's success; they therefore argue for cognitive restructuring efforts in behavior control of obesity programs in order to erase negative thoughts (for example, "I am a pig," "I have no will power") and instill positive ones ("I can handle this situation"). They counsel potential weight controllers to self-monitor their internal monologues, to evaluate the appropriateness of nasty self-statements to the situation in which they occur, and to praise themselves for efforts to improve. Likewise, Coates & Thoresen (in press), in the context of adolescent obesity care, advise patients to uncover thoughts that interfere with treatment and to replace them with adaptive cognitions, ones that foster compliance.

A major assumption underlying a cognitive restructuring manipulation is that thoughts can come to rule overt actions. This is plausible, but its usefulness in advancing a science of human behavior has been eloquently challenged (Skinner, 1977). More data are needed before the precise consequences of and most efficient procedures for having overweight adults, adolescents, and children alter their cognitive environments are understood.

The methods of the behavioral control of obesity have now been reviewed. Therefore following a brief discussion of problems in the field, we will see in greater detail the ways in which this technology is applied to children.

CHAPTER 5

Behavioral Treatment: Part III

The Overweight Child: Model for Treatment

Unanswered Questions

As suggested earlier, that which exists today for the overweight child in the area of behavioral treatment draws greatly from the study of the overweight adult. This is understandable. Age differences call for extensions of existing technology as well as for new technology; yet the literature that serves as the model for the behavioral control of childhood obesity is a literature having as many questions as answers—if not more. To be sure, the domain of behavioral control of adult obesity has many problems. Major problems are discussed below:

1. Results are modest. By treatments' end, weight losses are about 5 kg (Brownell, et al., 1978; Jeffery, et al., 1978; Wilson & Brownell, 1980). But as Wilson and Brownell (1980) state, this is predictable; average treatment times are not much beyond 11 weeks, and goals are usually under a .5 kg loss per week. A 5 kg reduction, therefore, is understandable, and it is likely to be statistically significant; but it is unlikely to be clinically significant, especially for a person with five or six times that amount of weight to shed (Wilson, 1978). More critical, however, than modest outcomes—critical for the investigator trying to predict the results of therapy and for the patient hoping to prosper from it—is the following problem.

2. Results are highly variable. Some patients lose much more than 5 kg. Some, unfortunately, fare much worse. And quite disheartening, some even gain weight. No one is certain why there is so much variability. Indeed, an understanding of the patient by treatment interaction, which this variability undoubtedly reflects, is absent despite several promising leads (Bellack, Glanz, & Simon, 1976; Carroll, Yates, & Gray, 1980; Gormally, Rardin, & Black, in press; Rozensky & Bellack, 1976; Weiss, 1977b). Nonetheless, today, predicting who should get what is still an art form more than it is a science (LeBow, 1981a); and equally foggy, if not more so, is matching therapist characteristics to patient characteristics in order to maximize efficiency.

3. Therapists train and hope. Few behavioral weight-control regimens, decidedly too few, ever attempt to program lasting change, let alone to accomplish the feat. Moreover, too few include measurements on post-treatment results beyond several weeks or months. Five years-afterward data on the outcomes of behavioral programs are scarce (cf., Levitz, Jordan, LeBow, & Coopersmith, 1980; Stunkard & Penick, 1979). Following their one-half decade post-treatment evaluation, Stunkard and Penick are pessimistic. They state, "clinically important weight losses achieved by behavioral treatments for obesity are not well maintained" (p. 805). The problem they identify lies, to a great extent, with the "train and hope" strategy (Stokes & Baer, 1977), a strategy that says one fails to plan for durability. Behavioral researchers and practitioners act as if teaching patients the how-to-reduce principles guarantees that successful users will reapply them when necessary, that is, when relapses begin. And behavioral researchers and practitioners act as if reapplication of these principles will assure weight losses. Neither assumption enjoys a wealth of data justifying it. Any belief that behavior therapy changes patients so that they will continue reducing is no more than that . . . a belief. Continuance and maintenance of weight loss, in other words, not to mention continuance and maintenance of the behavior modifications that presumably underlie these changes, are rarely witnessed.

4. Treatment is brief. Behavioral researchers and practitioners often end treatment at 4, 8, 10, or 14 weeks because the design of the regimen that they offer stipulates that they do so. It is the completion of an interval rather than the attainment of a goal weight (cf., Cautela, 1966) or a demonstration of 90 to 100 percent compliance with treatment prescriptions that signals termination. It is strange, from a logical perspective, to try to combat refractory obesity with short-term therapy; unhappily, the data do not suggest otherwise.

5. Too often only patients know if they have complied with the prescriptions of treatment. Sometimes therapists try to find out, too (see, for example, Brownell, Heckerman, Westlake, Hayes, & Monti, 1978; Pearce, et al., 1981; Stalonas, Johnson, & Christ, 1978). Their efforts to do so are increasing, although these are not matched by efforts to report the data obtained on compliance (Johnson, Wildman, & O'Brien, 1980). Yet reporting these data is vital, for without reliable information on whether patients carry forward the directives of treatment, conclusions about the merits of these prescriptions are impossible to make.

That patients stay in treatment and keep coming to sessions is no guarantee of adherence to its strictures. Hagen, Foreyt, and Durham (1976) indicate this after attempting to reduce attrition by paying patients for attendance. They collected $20.00 from each of their adult clients as a fee for service. Before beginning treatment, however, they gave one-third of the patients all the money back, another third $15.00, and the final third, nothing: The groups receiving nothing or a portion of their deposits were told that funds would be forthcoming if attendance reached 80 percent (10 out of 12 sessions). The group receiving everything—those receiving $20.00—were only to commit themselves to 10 sessions. The group promised the most money had the fewest dropouts and the lowest mean weight loss. Conversely, the group promised nothing for attending sessions had the greatest dropout rate and averaged the most weight loss. Perhaps, as Hagen and colleagues suggested, poor losers stayed in treatment because of the monetary privations they would have to face if they quit. Their peers, similarly unable to reduce, but not having to pay for quitting, left. And perhaps the poor losers who stayed to get their money were poor losers because they failed to comply with the methods of treatment; they attended sessions, and that was about all. Without data on whether or not these patients followed the advice of the therapists, it is difficult to know for sure what happened. When judging the value of treatment one has to separate the patient's application of methods from the worth of the methods themselves. Failing to do so may produce erroneous conclusions about the treatment's usefulness. Likewise, one has to differentiate between observance of directives and changes in treatment targets. Patients may or may not follow prescriptions, and adherence may or may not cause sought-after behavior modifications (see Mahoney, 1975a). Accordingly, no change may signify noncompliance with possibly influential techniques or compliance with useless ones.

6. *Too often behavior change is only presumed to cause body change.* Even the correlative relationship between behavior and body modification is infrequently tested (see Brownell & Stunkard, 1978). And when these tests are made (Stalonas & Kirschenbaum, 1980), methodological difficulties, arising from combining patients who may respond differently to different techniques and from failing to discriminate, as indicated, between observance of directives and alterations in target behaviors, are present (Lansky, 1981). An even more basic reason that adequate tests of the relationships between behavior therapy, behavior change, energy balance, and body differences are scarce is that usually only the body data are gathered.

7. *Dependent variables are narrowly conceptualized.* Weight loss is indeed the most frequently used barometer of progress. For many therapists and patients it is the exclusive concern. As a result, fat loss and the impact of behavior change on the energy equation are downplayed. Moreover, the health correlates of weight loss subsequent to behavorial treatment are neglected, although in recent years the neglect has diminished somewhat. Thus, there are now measurements of lipoprotein cholesterol changes (Brownell & Stunkard, 1981b; Coates, et al., 1982; Follick, Henderson, Herbert, & Abrams, 1980; Thompson, Jeffery, Wing, & Wood, 1979), as well as insulin sensitivity, and blood pressure differences (Gillum, Jeffery, Gerber, Elmer, & Prineas, 1980; Zegman, Lamon, Dubbert, & Wilson, 1980). When available, these factors give a clearer picture of what behavior therapy does. Likewise, when measurements are taken on how the patient's peers see him before and after treatment, the effects of behavioral treatment may be better judged. Social validations, evaluations that bespeak these measurements of clinical significance (Baer, Wolf, & Risley, 1968; Kazdin,

1978; Wolff, 1978), however, are lacking. In a preliminary attempt to acquire such information (LeBow & LeBow, 1981) asked each adult patient to list business associates, neighbors, and friends who could be contacted before treatment began and afterwards. Questionnaires were sent to these people. This can be found in Table 5.1; patients read it before agreeing to its use.

Making this evaluation and determining if patients reach the weight and fat ranges of their leaner peers is informative. Also informative is determining after treatment if patients see themselves as having improved their bodies and behaviors. By collecting such data, investigators will be able to look at the significance of treatment and better rule on its limitations and meaningfulness.

8. Reporting methods vary. Even when noting progress in terms of weight loss, data are handled differently by different reporters. Percent of body weight lost, kilograms lost, percent of overweight change, rate of loss, the weight reduction quotient (Feinstein, 1959) are not identical measures of effectiveness. Recommendations for uniform and complete reporting have been made (Gormally et al., 1977), and the problem appears to be diminishing.

9. Few well-described and well-executed comparisons and component analyses are performed. Studies comparing different behavioral strategies are more plentiful than are those comparing behavioral with other types of treatment. And studies pitting behavioral methods against one another are done mainly on short-term therapies that leave long-term consequences in doubt. Similarly, component analyses are done on short-term therapies (Miller & Sims, 1981).

As said in Chapter 4, behavior therapists favor a package strategy in which multiple procedures are combined into one, often large regimen of treatment. Then, if overall tests of effectiveness are made, the package is compared to a control group, for example, an attention-placebo condition (Wilson, 1978). The rationale of the package strategy is that no single method appears as sufficient, and that more is better. True, no particular behavioral method has as yet distinguished itself as universally effective; probably this never will happen because patient differences outnumber similarities. But more is not always better, especially when complexity confuses and multiple interventions mean untailored care that results in the patient's rejection of the entire therapy package as impersonal. Provided the package appears to work, however, tests of its contents may be attempted. Wilson (1978) offered two procedures for doing so. First, he suggested that the investigator could systematically add in treatment elements so that one cohort of patients received one well-described component, a second cohort this component plus another, a third cohort both of these components and yet another, and so on. Sash (1975) did this in his study of overweight youths in a boarding school. One group of boys received moderate calorie restriction, another group received this restriction plus instructions to schedule consumption, a third group received both these components plus exercise, and a fourth (the final group) all the above treatments and eating-pace reduction (see also, Romanczyk, et al., 1973). Second, Wilson suggested that the investigator could dismantle treatment piece by piece and by so

Table 5.1
Social Validation Inventory

This questionnaire is being sent to you with the permission of _____ .
Your honest answers will help us evaluate our program. All statements made by
you will be held in the strictest confidence. Under no circumstances will they be
revealed. Please return in the self-addressed stamped envelope.

1. How fat is _____ ?
   a. very, very fat
   b. very fat (fatter than most people I know)
   c. fat (fatter than he/she should be)
   d. not that fat
   e. not fat at all

2. How enjoyable is it to be with _____ ?
   a. very, very enjoyable
   b. very enjoyable
   c. enjoyable usually
   d. not very enjoyable
   e. rarely, if ever, enjoyable

3. Does _____ discuss his/her being fat?
   a. all the time
   b. most of the time
   c. some of the time
   d. rarely
   e. never

4. Is _____ uncomfortable about the way his/her body is
   shaped?
   a. very, very uncomfortable
   b. very uncomfortable
   c. uncomfortable
   d. not too uncomfortable
   e. not at all uncomfortable

5. How personable is _____ ?
   a. very, very personable (a real charmer)
   b. very personable (has excellent social skills, can get along with almost
      everyone)
   c. personable (there are a few that may not like her/him, but by and large
      she/he is well thought of)
   d. not very personable (most never like or dislike her/him)
   e. a real zero

doing uncover the individual effects of each element; the best mix of elements could then be revealed (see Lang, 1969).

10. Single-subject researches are lacking. Too little is known about how individual patients respond to treatment elements because fine-grain analyses of patient response are rare; Coates' (1977) dissertation (see Application 7, Chapter 7) is a notable exception. The designs advocated by the research strategy yielding such information—for example, the multiple baseline design in which intervention could be applied sequentially to several behaviors whose baselines are gathered until intervention commences or the reversal design in which baselines are recaptured following an intervention—are useful in the clinical setting. For here, matching and random assignment of patients to treatments is often unfeasible. Hayes (1981), Hersen and Barlow (1976), Kazdin (1978), and Leitenberg (1973) thoughtfully discuss these and similar designs.

11. Assessment is deficient. Defining, observing, and recording the patient's behavior and delineating demographic and historical factors related to the onset and perpetuation of his obesity has played second fiddle to treatment. Consequently, we know far less about assessment than we do about intervention (Brownell, 1981). The assessment deficiency contributes to and expresses the bag-of-tricks notion that undermines behavior therapy. Wrongly, intervention may be seen as the behavior therapist's total contribution, as the sum and substance of what the behavior therapist has to offer the overweight. Those holding this view often deal with the overweight as if they were all alike (cf., Kiesler, 1966), instead of articulating differences and designing treatments accordingly. Packaging behavioral strategies based only on what the recipients weigh fails to consider patient needs, preferences, and customary actions.

12. Monitoring is deficient. Failing to consider patient differences when designing treatment is much like failing to recognize the continuous changes among them that treatment brings. Alterations in behavior, metabolic rate, calorie intake and outgo requirements, and attitudes about the treatment's components are usually not monitored, and it is thus difficult to refine therapy as it progresses.

These problems discussed above, many of which are interdependent, are not irremediable. If the full potential of behavior therapy in helping obese adults is to be realized, they will have to be addressed. They are issues facing present-day investigators of adulthood obesity treatment, and more important to this narrative, they are warnings to researchers and practitioners of childhood obesity treatment.

Approaches to the Overweight Child

As will be evident, behaviorists employ one of several approaches to treat obese children, and each approach uses one or more of the procedures discussed above. Each approach, however, differs in focus of change and how completely dietary and activity teachings are woven into the fabric of treatment.

Focusing on Weight Loss

Most attempts falling under the rubric of the behavioral control of obesity do concentrate on weight reduction, but they also tell children or parents or both how that reducing is to be accomplished; that is, they give behavior-change prescriptions, such as those embodied in the stimulus-control and eating-speed technologies. In the weight-loss focus approach, however, information of this sort is not provided in any great detail. Instead, emphasis is placed on the power of positive consequences; the patient is told that if weight is lost, he will receive a positive reinforcer (positive-reinforcement procedure) and, at times, if weight is gained or not lost, he will forfeit something valued (response-cost). The weight-loss approach could be bolstered by giving dietary or activity information or both, but its essence, as it currently exists, is to apply behavioral principles to events, best seen as the outcomes of behavior changes. They are not themselves behavior changes. In other words, users of this approach do not say much about what actions must be modified.

Not being told much about how to reduce tells patients, in effect, to resort to their own methods. And if the contingencies are powerful, if the reinforcers for losing and the punishers for gaining are potent, as well they should be in order that the approach work, children may adopt unwise methods (see Chapter 4). How likely abuse will be if contingencies are powerful depends in part on how old the child is; older children, having greater control over their food supply, are more likely to use abusive measures to lose weight. The ensuing application documents one potentially injurious practice. This application is the only illustration of the weight-loss focus approach with children that was available. Undoubtedly, the reported use of this method, the simplest of all the behavioral maneuvers, does not reflect its actual use by practitioners, parents, teachers, counselors, and others who labor on behalf of overweight children.

Application 1: Contracting With An Obese
10-Year-Old

Dinoff, Rickard, and Colwick (1972), in an early investigation of behavioral principles to treat obese children, applied contracting in a therapeutic summer-camp setting. Their patient, a boy, began their seven week program weighing about 88 kg and standing about 157 cm. He was described as bright but immature and manipulative; also, he was described as grossly obese, having "large rolls of fat (hanging) from his waist and neck" (p. 110). He was somewhat of an outcast at camp; he was teased for being fat. His obesity led not only to ridicule but also, and perhaps exacerbating the ridicule, diminished his athletic prowess. This youngster's difficulties, like the difficulties other obese children bear, may have been compounded by the contradictory message: "Play with us to be one of us, but we don't like fatties . . ." (see Chapter 2).

To help him, the investigators simply made him a deal. The negotiated contract stipulated that when he lost 4.5 kg, he could satisfy his curiosity about the goings on in a research area at the camp; he could explore a one-way mirror arrangement. The contract, an event-limited agreement, operated until the weight vanished. Apparently the boy had free reign on how he could reduce, and thus earn the activity reinforcer; yet, since the camp was a controlled environment, there were limits on unwholesome weight reduction practices, although he did try one. He and his counselor, who acted as a model, were to lessen the number of servings each customarily enjoyed at meals. Evidently the boy adhered to the letter of this law, not its spirit, for he took fewer servings but selected carbohydrate-rich foods; by so doing he excluded other foods he needed. He chose what he liked. Soon he lost weight and earned the activity reinforcer.

A second contract was then put into operation. The criterion for reinforcement was the same, 4.5 kg loss, but there was a new activity reinforcer—the opportunity to run a videotape machine; also, checks on food choices were made, at which the boy had to show his servings to a monitor and limit his desserts. After some difficulty, the youngster managed to lose the required weight, whereupon another, final, contract was devised. This time the activity reinforcer was the opportunity to use a dictaphone. And, as before, he lost the 4.5 kg.

In all, the child reduced 13.6 kg. He did so under the incentive conditions created by the three contracts with, according to the authors, daily weight checks strengthening his adherence to these agreements. If the boy was in a sense entrapped by these contracts, it was through the addition of luxuries and praise from peers and directors, not through the fear of losing surrendered valuables. The boy could have extricated himself from each contract without suffering more than loss of the activity reinforcer; also he could have refused to negotiate new agreements. Thus, as Dinoff and associates indicate, the child was not constrained to live up to the contracts.

Therapy in a summer camp is therapy in a controlled setting that, in and of itself, may contribute to favorable results; opportunities to snack and to be sedentary are regulated. In homes such practices are less controllable, but it is when the child refuses snacks and seeks more play, when he could do otherwise, that weight loss is most meaningful. It is in the home and nearby that bad practices have likely arisen in the first place and are likely maintained, and it is in the home and nearby that they have to be resolved. Without mounting an effort against the problems that exist at home and on the way home from school (for example, visiting candy stores), at the school vending machines, at the movie on Saturday afternoon, at the school cafeteria, and so on—the problems that contribute to overeating and underexercising and that prevent therapeutic change—the durability of weight loss is in jeopardy. Dinoff and colleagues did not indicate the durability of their results. Even a case study, such as theirs is, can be helpful to researchers and practitioners by illustrating potentially useful treatments and by suggesting research directions (Wilson & Brownell, 1980); but to be at its best it should be well-detailed and its results well-displayed.

Focusing on Environment Alteration

Behavioral researchers and practitioners have more to offer the overweight child than what is incorporated in the weight-loss focus approach. They have technology for modifying the world of the child, so that weight will be more controllable, at least that is the hope.

Tactically, users of the environment-alteration approaches most often dwell on engineering eating behavior changes and, to a lesser extent, on engineering activity behavior changes; but they primarily evaluate by tabulating weight or overweight changes. Procedurally, they combine the methods discussed in Chapters 3 and 4; any number of antecedent and consequent control procedures may be joined and accompanied by behavior-initiating techniques. The objective is to alter body shape by teaching children or their representatives to alter behavior— thus, the how-to counsel or what is believed to be the how-to counsel, is provided (for example, Jonides, 1982).

Two environment-alteration approaches exist. I have drawn a distinction between them based on the extent of nutrition and activity information they contain. With each ensuing application, therefore, I have asked how much information about nutritious and low-calorie diets as well as about calorie expenditure planning do practitioners and researchers supply their patients. Admittedly, my classification scheme is arbitrary, and my selection of reports to include within each category, at times, debatable; even under the same category the reports vary as to how much they emphasize this information. When deciding how much dietary and activity teachings are in fact stressed, I have relied on discussion in the studies, realizing that for several reasons (for example, space limitations) some authors may not have mirrored the actual emphasis given. I apologize for placement errors. Notwithstanding these mistakes, I do feel my ordering helps to depict ways that behavioral researchers and practitioners go about the task of treating obese children.

Environment Alteration: Nutrition and/or Activity
Advice Not Integrated

Two reports are included here. The first tries in vain to eliminate a child's food abuses and the second, more comprehensive and more successful, pits behavioral methods applied to obese children against a no-treatment control group. Nutrition and activity teachings are not integral parts of either investigation, although the second addresses these components at times.

Application 2: Behavioral Care for a
Prader-Willi Child

The patient in Skopec and Cassidy's (1976) case study, carried a diagnosis of Prader-Willi syndrome. Such a child suffers from a congenital defect characterized by hypotonia, hypogenitalism, mental deficiency, and obesity; in addition, such a child is usually short, with small hands and feet, often lacks emotional control, and eats excessively (Coplin et al.,1976). The 12-year-old boy, whom the second author attempted to help, conformed to this description.

At the time of treatment, he was diabetic, retarded, and extemely fat; he weighed 104 kg and stood about 152 cm. At the age of 6, he was already 50 kg and by 9 he tipped the scales at 75 kg. At this time he was hospitalized for congestive heart failure, which fortunately was successfully treated. Though many diets had been attempted and different medications prescribed to control his voracious appetite, none was successful. He had developed a surprising ability to snitch forbidden food without getting caught.

In June of 1973, after the boy was again hospitalized, a behavior modification program was attempted. Problems began immediately. For one, it was a 70-mile trip to the mental health center where behavioral treatment could be conducted, and the boy's mother generally found it difficult to arrange for transportation. In addition, family finances were tight despite father's working two jobs. Consequently, a registered nurse of a nearby visiting nurse association was asked to help in developing and monitoring a behavioral program for the youngster at home.

Several weeks later the nurse visited the child's mother in order to construct the behavioral plan. Behaviors to be changed involved eating and tantrums. The child (as the nurse describes) was to be awarded a star each hour that he did not steal food or otherwise go off his low-calorie diabetic diet. Fifty stars bought a back-up reinforcer such as a trip or an activity. Time-out was to be applied contingent on tantrums. Mother chose a time-out room for her son where he was to sit quietly for a specified length of time whenever he was being punished for misconduct.

Being in charge of the home, she did all the cooking, cleaning, ironing, mending, shopping, budgeting, and bill paying for this family of nine (mother, father, and seven children, ages 11 to 21 years). The atmosphere was loving but boisterous and hurried. The father most often was either working or sleeping. The children were in school, and several of them also worked at part-time jobs. Mealtimes were irregular because of everyone's varying schedules. Since other family members were so busy, the mother became wholly responsible for her son's program; this seemed to add many duties that she did not have the time or stamina to carry out consistently.

She found it difficult to cope with his tricks to obtain edibles. He would climb to precarious positions to get food hidden on high shelves. He would often sneak to the refrigerator while she was busy in the same room and gobble food until he was caught or until everything he liked was consumed. Mother would find empty containers neatly replaced in the refrigerator. Even if she caught her boy with a mouthful, he denied responsibility. She was angered by his frequent night raids on the refrigerator; his bed was beside hers, and he was stealthy enough not to awaken her.

Another irksome circumstance was that the child usually had money in his pockets when she noticed her loose change disappearing. He denied taking money and when questioned, would say that he found it. On occasion, he was seen by neighbors buying candy at the corner store. Whenever he came home from day camp, mother would check his lunch pail and frequently found wrappers of things she had not packed. When confronted with these acquisitions, the boy steadfastly claimed his innocence.

Yet another source of irritation for the mother was the boy's frequent tantrums. Because of them no one would babysit, tying her to the home. If she did go somewhere, she had to take the child with her. And when with him, she was continuously on edge, worried that he would become unmanageable. She felt constrained by her son and by the program, too.

About the program, indeed many problems arose. During home visits, these difficulties were examined, and solutions were suggested. Often, however, the best that could be accomplished was a compromise. For instance, the mother complained of little time to make the detailed records of behavior that were needed. I attempted to work around the problem by having her keep just an outline of foods consumed and behaviors performed (for example, tantrums, stealing). At our meetings, I would survey the data and ask for more complete explanations where necessary. Furthermore, I encouraged her to discuss the problems she was having and stressed that she should call me any time she wished. After each activity, I would total the boy's caloric intake and write progress notes.

Another major problem involved delay of reinforcement. It was as if the child could not keep long-range goals in mind. Food, to which he had easy access, was rarely avoided, even when he knew that eating in the present meant no movie, and so on, in the future. That is, eating at unscheduled times was highly probable for the boy even though it meant the eventual loss of something he enjoyed—the positive backup reinforcers were distant in comparison to the immediate positive consequences attendant upon eating.

And yet another difficulty involved the family and school environments. Mother could not always alter family situations in her son's best interests. For example, birthday parties were frequent because there were so many children. Also, there were many such get-togethers at the child's school—he attended a small public school for the mentally handicapped. He loved these parties, so mother tried to use them as incentives. At each party, he was allowed a small piece of cake contingent on previous good behavior. But this procedure failed because he seldom was good long enough to be entitled to the treats, yet managed to sneak at least one or two pieces of cake anyway.

The mother made other modifications in the program from time to time. For example, on one occasion she tried to deal with situations of high temptations, such as holidays. The child was to earn extra stars for no illicit eating. But this alteration failed because whenever he saw food, nothing else mattered to him. Though the mother did take efforts to keep food out of his sight, she could not entirely accomplish this feat. With so many hungry mouths to feed in the family, she could not lock the refrigerator or the cupboards.

She and I embarked on a program of small daily reinforcers for the boy's daily good behavior, in addition to the bigger payoffs for weekly good behavior. Events each day, such as a special television program or a game with a family member, were used, but often these consequences had no effects, perhaps because mother had no time to be vigilant in monitoring her son's activities or to be judicious in applying the techniques.

The boy's tantrums posed special problems. His worst ones often occurred early in the morning while he was getting ready for school. Time-out was not employed because this would make him tardy. I suggested using a favorite television show as a reinforcer for good behavior in the morning. The boy watched this program as soon as he came home from school. Agreeing that this idea was sound, mother nevertheless forgot to follow through with it. Again, she was usually so busy when her son returned from school that his behavior in the morning, good or bad, was forgotten. Tantrums also came at bedtime when he wanted to stay awake longer. Feeling it was inappropriate to apply time-out when he, in fact, wanted more time up, she would spank him and then send him to bed.

I tried to involve others in the attempt to help the boy. At one point during the program, he attended a summer day camp for mentally retarded children. I visited this camp to discuss his behavior and the program with the camp administrators and counselors, so that we could coordinate our efforts. The program was well received by most; however, the counselor who was very close to the child was opinionated about behavior modification in general and disapproved of what we were trying to do . He never really gave us his assistance.

Eventually, the mother became quite discouraged with the program. To her, many of the child's handicaps appeared to be beyond control. I tried being supportive in spite of my own disappointment that the plan was failing. Yet, there were some positive things that had happened since the program had begun. For one thing, the boy had not gained weight—his rate of gaining in previous years was high. Also, he had not shown sugar in his urine, indicating that his diabetes was under control.

In early December, the mother and I met with the boy's school principal, teacher, and counselor. We pooled all our ideas about him and constructed plans for more control over his diet at school and for extra reinforcers there and at home. But again, despite everyone's efforts, he did not lose weight. He frequently was able to steal large amounts of food, and the only consequence of this pilfering was losing a star for that hour. The mother decided that if there were any large infractions—he had devoured a pie in a few minutes—he would get no stars for the whole day. This tactic worked only in slowing down reinforcement; he did not seem to care what happened and this apathy upset his mother more than anything else. In March, she had an attack of rheumatoid arthritis. (She had had a severe attack a few years before and had been barely able to get about on crutches.) She was quite ill for a week and then was left incapacitated, needing daily rest periods. By the end of this month, she decided to discontinue the program; it was not really helping the boy enough to make it worth the effort to continue. He weighed 103 kg at this time. After the behavioral plan was abolished, he gained weight, and his diabetes zoomed out of control. He was sneaking food frequently night and day without being caught. Because his urine tests for sugar were high, his physicians increased his Orinase, and not long thereafter he was on maximum dosage.*

*From H. M. Skopec and A. Cassidy, Sometimes our plans go awry. In Michael D. LeBow, *Approaches to Modifying Patient Behavior* (New York: Appleton-Century-Crofts, 1976, pp. 357–360). Copyright © 1976 by Appleton-Century-Crofts. Reprinted by permission of the publisher.

The value of the above report lies in its narration of difficulties. The behavioral program, when it was operating at its best, acted as a brake on uncontrolled eating, weight gain, and diabetes. Its ultimate failure may have been due to a combination of problems: insufficient analyses of behavioral difficulties and their connections with the environment; insufficient reinforcement for the mother; insufficient numbers of other helping agents (family members, school officers); lack of powerful consequences that could be delivered immediately and contingently; poor targeting in general; competing positive reinforcers. Had these problems been solved and had a dietary plan lower in calories and carbohydrates been used (Coplin, et al., 1976), results might have been better.

Application 3: Reducing By Problem-Solving

This report by Wheeler and Hess (1976) is a controlled study that, as indicated, compares treated children to those neither treated nor contacted. All the young-sters ranged in age from 2 to 11 years, and all were referred by pediatricians. Therapy, over seven months for some, occurred at an out-patient medical facility and was free to health-plan subscribers. Sessions with mother and therapist lasted about 30 minutes each; they took place bi-weekly at first but then, depending on need, at longer intervals. Height, weight, skinfold thickness (site unmentioned), blood pressure, and serum cholesterol were measured; also photographs were taken. Behavioral data on eating were gathered for two weeks before as well as throughout the program; parents or children completed food records. Further-more, in an attempt to maintain motivation, attitudes about intervention were monitored.

Instead of receiving a previously formulated treatment package, Wheeler and Hess' patients received a decidedly more tailored therapy. That is, instead of being the subjects of a cover-all-bets type of behavioral strategy in which compliance with a list of pre-set directives was requested, they underwent a cover-best-bets strategy. Interventions were devised as problems were uncovered. Therefore, different children had different programs.

Difficulties were attacked as they surfaced, and the attack lasted until they were solved. Yet, allegiance to procedures used to remedy problems was not blind. If prescriptions appeared to be wrong, as indicated by verbal reports and other data, they were modified or rescinded. Those tried included stimulus- and consequence-control methods; Table 5.2 (Wheeler & Hess, 1976, pp. 237–238) illustrates application to eight commonly seen difficulties. Note that prescriptions involved both eliminating and controlling inappropriate antecedents, building (when possi-ble) appropriate antecedents, and providing positive reinforcers to parent and child for behavior changes. Thus, to handle overeating at scheduled meals, parents were told to serve food from the kitchen, to allow for seconds but to give vegetables before the main dish, to start the meal with less-preferred foods, and to reinforce their children for failing to be plate cleaners. By interviewing children and mothers and by scrutinizing food records, the authors were able to identify the problems; gradual change was emphasized.

Not all variables originally assessed were evaluated after treatment. Percent overweight was the barometer. Those youngsters given therapy (9 girls, 5 boys) reduced their average percent overweight from more than 40 percent to less than 35 percent. Control subjects displayed the reverse pattern, becoming more overweight with time, nearly 6 percent more. Twelve children from the original treatment group of 26 dropped out within the first four sessions; nevertheless, some of them still fared well. For another analysis, Wheeler and Hess matched 11 pairs of treated with untreated children on ages, degrees of overweight, and lengths of therapy. As before, Wheeler and Hess confirmed that the problem-solving maneuver was better than no treatment at all—10 percent of overweight-change better. It would have been valuable had the authors also documented changes (if any) in fatness, blood pressure, and cholesterol, and had they provided data on individual response to treatment and follow-up.

They did try to identify characteristics of their sample that could eventually predict successes and dropouts. Younger children (those under 8 years of age) seemingly did better. More males than females dropped out. And dropouts were also bad record keepers, among the heaviest or the lightest, and more likely to have fat parents. Corroborating some of these trends from a sample of 102 overweight children, Wheeler and Hess (1977) found that more of the dropouts were younger, male, and less obese. But those having these dropout characteristics yet staying in therapy are likely to prosper from it, many doing the best of all.

Environment Alteration:
Nutrition and/or Activity Advice Integrated

Although varying in emphasis given to nutrition and activity, each of the six applications in this section appears more than do the two above to be concerned with supplying these teachings. Nevertheless, each views the child to be plagued by bad behaviors, behaviors that fatten him and that prevent him from becoming thin; the stress is on controlling behavior. But giving equal status to behavior and each of the energy components has been argued (Stuart, 1971), and that behavior modification is the way to make the energy teachings work has been reasoned (for examples see, Blackburn & Greenberg, 1978; Coché, Levitz, & Jordan, 1979; Collipp, 1980c; Epstein, Wing, Steranchak, Dickson, & Michelson, 1980; Merritt & Batrus, 1980; Mitchell & Fiser, 1978; Schwartz & Sidbury, 1974).

Application 4: A Behavioral Package for the Retarded

Rotatori, Parish, and Freagan (1979) devised a multimethod behavioral weight-reduction regimen to be applied to six mildly retarded school children (ages unstated). A school nurse conducted the seven-week program and parents of the

Table 5.2

Changes in Eating Made During Treatment

Problem behaviors	Situations			Consequences
	Eliminate inappropriate	Control inappropriate	Provide appropriate	Provide positive
Child consumes large amounts of candy, cookies, and ice cream	Eliminate such foods from home	Buy food in portion controlled sizes for clear record of amount Use outside source (ice cream truck, walk to store) for treats	Less caloric but attractive snacks	Select one food as daily treat for appropriate eating
Child eats "on the run"; snacks from kitchen	Kitchen off bounds Tempting foods locked away or eliminated	Set times for snacks same time every day Child given "out of house" activities during difficult times	Bin of snacks easily accessible and of low calorie content Substitute lower-calorie snacks	Occasional favored snack placed in bin
Child eats overly-large quantities of food at meals	Mother serves portions in kitchen	Mother provides seconds of vegetables and salads first	Meal begins with child's less-favored food (salad first)	Child gets money or token for leaving food on plate
Child must prepare own food (changes difficult)	Child's responsibilities change	Mother prepares frozen dinners or buys low-calorie ones Child cooks with sibling	Child cooks low-calorie foods	
Child consuming food for which less-caloric substitutes are available	End purchases of high-calorie foods		Buy lower calorie foods Educate concerning the problems or possibilities of alternate foods	Reward mother for following suggestions and devising her own

| Problem behaviors | Situations | | | Consequences |
	Eliminate inappropriate	Control inappropriate	Provide appropriate	Provide positive
Child gets no exercise	Curtail TV and other sedentary activities	Schedule TV viewing	Develop new exercise child enjoys Revise family activities	Make treat contingent upon certain countable activities Involve parent in shared activity
Parents are "fair" and share with child their inappropriate eating	Eliminate inappropriate food from child's world	Parents inappropriate eating changed to outside home	Parent cooks special treat for special child Incorporate low-risk foods into family diet	Reinforce "different" treatment
High incidence of party or out-of-home eating (baby-sitter)	Restrict parties	Have mother inform others about child's difficulty or have office visit Request limitations of availability of inappropriate food	Select and save for treat at home one special food	

The problems listed are the eight most frequent problems listed in all records, both treatment and dropout.

From Mary E. Wheeler and Karl W. Hess, Treatment of juvenile obesity by successive approximation control of eating, *Journal of Behavior Therapy and Experimental Psychiatry*, 7 (1976), pp. 237-238. Copyright ©1976 by Pergamon Press. Reprinted by permission of the publisher.

children participated as agents of reinforcement in it; they also studied the methods taught to their youngsters, received nutrition instruction, and learned about their youngsters' dietary deficiencies. Although modifications in the dietary problems were attempted, aided by modifications in the school breakfast and lunch programs, these results were unreported. The children had seven behavior-change lessons, one lesson three times weekly, beginning with record keeping and ending with elimination of unwanted, between-meal eating; other lessons comprised eating-urge reduction, serving reduction, place-of-eating reduction, consumption pacing, leaving leftovers, and exercising. There was more to the training than instruction, however. The children heard a taperecording of the lesson, saw it demonstrated, practiced it, and finally received feedback on the practice.

Weekly weight losses were followed by activity reinforcers; evidently the nurse, parents, or children themselves administered the reinforcers. Children rated their own compliance with the behavioral techniques and after grading themselves exchanged marks for envelopes containing activity or "covert" (p. 34) reinforcers. Outcomes were modest, a mean weight loss of 1.68 kg in almost two months—.27 kg every seven days. Follow-up data as well as basic demographic information were undisclosed in this brief and anecdotal, albeit suggestive, report (see also Application 3, Chapter 7; Rotatori, Fox, & Parish, 1980; Rotatori & Rotatori, 1979; Schoenwetter, 1978; Staugaitis, 1978).

Application 5: Contracting with Parents of Overweight Girls

Aragona and colleagues (1975) presented a well-controlled study comparing two behavioral interventions against a no-treatment group. Fifteen 5- to 10-year-old girls, judged to be overweight by their physicians and parents, were assigned to one of three conditions: response-cost, response-cost-plus-reinforcement, and a minimal-contact control. The two behavioral groups had several treatment components in common:

1. Contracts. These documents were signed by the child's parents and fueled by financial deposits. Parents could earn back the money weekly for attending, for record keeping, and for demonstrating that their children lost weight—the magnitude of reinforceable loss (from .45 to .91 kg) was negotiated in advance. Bonuses from unearned funds that accumulated were dispensed contingent on the children's weight changes. Significantly, the contracts targeted not only weight loss but also presumed contributors to it, such as exercising and calorie-intake monitoring. Parents had to ensure that their children followed the program, and had to collect the data.

2. Stimulus control. Customary directives were applied. For example, parents were taught to teach the children to snack on low-calorie foods, to eat slowly, to dine in one place, to stop being plate cleaners, and so forth.

3. Exercise. Thirty minutes of daily calesthenics were required. The children were to reach this level within the initial three weeks of intervention and to keep to it throughout.

4. Nutrition education. Parents were taught about the relationship between good foods and weight. Sources of nutritional information were *Food and Your Weight* (USDA, 1967) and *Nutrition* (USDA,1971).

There was one essential difference between the two behavioral groups: parents in the response-cost-plus-reinforcement condition were taught to be reinforcing agents, to reinforce their children materially and socially for complying with the methods of treatment and for reducing; they were, in brief, taught to praise their children and give them money or tokens (presumably backed up by other positive consequences) for losing specified amounts of weight, exercising, reducing calorie intake, and practicing stimulus control. In order to become increasingly effective at these tasks, parents read and discussed Patterson and Gullion's (1971) *Living With Children* and recorded their daily reinforcement practices. Notably, children were excluded, except at weight checks, from the actual treatment sessions; what effects teaching parents alone had is unknown (see Kelman, Brownell, & Stunkard, 1979; Kingsley & Shapiro, 1977; Chapter 6). Girls in the control group were weighed initially, at the end of treatment, and six months after treatment, whereas those in the behavioral groups were weighed at each session. Therapy lasted for 12 weeks, succeeding a two-week baseline; additionally, the program included two follow-ups—8 and 31 weeks post-treatment.

Three youngsters dropped out of the study, two before intervention and one after the second week of it; one of the dropouts was from the response-cost-plus-reinforcement condition; the others were from the response-cost group. Other results unfortunately expressed only weight changes, even though data that allow for compliance determinations were collected. Treatment was significant, both experimental groups doing better than the control group but not better than each other. Weight losses in therapy averaged about .36 kg weekly (response-cost-only) to just over .42 kg weekly (response-cost-plus-reinforcement). By the first of the follow-ups, two months later, greater differences emerged between these treatment groups. The girls in the reinforcement cohort kept off an average of about 3.6 kg, whereas their response-cost-only counterparts managed to sustain an average reduction of just 2.3 kg; controls gained 1.6 kg. Thus, at this evaluation the response-cost-plus-reinforcement group appeared to be holding better; both therapy conditions still were superior to the control, although only the reinforcement one was significantly superior to it.

At the second of the follow-ups, there was even a larger difference between the therapy groups; comparisons with the control were not made because of attrition in this group. Reinforcement children regained, yet still showed a mean loss of approximately .32 kg. Response-cost-only children, in contrast, put on an average of 3.3 kg above their pre-treatment weights. Therefore, the regaining trend was less for those girls whose parents were taught to be reinforcing agents. Commenting on this progression—that is, both therapy groups relapse but response-cost only children relapse more and sooner—Aragona and colleagues speculated that directly teaching reinforcement skills prolongs progress.

This is a well-executed study. Nonetheless, as noted, much information remains undisclosed. Behavioral, energy, and fatness data would be useful. Furthermore, it would be valuable to know what the expected increases in weights of the children were in comparison with their actual increases. The authors do tabulate height changes, along with the weight changes, so half the information needed to make this determination is available there.

Edwards (1978) provides the other half. He recomputed Aragona and co-workers' data to find out how much of what appeared to be relapse in the therapy groups could be accounted for by linear growth. Using the weight index, which compares weight-to-height ratios of individual children with weight-to-height ratios of children at the 95th percentile in a normative sample, he showed that the response-cost-plus-reinforcement group did indeed outperform the control. Weight index scores for the girls in the control condition varied little during the study. Weight index scores for the treatment groups, however, indicated that the relapsing Aragona and colleagues said occurred for both these groups was visible only for the one without reinforcement. The maintenance picture for the response-cost-plus-reinforcement subjects, in other words, was much improved over what Aragona and colleagues had seen. Thus, as has been said, it is imperative for researchers and practitioners to consider height changes when interpreting weight changes, if growing children—children who according to Edwards are likely to gain in height and weight during any six-month interval—are treated for obesity.

Application 6: A Pediatric Nurse's
Three-Pronged Weight-Control Program

Like Aragona and co-workers, Carman (1976) joined three major elements to treat obese children. Her report is demonstrational, providing data that only hint at effectiveness; there is no control group or single-subject evaluation of treatment methods; there is no attempt to show (like Aragona also failed to show) that behavior changes occur and correspond to body changes; there is no comprehensive presentation of fatness or other (other than weight) body data; there is no detailing of methods to permit replication. Carman's study is of interest because it blends nutritional information, exercise, and behavior modification to reduce overweight children, and because, like Application 4, it demonstrates a meaningful extension of obesity control programming. The programmer is a nurse.

She and a pediatric nutritionist held the weight-control classes for 11 children, seen together, ages 7.5 to 13.5 years—one participant was 16-years-old; the program, 10 weeks, was comprised of weekly, hour-long lessons. The parents of these children also met in a class but separate from the children. They received the same information as did their youngsters, and furthermore, they learned to stop bickering with them and to start praising efforts to improve.

The nutrition component of the program, the goal of which was to teach a working knowledge of good nutrition, entailed lecturing on how to lower calories in snacks, how to recognize high-calorie foods, and how to plan menus. Counting calories was encouraged among older children (ages unstated). The activity component also was conveyed by instruction, but it included practice; a different child led class exercises at each session. Again, older children were taught to count calories—calorie expenditures.

The behavioral component was mainly comprised of stimulus-control information, such as finding a personal eating place, reducing junk-food accessibility, reducing plate sizes, and serving food only from the kitchen area. Also included were self-monitoring and reinforcement; students made food records and earned points backed up by a field trip for record keeping, attending, completing homework, losing weight (no more than 1 kg a week), and maintaining losses week to week. Furthermore, they had feedback from weight-loss progress graphs, and lastly (upon graduating) they received a rather fancy, frameable diploma.

Results principally described changes in weight. In addition to excluding behavioral and energy data, Carman also neglected to discuss the blood test data that were gathered both before and after treatment. She indicated that there was an average weight decline of about 2.7 kg by the time classes ended and that losses varied from approximately 1.4 kg to 4 kg. A month and a half later, Carman did a follow-up and found that attrition from the end of treatment to this checkup was over 45 percent, despite her offering the students money for returning; only six children came to the follow-up meeting. She detected continuance, maintenance, and relapse—one youth regained some weight, one regained everything. At eight months, she followed up again. Attrition had jumped to 55 percent and weight changes now ranged from a gain of 4 kg to a loss of about 7.3 kg. Thus, variability evident at post-treatment had increased by the final checkup; perhaps height changes, from approximately 1.3 cm to 12.8 cm, accounted for part of it.

Repeating her study on another group of overweight youths, Carman found again that attrition increased over time, from about 30 percent during intervention to almost 65 percent five months afterwards; also, she found that weight changes varied at each evaluation—more variability with ensuing evaluations—and that height changes of about 1.9 cm to 7.6 cm occurred by the last follow-up.

Like the authors of Application 3, Carman searched for characteristics of her sample that were associated with weight changes. She discovered, as did they, that the younger did better; children with two fat parents did poorer than those with one or none; sex of the child was not a factor, but degree of heaviness was; the heaviest did the poorest, although they were also the oldest. Unlike Wheeler and Hess, however, she did not evaluate dropout variables, but she did note that faulty

scheduling—for example, requesting summer checkups when families were vaca-
tioning—might have caused attrition.

*Application 7: Long-Term Results and
Behavioral Treatment*

Follow-up evaluations of over one year are infrequent in the literature in adult
obesity treatment and decidedly rare in the child literature. Rivinus, Drummond,
Combrinck-Graham (1976) provide an exception. They not only disclose two-year
findings but, in a separate report (Rivinus cited in Israel & Stolmaker, 1980) state
five-year post-treatment results. But their data only suggest the value of behavioral
methods for overweight children. Like most researchers and practitioners, Rivinus
and colleagues remain silent about the fine-grain correspondences between
behavior changes and weight changes. Essentially, they apply a behavioral treatment package accompanied by nutritional and exercise advice, positively reinforce compliance with teachings, and tabulate weight losses against height
increases.

Ten economically deprived, overweight Black youths, 8.5 to 13 years old,
received 10 weekly sessions (one other meeting occurred at the fourteenth week)
of behavior therapy, exercise encouragement, and dietary supervision; staff were a
pediatrician, psychologist, psychiatrist, nurse–practitioner, and dietician. Seven
girls and three boys met as a group accompanied by parents; one family dropped
out. Meetings lasted two hours, during which parents and children discussed
problems, progress, and new prescriptions to reduce safely.

A third of each session was a group supper. Parents and children ate at separate
tables, as staff sitting with them watched their actions. Evidently appropriate food
selections and styles of eating were in this way monitored, modeled, and positively reinforced. The generalization potential of this practice opportunity remains to
be seen; at present, though, it does seem to be a logical way of extending *in vitro*
treatment lessons to the home. Coupling instruction with practice, as suggested
previously, is productive in initiating and strengthening lessons on behavior,
nutrition, and exercise.

Rivinus and colleagues gave an array of behavioral teachings. Among them
were self-monitoring of intake, stimulus control, and reducing eating speed; some
were specially developed in response to the needs of specific individuals. To
motivate parents and children, the authors devised contracts at the outset. These
documents specified a money-return contingent on weight loss—one dollar per .5
kg; funds were obtained from parents ($1.00) and child ($1.00) each week and
dispersed to the child. Relatedly, points were given to the children for complying
with stimulus-control teachings, pacing directives, and caloric intake limits;
points were lost for surpassing these limits. Back-up reinforcers were available,
such as bowling tickets or dancing opportunities; children earning the most points

each week became King and Queen for that week. Notably, as Jordan and Levitz (1975) comment, some of the back ups in this study encouraged behavior changes in line with program goals—for example, bowling increases activity.

Rivinus and associates also attempted to build a weight-maintenance system. Presents were to be given to the child for sustaining progress. Questionnaire responses indicated that even after two years, families still followed this suggestion and relatedly still applied the behavioral principles they had been taught. Testimony like this is important, but more than testimonials are needed to document maintenance practices.

Nine children finished this 2.5 month interdisciplinary program, all the finishers reaching an attendance level of 91 percent and reducing an average of more than 2.7 kg; losses ranged from about .5 kg to 9 kg. These youngsters started treatment at least 35 percent overweight. Ten weeks after it had ended, eight of the nine finishers were still progressing; the one who wasn't (an 8-year-old girl) nevertheless, was still close to her post-treatment loss. The average reduction had increased to nearly 4.2 kg. Then, almost two years after this checkup (120 weeks after intervention had started) the authors again evaluated. They were able to report on all nine children. Six were still lighter than they had been before treatment. In fact one, originally the best loser, was 15.9 kg lighter. The average loss at this time, even though three children had gained, was somewhat greater than it had been at post-treatment.

Looking at the more informative measure, percent of overweight change, the authors disclosed a mean reduction of 51 points; while before intervention the children had averaged 72 percent overweight, at the 120 week checkup they averaged 21 percent. Moreover, three no longer were overweight at all, and everyone else was lighter, too. Height increases in this sample of growing children were normal, a mean 11.2 cm. At five years, the mean amount of overweight reduction climbed by 5 percent from the previous follow-up to 56 percent; corresponding with this change, the average degree overweight fell by approximately 4 percent (Israel & Stolmaker, 1980). Thus, the children had continued to progress.

As in Application 5, however, the precise impact that parents made on their children's progress is unknown. Possibly, mother's weight and her ability to self-apply therapy affected her child's success, for as noted in the report, overweight mothers, failing to reduce in treatment, had overweight children who did the poorest. Possibly, the degree of social support she provided for her child was also a factor.

The potential of social support as a tactic in treatment and maintenance has been briefly addressed in Chapter 4. Systematic inquiry into it is missing in childhood obesity research, although several investigators including Rivinus and co-workers (see Brownell & Kaye, 1982; Coles, 1982) have noted its probable significance in alleviating the weight control dilemmas of the young. Capell and Martin (1975), for instance, in addition to using stimulus control procedures for obese handicap-ped juveniles, taught the families of these youths to reinforce progress. Gross, Wheeler, and Hess (1976) likewise promoted the idea of family support in their study of older, physically unimpaired adolescent girls, and so also did Epstein, Wing, Steranchak, Dickson, and Michelson (1980) in the application discussed next.

Application 8: Behavior Modification
for Overweight Parents and Children

Epstein and colleagues recruited 18 families for this treatment study; two dropped out before the second session, one after the third, and two before the program commenced. Mother and child were evaluated following seven weeks of treatment and then for three months afterwards. At the outset, the children, eight boys and five girls between 6 and 12 years of age, ranged from 42 to 100 percent over-weight; the average was nearly 65 percent overweight. Their mothers, definitely less overweight as a group (average over 35 percent), varied between −15.5 percent and +121.2 percent. Sessions occurred weekly during treatment and monthly during follow-up.

Like Carman (Application 6), Epstein and associates saw mothers and children separately, and like Aragona (Application 5) they developed a multi-element intervention coupled with nutrition and exercise education. But in contrast to these investigators, or any others mentioned in the Approaches section, they compared nutrition education to behavior modification. They did so using an additive design that permitted everyone to receive nutrition and exercise instruction while some also received behavioral lessons. In other words, for one group of children and one group of mothers there were two interventions—nutrition and exercise teachings—whereas for comparable groups of parents and children there were these interventions plus behavior modification. The nutrition component of ther-apy included lectures on counting calories and following a diet. The authors applied the color-coded food system described in the self-monitoring part of the previous chapter (see Dickson, Szparaga, Epstein, Wing, Koeske, & Zidansek, 1981; Epstein, Wing, Koeske, Andrasik, & Ossip, 1981). Recall that with this method foods are coded primarily according to their caloric densities with-in a particular group—green foods may be eaten ad libitum, yellow foods sparingly, red foods even more sparingly or avoided entirely. For example, within the vegetable grouping, as the authors say, asparagus is a green food, corn a yellow food, and potato salad a red one. Patients were restricted to four or less red foods weekly; also, they were restricted to an intake of 1200 kcal or 1500 kcal daily.

The exercise component, like the nutrition, was directed at teaching children and parents what to do to reduce, namely what to do to remove the calorie surplus. Toward this end, lectures on aerobics and calisthenics and practice in doing activities within these categories took place; also continuous sitting in front of the television was discouraged. The exercise component was not manipulated; all groups received it.

The behavioral component was the how-to part—the way to make the recommended changes in energy balance happen. Tactics, such as stimulus control, eating pacing, modeling, praising, and monitoring, accompanied by between-session telephoning to give instruction and support, were used. Contracting also was applied. Families deposited funds and earned them back contingent on monitoring calorie intake and weight, adhering to red food proscriptions, and losing weight; the child received money for complying with monitoring and eating directives, whereas both parent and child earned it for reducing. Nutrition groups received money from deposits only for attending.

Even though attendance was not specifically contracted for in the behavioral group, it was highest in this condition (89.3 percent). The nutrition group, however, attended reliably as well (71.9 percent). Weight declined for all groups from pre-treatment to follow-up, about 2.7 kg on the average for the children and about 3 kg on the average for the mothers. Children and parents in the behavioral groups lost the most, means of almost 4 kg for the youngsters and over 4 kg for the mothers. Furthermore, the weight losses of the children resembled those of the parents more so in the behavioral than in the nutrition groups. This result suggests that the behavioral teachings may have helped mother and child unite in their mutual efforts to reduce (see Epstein, Wing, Ossip, & Andrasik, 1981). If they did, this indicates a great advantage of incorporating behavior modification principles into the treatment programs for obese families.

But what effects the particular behavioral teachings given had on the body changes found remains a mystery, for the relationships between behavior and body modifications, the extent of compliance with the teachings, and the extent of changes in behavior, are all undocumented. What is clear is that the behavioral group, parents and children together, significantly outdid the nutrition group. To reach this conclusion, Epstein and colleagues evaluated percent of overweight changes from the start of treatment to follow-up. Children and parents receiving behavioral care in addition to nutrition and exercise instruction reduced an average of almost 13 percent, whereas their nutrition education counterparts reduced less than 5 percent. For the youngsters treated behaviorally, there was a 17.5 percent drop in degree of overweight; for those treated without this component the comparable figure was 6.4 percent. Likewise, parents given behavior modification changed over twice as much in percent overweight as did parents not receiving it.

Application 9:
Controlling Weight-Loss Plan Violations

The rationale of this program, suggested in Chapter 4, is that for children to become thinner they need to solve difficulties they encounter while trying to follow an obesity-control regimen (LeBow, 1981a; LeBow & Perry, 1977;

Mahoney & Mahoney, 1976a). They need to lessen the deviations they commit from plans to eat specified types and quantities of food and to perform specified amounts of activity; therefore, the target behavior class is deviations from obesity reduction plans. Typically the program lasts about five months. Assessment is continuous and thus deviations along with their underlying themes (explained below) are identified as they arise and then modified by behavioral procedures as required; accordingly, treatment follows assessment and is tailored to the child's changing requirements.

Session 1. The initial three of the first meeting's seven objectives are to determine if the child really wants to undergo treatment for obesity, to overview the program for him, and to search out potential reinforcers (to start a reinforcer menu). The interview found in Appendix G is administered; the number of questions asked depends upon the child's age and verbal skills; parent(s), usually accompanying the child every session, supply missing information by discussion during the meeting or by completing the interview at home.

The fourth objective is to begin a weight and height chart. As shown in Table 5.3, the child's name, age, and birthdate are entered in the upper left-hand corner. Further to the right, eight measures are listed: pre-baseline weight, height, and percent overweight, pre-deviation-baseline weight (taken the following week usually), starting weight (taken two weeks after the first session), and termination weight, height, and percent overweight (taken approximately five months after the first session). Reduction goals (weekly, monthly, overall) are unlisted, but weekly ones are discussed by the third session. They vary from no change to just under 1 kg, depending on the child's age and percent overweight; reduction goals may be modified during the program.

The six columns on the table permit tabulations of the child's weekly weight changes and monthly height changes. On February 23 for instance, John S., an overweight 10-year-old boy weighs 55.5 kg. He does not lose or gain from his starting weight taken on February 16, so zeros appear in the next three columns. Height is not measured; it will be taken, however, the next week, and each month thereafter. On March 2, John weighs 55 kg. Thus, an "L" is placed in the loss/gain column, the amount of change for the week is .5 kg, and the total amount of change thus far is .5 kg; height on this date is the same as that on February 2—145 cm. Weight and height are tabulated in this way throughout; midweek checks on weight, if any, are similarly documented.

Fifth, a standards chart, Table 5.4, is started. On it, corresponding to the sessions when gathered, are body and energy data. The calorie intake allotment is formally set after baseline terminates; it may be revised later. The calorie expenditure objective is written following the eating control component and activity baselines, about session 12. Body circumference and skinfold data are taken during sessions 1 and 3 (start of program), and monthly from then on.

Sixth, a pediatrician's or family physician's consent form (see Appendix F) is handed out; it is to be completed within three weeks. The form should specify a level of calorie intake (see Table 6.1); lowering the intake level further may be necessary at some point during the program, and if done the child's physician should be notified.

Seventh, homework is assigned. The child with his parent(s)' assistance (amount of assistance varies with the child) is to gather baseline data on eating. Seven forms, analogous to Table 4.3, are provided; calorie counts are done subsequently by the therapist.

Session 2. Occasionally, the child's day-to-day consumption is so blatently variable that a second week of intake baseline is requested. Usually, however, the request is for a baseline on deviating. Children are to plan five days of eating, one day at a time, to a calorie intake level approximating the one they will be formally assigned at the next session; parent(s) help in this step, as they have before. Table 4.4 is to be filled out ahead of the meal and Table 4.5 after it. By accomplishing these tasks, children can pick out where plans and performances disagree; with their parent(s), they are to describe the kinds, amounts, and preparations of the foods the plan violation involves as well as the situations in which it occurs. Data are to be brought to the next meeting.

Session 3. Formal intervention begins. Four eating control steps are explained and two days of doing each of them assigned. During the five unassigned days, children are told to watch their eating as best they can; as important as meeting the weekly weight-loss or no-change objective is following assignments. Step one (already discussed with parent and child during the baseline stage) is meal planning. Using Table 4.4 the child and his parent(s) forecast foods, calories, and so on. Allotted daily calorie intake (top of form) is to approximate total calories planned (bottom of form). A calorie intake slush fund, to cover unplanned consumption, is stipulated, about 10 percent of the child's intake objective; it is the slush fund plus the planned consumption that is to approximate the allotted number of calories.

Step two is meal recording. As described in Chapter 4, this step involves documenting for the planned days what in fact is eaten. Table 4.5 is used or, if the child is on an exchange diet, Table 4.6, the card system, is employed.

Step three involves comparing proposal with performance and locating disagreements, identifying deviations. Failing to eat a proposed food is not deviating. Making substitutions to recover from a deviation is to be praised as a sign of adaptive replanning—for example, substituting fruit for planned pie at dinner because of deviating at lunch. But frequently undercutting the daily calorie allotment is to be discouraged. Locating deviations that occur during intervention is like finding them during baseline. Now, however, the child and his parent(s) note (Step 4) in a diary or on a special form provided not only the same details recorded in baseline but also the calories acquired from each deviation; this is

Table 5.3
Weight and Height Chart*

Name: John S.
Age: 10

Birthdate: 2 Jan 1971						Date
	Prebaseline weight = 56 kg					2 Feb
	Prebaseline height = 145 cm					2 Feb
	Prebaseline percent overweight** = 27%					2 Feb
	Predeviation baseline weight = 56 kg					9 Feb
	Starting weight = 55.5 kg					16 Feb
	End of program weight =					
	End of program height =					
	End of program percent overweight =					

Date	Wt (kg)	Loss/Gain	Weekly Wt. Change	Cumulative Wt. Change	Height cm
23 Feb	55.5	0	0	0	
2 Mar	55	L	.5	.5	145

*Fictitious data

**Calculated from Fig. XIV, 90th percentile, of NCHS Growth Curves (1977).

128

Table 5.4
Standards Chart

	Sessions:	1	2	3	4 ... 20
Daily calorie intake				1600 kcal	
Weekly calorie expenditure					
Waist size		73 cm		73 cm	
Chest size		78 cm		78 cm	
Hips		79 cm		79 cm	
Thighs					
R		46 cm		46 cm	
L		45 cm		45 cm	
Triceps skinfold		23 mm		23 mm	

calories resulting from the foods involved in the deviation minus calories remaining in the slush fund. What's more, child and parent(s) note the theme or combination of themes underlying it. Table 5.5 lists possibilities, a list the child is given ahead of time. Suppose, for instance, John eats an unplanned for, three ounce (85 g) slice of pecan pie while out to dinner with his family. Having 100 kcal left in his slush fund, he would record a 250 kcal deviation. Furthermore, he would write that themes one and six played roles in the deviation, if he feels that knowing desserts are available at the restaurant and watching others still eating fanned his appetite.

Session 4.   Homework is handed in at the start and three days of record keeping is requested at the end. Data are scrutinized, praise for compliance given, and weight taken.

In addition the child is taught how to recoup from a deviation and to reflect on ways to prevent its reoccurrence. He can try to make up for a deviation by dividing the calories from it by the remaining days of the week in order to calculate the daily recouping problem. Thus, John's 250 kcal deviation, if happening on the first day of that program week, would be divided by six to equal 42 kcal. The child is encouraged to recoup by increasing exercise—calorie expenditure suggestions are given. Although recouping completely really becomes a possibility only as a full week on the program is shaped, even in the early phases attempting to recoup is a good experience.

Reflecting, the second new practice discussed in this session, is thinking about ways to deal with plan-violation themes (see Mahoney & Mahoney, 1976a, step

Table 5.5
Common Themes of Violations in Eating Plans

Number and Title	Description
1. Food probably there	You are fairly certain something delicious is there, but you do not actually see it.
2. Food definitely there	You see the treat and lots of other food, perhaps.
3. Food on my mind	You keep thinking about a certain food or about food in general.
4. Clean my plate	Your parents or someone else tells you to not leave food on your plate. To do so is wasteful.
5. Finish before dessert	This is like the theme immediately above, except you are told no dessert unless you clean your plate.
6. People eating	This involves a situation in which you see others eating and you join them. These others may be people you know or just strangers.
7. Friends offer food	People you know bring you things to eat— just to be nice. Some of these friends are relatives.
8. Friends suggest food	Someone says let's get some candy. Or, someone says let's go to —— (the fast food restaurant).
9. No choices when out	You are at a restaurant that has a menu with nothing you have planned to eat on it. Or you are at your Aunt and Uncle's or Grandparent's home.
10. Second, thirds, and so on	You take additional helpings.
11. I've been good	You reward yourself by eating. Perhaps you say, "I avoided something rich earlier during the day so I deserve a treat."
12. I'm no good	You have gone off your diet a bit and you feel you have already blown it, so why not enjoy.
13. I'll never make it	You don't think you will be successful because you see yourself as weak when it comes to food, so you eat.

Themes are sources of deviations. Other themes are possible, as are combinations.

4). Future sessions examine and amplify these reflections. For example, if watching others eat is a problem, John, his parent(s), and the therapist could design a short-term behavioral contract whereby the boy receives points redeemable by parent-sponsored trips and prizes for restraining himself in problematic settings. Simply by seeing his deviations and analyzing their sources, he may be able to overcome them. Relatedly, he may learn to plan for some of them. If going to a restaurant on Friday night is a regular event and watching others eat desserts unavoidable, John may be advised to include dessert in his meal plans for Friday night. By doing so, he makes eating dessert no longer a deviation on Friday night — accommodating new plans to past transgressions eliminates deviations.

Sessions 5 through 10. Homework assigned during these meetings eventually brings data collection to a full week—five days at the end of the fifth session and seven days at the end of the sixth. A bar graph of deviations is started and posted, usually in the child's bedroom; frequency is on the ordinate and sessions (sessions including baseline where deviation data are collected) is on the abcissa. At the top of each bar, calories are written to denote whether the child has equalled his weekly (for example, two days) allotment (that is, daily intake goal times number of days of data collection for the week), exceeded it, or undercut it. Homework requested at the tenth session includes not only food planning, and so on, but also a one-week activity baseline (see Chapter 4); data collection on eating may be temporarily stopped at this time, if the recording assignment appears to be excessive.

As indicated, during every session the child is weighed, records are collected, problems discussed, behavioral programs checked, and progress positively reinforced. Also, practice in completing forms is provided and compliance with prescriptions is measured. Points are assigned from zero to one (fractions between), according to percent of compliance with the prescriptions given (for example, planning, recording intake, recording and categorizing deviations, recouping from deviating, graphing, following behavioral programs). Sometimes it is apparent that returning to the tasks of earlier program weeks or slowing advancement is required.

In addition to helping their youngsters by explaining practices, constructing menus, and so forth, parent(s) may act as reliability checkers. Also, during treatment, the therapist may visit the home to gain a better picture of how the child lives (food cues are inventoried, for example). Furthermore, the child and parent(s) are given suggestions about tasty lower calorie treats and told about the importance of a balanced and varied diet. They are helped to learn nutrition principles by reading recommended texts, such as Selph and Street's, *Alphabet Soup* (1975), which contains prose and poetry dealing with foods. They are also helped by seeing filmstrips accompanied by audio cassettes, such as "Break the Fast," "The Nutrient Express," "George Gorge and Nicky Persnicky" (Polished

Apple, 1976). Finally, becoming more active is encouraged, but is not formally addressed until after the eleventh session.

Session 11.   An activity-deviation baseline analogous to the eating-deviation baseline is requested following a review of the activity baseline data. Instructions are similar to those given in the second session; calorie expenditure levels are not stipulated. The task, briefly, is to plan activities and describe violations from plans.

Session 12.   The activity phase formally commences with lecturing and discussion about the value and kinds of activities and about obstacles to becoming more active that baseline data identify. Activities for the ensuing week (two days) are, using Table 4.7, forecasted; planning during the session occurs and calorie expenditure equivalents are given. Data-keeping on eating is temporarily suspended to lessen the recording chores. Also, during this meeting, a list of activity-deviation themes (Table 5.6) is provided. The child uses this list like he uses the eating-deviation themes listing.

Session 13.   The "accomplishments" part of Table 4.7 is explained (see Chapter 4), as is recouping, (becoming more active on planned and unplanned days), reflecting, and activity-deviation graphing (with calorie expenditure evaluation). Behavioral programs for activity problems begin if needed, and homework assignments (five days) continue.

Sessions 14 through 19.   Program days increase to seven and compliance evaluations resume. And for at least two weeks, homework becomes recording both eating and activity sequences.

Session 20.   Maintenance starts. For the still obese child, however, this meeting starts continuance. Standards are reassessed and a new calorie intake level assigned. Also, an arrangement whereby the child will be seen intermittently is proposed—biweekly, then monthly, then bimonthly, then semiannually.

Vigilance in monitoring behaviors, weight, and the fit of clothes is stressed and reinstituting the eating and activity sequences as soon as relapsing begins advised; a week-on, week-off data-keeping strategy is valuable during the first few months of maintenance/continuance. Among the signs of relapsing are weight gain for already overweight children, increasing flabbiness, increasing television, and snacking. The eating and activity sequences are reviewed with child and parent, and telephone contact is encouraged. Also, the next formal appointment is made.

The 11-year-old boy discussed in Chapters 3 and 4 received an approximation of this program. He was taught to find discrepancies between his plans and performances and he became adept at doing so. Four months after treatment started his weight was 9 kg less; his losses at the three-month follow-up exceeded 9.5 kg and by six months were approximately 10 kg. He began to relapse at nine months, still showing a reduction of almost 8 kg, but by 19 months he was 2.7 kg

Table 5.6
Common Themes of Violations in Activity Plans

Number and Title	Description
1. No time	You feel you have too many other things to do first. Sometimes, you are involved in something that you feel you cannot leave.
2. No alternatives	Something happens, such as rain, that spoils your plans to be active, and you have no alternative activities on hand.
3. Someone does it for you	A parent drives you instead of letting you walk or does something that takes effort to save you the job.
4. Someone warns you not to	You are warned about the dangers of an exercise and you decide to heed the warning.
5. Friends and family rest too much	No one close to you will exercise with you.
6. I hate it (Coles, 1982)	Exercise becomes boring or painful.
7. People will laugh (Coles, 1982)	Others, you have reason to expect, will ridicule you when you exercise.
8. I failed already	Like the eating-deviation theme (Table 5.5, theme 12), you have violated your plan, so you quit trying.

Themes are sources of deviations. Other themes are possible, as are combinations.

heavier than his pretreatment weight of 80. 4 kg; at this time, however, he was 10.2 cm taller, indicating a decline in percent overweight. Also, his interactions with others had improved. The boy's mother, who participated with him in therapy, increased the 10 kg loss she had managed by the end of treatment to approximately 11 kg by the 19 month checkup. Thus she was more successful than her son at maintaining progress. Three other families treated the same way posted similar results; that is, parents were better maintainers than were children (Levitz et al., 1980).

Conclusions

As said at the end of Chapter 2, these are indeed the early days of the behavioral control remedy for obese children; some reports are uncontrolled clinical trials, others more rigorous tests. Such methodological flaws as failing to control for attention, maturation, and expectancy are rife. So are such reporting shortcomings as failing to say whether engineered behavior changes endure, whether new ones arise after treatment, and whether body changes last; furthermore, energy data are absent, and too often treatment procedures are insufficiently described for replication. Thus, by and large, the deficiencies of this literature resemble those of the adult literature:

1. Treatment lengths are pre-set. A brief-treatment policy seems to exist in which treatment ends before many of the children attain goal weights or demonstrate sufficient behavior changes; criteria for handing children's self-care credentials, or handing their parents credentials as caregivers have not as yet been put forth.

2. Variability in response to treatment is pronounced. Few leads exist about reasons for this variability or about guidelines for directing specific therapies to specific children or relatedly about predictors—demographic, personality, behavioral—of response to treatment (see Geller et al., 1981). What are the expected effects of the various behavioral tactics for children who differ in weight, fatness, social skills, socioeconomic background, health problems, and physical disabilities? Is there less variability when other therapeutic methods are applied, and how valuable is behavior therapy compared to these other methods (see Application 8)?

3. Follow-up evaluations and follow-through strategies are in short supply. Although there have been evaluations of a year and more (Colletti, Savrin, & Stern, 1979; Application 7), the practice is not routine. Durability usually exists more in the hopes of researchers and practitioners than in their plans.

4. Clinical significance needs to be demonstrated more often. Data on fatness changes and the social impact of weight and fat reduction are missing.

5. Behavioral data are frequently lacking. Do successful youngsters succeed because they follow behavioral prescriptions? Do those who fail, fail because they do not comply? Do behaviors change? The relationships among taking behavioral advice, changing behavior, changing the ratio of calorie intake to outgo, and changing body shape need articulation; fine-grain analyses are required. More single-subject strategies of evaluation would be welcome (see St. Charles, 1981).

6. Dependent variables are too few. This problem relates to the two previous issues. Not only are fatness data, behavioral data, and social validations missing, but also health status changes frequently are not calibrated; and when they are assessed, they may go unreported (see, for example, Application 6). Moreover, still unclear are the far-reaching consequences of offering or not offering behavioral treatment to overweight children (see Baer, 1974; Willems, 1974 for discussions of behavioral ecology).

7. Assessment and monitoring are neglected. The outcome of inattention to these parts of the behavior modification process is dearth of individualized programming. Data retrieval strategies, other than having patients self-report food ingestions and exercises, are needed, if therapists and researchers are to initially tailor prescriptions and then to refine them as treatment proceeds. We need to know about the obese child's world before we embark on and polish regimens to alter it.

The future of childhood obesity research and therapy requires that attention be paid to the aforenamed issues. Needing scrutiny are the process concerns noted and others, such as how often to see the child in therapy (Coates et al., 1982); how to maintain the child's participation; whether to offer treatment to groups or to individuals; how best to convey prescriptions; whether, when, and how to enlist helping agents, including who to enlist as well as what and how to teach them. Also in need of scrutiny are outcome issues, such as the cost effectiveness of the various treatments and approaches, and what the long-range impact is of body changes and behavior changes on the child's self-perceptions as well as on others' perceptions of him. Furthermore, there is need for in-depth study of behavioral practices coupled with the best of the dietary and exercise regimens for children (see Rosenbaum, Faris, Shriner, Blankenship, & Suskind, 1982; Rosenbaum, Faris, Shriner, & Suskind, 1981). For it is through this combination that behavior therapy may have most to offer obese children toward making them healthier and happier.

These and other related topics will be addressed again in the next chapter, primarily within the framework of obstacles to remain cognizant of when attempting to aid the obese child.

CHAPTER 6
Obstacles

What makes the task of improving the lot of the obese child so difficult? This chapter names problems, formulating them as obstacles, that are common. In principle all of these obstacles are removable, but in practice some or all often thwart researchers and practitioners. One potential problem for instance, already examined in Chapter 2, has to do with messages the child receives that interfere with treatment's objectives. When parents refuse to alter an environment of food splendor or continue to force dinner down their child's throat by threatening him with a loss of dessert, they create obstacles to effective, meaningful care.

That such actions need to be unmasked signifies that more than a child's body weight needs to be assessed and monitored. Figure 6.1, the obesity triangle, lists some of these other components in three groups. Each heading includes variables of potential significance to researchers and practitioners who wish to more fully assess the child before treatment, monitor him during it, and evaluate him at its end and afterwards. The arrows on the diagram mean that Points A, B, and C are interrelated; these interrelationships need to be articulated and the directions of their effects explored.

For instance, does following activity prescriptions decrease calorie intake (Epstein et al., 1978)? If so, does the intake decrease and calorie expenditure increase resulting from activity changes promote body fat decreases, plasma lipid changes, and blood pressure reductions? And when body fat decreases temporarily mask weight decreases, does the failure to lose weight inhibit further compliance with activity prescriptions? The presumption is that one or more changes at the behavioral point (Point B) affect the balance of energy (Point C) to cause changes in one or more of the elements of the body (Point A). There is a long history to describing weight and fatness change as the outcome of prolonged energy imbalance—that is, that Point C affects Point A. Of more recent vintage is the idea that certain modifications in behavior underlie these energy changes—that Point B affects Point C.

The idea appears to be sound (LeBow, 1981a); tests of it, however, have been criticized, and proof of it has been challenged (see Brownell & Stunkard, 1978;

Much of this chapter is adapted from LeBow, M. D., "Obstacles to effectively treating obese children," *Child Behavior Therapy,* 1981.

136

Figure 6.1
The Triangle of Obesity in Juveniles

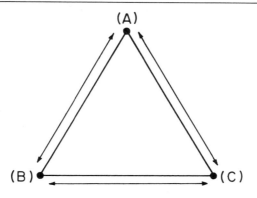

A. Body Measures
   Weight
   Fat
   Height
   Percent Overweight
   Blood Pressure
   Plasma Lipid Levels
   Glucose Tolerance
   Aerobic Fitness
   -Heart rate at rest and
    at work
   -Maximal Oxygen Uptake[*]

B. Behavioral Measures
   Eating and its Con-
    comitants
   Activity and its Con-
    comitants
   Athletic Skills
   Social Skills
   Bickering
   Contradictory Messages
   Family Perceptions of
    Obese Child
   Peer Perceptions
   Self-Perceptions
   Self-Statements
   Deviating From Plans
   School Performance
   Attendance
   Compliance with Directives

C. Energy Measures
   Calorie Intake
   Calorie Expenditure

Dependent variables listed are not exhaustive of all possibilities. Also, it is not
intended that each one be included in every treatment program. The triangle is a guide to
variables of concern and a prompt that single-point measurement is limiting.

*Maximum rate of oxygen consumption in ml/kg/min (max VO_2) is predictable from submaximal
exercise data.

Lansky, 1981; Chapter 5). Today, major problems confronting the behaviorist
working with the obese child involve understanding which behavioral prescriptions produce energy changes safely and economically, what effects these energy
changes have on the body, and what effects both energy and body changes have on
continued behavior change. Calorie intake must eventually be balanced with
calorie outgo, and caretakers and the child must be taught to renew effective
practices when facing the prospect of a relapse into positive energy imbalance. To

address these problems in the hope of solving them, investigators need more comprehensive measurement practices than exist at present, as the obstacles to be discussed below and the previously discussed issues related to them reveal.

Devising the Negative Energy Equation

For the child to change the shape of his body, he must make the energy equation negative. This means that he must somehow make the ratio of calorie intake to calorie outgo stay at less than one for some length of time; he must reduce calorie intake, increase calorie outgo, or do both. Where the emphasis is placed, on which Point C term, should depend on which term is most awry, most different from normal (Brownell & Stunkard, 1980b).

Are Obese Children Consuming Too Many or Ex-pending Too Few Calories?

Studies disagree. Some find obese youngsters to be less active than their nonobese counterparts (Bruch, 1940; Mayer, 1975; Rose & Mayer, 1968; Waxman & Stunkard, 1980). Others find them not to be different (Stunkard & Pestka, 1962). Thus, Corbin and Pletcher (1968) show that fat children, fifth graders, are less active than are thin ones, whereas Wilkinson, Parkin, Pearlson, Strang, and Sykes (1977a), working with 12-year-olds, do not. In the Corbin and Pletcher study, the activity levels of 50 children were evaluated through motion pictures taken during physical education periods; 40,000 analyses of the pictures were made. In the Wilkinson and co-workers' study, pedometers, instruments permitting distance measurements, were used with forty youngsters.

In relation to amount eaten, contradictions also exist. Corbin and Pletcher find nonsignificant calorie intake differences (Cahn, 1968; Morgan, 1980; Poskitt, & Cole, 1978; Vobecky, Demers, & Shapcott, cited in *Obesity and Bariatric Medicine*, 1981). Bernfeld and Lesieur (1976), on the other hand, find pro-nounced differences; they cite gluttony as characterizing three-quarters of their 100 obese youngsters. And Huenemann (1974a) reports no distortion in either the calorie intake or expenditure terms in her sample of obese and nonobese six-month-old children.

Why the disagreements? Perhaps differences, in part, result from how the terms of the negative energy equation are estimated (Brownell & Stunkard, 1980a, b). Some investigators employ subjective data-retrieval methods (for example, Cor-bin & Pletcher, 1968), whereas others employ more objective ones (Wilkinson et al., 1977a). In terms of measurement differences, less activity among the obese when compared to the nonobese should not be construed to mean fewer calories expended (Brownell & Stunkard, 1980b). Weight of the performer, as well as the kind and amount of activity, must be considered.

Waxman and Stunkard (1980) illuminate this point while trying to answer which term of the energy equation is most awry. They offer an in-depth analysis of activity levels, calorie expenditure levels, and calorie intake levels on a small sample of overweight and nonoverweight youngsters, ages 6 to 13 years; all were boys. Each overweight boy had a nonobese brother and classmate as controls. Trained observers collected the data in the home and school. Information on calorie intake was gathered at selected meals, whereas activity was rated at other times in 15-second blocks during 15-minute periods; the children were categorized as either sitting, standing, fidgeting, walking, running, or running fast. Calorie expenditure estimates were obtained from oxygen consumption analyses carried out no less than two hours following lunch; these analyses were done for four of the categories sampled during activity measurement.

Setting affected activity and calorie outgo ratings.   At school, overweight children were about as active as the nonoverweight. Inside and outside the home (at play), they were not. But as the activity gap closed between the heavy and light children, the calorie expenditure levels for the overweight rose above those of the controls. When least active, the overweight expended approximately as many calories as did the nonoverweight. When as active as the nonoverweight, the overweight children expended far more calories.

Waxman and Stunkard report that overweight boys consume more than do others. Summarizing, they argue that heavy youngsters in the study take in more and take it in more quickly than do their lighter peers. Excessive calorie intake is their problem.

As Waxman and Stunkard indicate, replication and extension of this study is needed. Conclusions are not as yet possible. If the problem is one of excessive intake, why is that? What forces existing in the obese child's environment affect the magnitude of each term of the energy equation (Bridgewater, Walsh, Jeffrey, Ballard, & Peterson, 1981; Jeffrey, Lemnitzer, Hickey, Hess, McLellarn, & Stroud, 1980)? Is the obese child overly responsive to external cues to eat (Costanzo & Woody, 1979; Geller et al., 1981; Gordon & Boulton, 1978; Isbitsky & White, 1981; Johnson, Parry, & Drabman, 1978; Lechowick, 1981; Milstein, 1978; Naiman, 1978; Rodin & Slochower, 1976; Stager, 1981; Wagner & Schumaker, 1976)? Is there a response inhibition deficit (Bonato & Boland, 1982)? How powerful a determiner of the obese child's leftovers is food palatability (Ballard, Gipson, Guttenberg, & Ramsey, 1980)? Studies of obese and nonobese boys and girls differing along an array of demographic and lifestyle characteristics will precede the answers to such questions.

Energy Imbalance and the Child's Physical Health

The issues to be discussed here and in the section following concern the settings of the two Point C (energy) terms and how these settings affect Point A (body) measures on the obesity triangle. Although moderated by the degree of each child's obesity and healthiness, reducing calorie intake becomes progressively less wholesome as the level of restriction intrudes on basic nutritional requirements (see Appendix A). However, in order for the weight and fat loss to occur, the energy equation has to become negative. By elevating the calorie expenditure term, however, therapists need not ask for a dramatic reduction in calorie intake. Thus, if a calorie deficit of 300 kcal is sought, the child may reduce his intake by 300 kcal, or by 200 kcal, or by 150 kcal, or by less, depending on how much his calorie outgo is stepped up—zero, 100 kcal, or 150 kcal, or more. Such compensation is an advantage of raising calorie expenditure.

Another advantage is the body changes brought about by doing so. Evidence exists that increases in calorie expenditure through increases in activity heighten fat loss and diminish lean tissue loss. Accordingly, while studying adults, Johnson, Mastropaolo, and Wharton (1972), found significant reductions in fat without reductions in weight. Twenty coeds, averaging 163 cm and close to 61 kg, exercised 30 minutes daily for 10 weeks. By the end of this 2.5 month period, the women had lessened their overall calorie intake but had not become lighter. Fatness had, however, decreased (skinfolds); body density had increased. Similarly, Zuti (1972) disclosed that by elevating calorie expenditure he could promote reductions in fat and gains in lean tissue (Dressendorfer, 1975). Instead of simply evaluating what happened to those who had exercised, he compared exercisers with nonexercisers; he did so using heavy women between approximately 7 kg and 18 kg overweight. In his weight-control program, 16 weeks long, his patients had a negative energy equation calling for about a 500 kcal deficit per day. Notably, he devised the equation differently for different groups of patients: only calorie restriction for one group, only calorie expenditure increments for another, and changes in both terms for the third cohort. By the end of treatment each of the groups had lost a mean of roughly 5 kg. Yet those having had a negative energy equation with a calorie expenditure focus—two groups—had lost 35 percent more fat than had the diet-only patients (see also Brownell & Stunkard, 1980b; Brozek, Grande, Anderson, & Keys, 1963; Buskirk, 1974; Keys & Brozek, 1953; Oscai & Williams, 1968; Pollack, Cureton, & Greniger, 1969). Hence, a negative energy equation that does not forget the calorie expenditure term appears to have advantages for adults.

Advantages appear to accrue for children as well (see Peña, Barta, Regöly-Mérel, & Tichy, 1980). Pařízková (1973, 1977), for instance, reporting on the body composition changes of obese youths losing weight at a summer camp, notes that they reduce weight and fat and gain in lean body mass. Children in the camps, which last seven to eight weeks, exercise daily (sports, games, dancing, walking) and diet (1700 kcal/day); the diet limits carbohydrates and fats, not protein. In one study, Pařízková (1973) shows average weight reductions of about 7 kg for 18 boys and 15 girls with lean body mass increases of 6.2 percent for the boys and 4.8 percent for the girls. Pařízková (1977) summarizes later work, and indicates that seven boys (11.8 years on the average) lost a mean of 11.4 percent body weight. Fat decreased by an average of 5.3 kg, while lean mass in increased by 6 percent; other positive changes (aerobic capacity improvements) also are described. As Pařízková (1973) writes, "A physically active life develops lean body mass at the expense of fat both in boys and girls" (p. 122).

The import of such modifications, as noted earlier, is easily overlooked if weight is seen as the essence of a successful therapy; as a result, researchers and practitioners fail to collect fat-change data. The omission restricts interpretation. It also reinforces an erroneous conception that many children and parents hold: that is that a bathroom scale difference is what to watch for and dieting, the quickest way to cause it, is what matters most.

Energy Imbalance and the Child's Stature

Stature represents a special concern when examining the impact of treatment on the child's well-being. Previously (see Chapter 1; Application 5), the importance of evaluating the effects of growing taller on losing weight was noted. The converse is important too: that is, evaluating the effects, if any, of losing weight on growing taller; that is a Point A to Point A issue. Continuing with the examination of the Point C (energy) impact on Point A (body), most of the ensuing discussion addresses a related topic: Does a negative energy equation created mainly or exclusively by diminishing the calorie intake term alter the child's rate of linear growth?

Answers are divided. For example, after reviewing the literature on treatment of childhood obesity, Merritt (1978) concluded that slowed growth is to some extent a likely byproduct of losing weight. Yet he found no apparent long-term growth retardation among very obese juveniles (9 to 16 years old) given a protein-sparing-modified fast consisting of lean meat protein from 1.4 g to 3 g per kg of ideal body weight. Likewise, Rivinus and colleagues (Application 7) reported normal height changes among their sample.

Similarly, Schwartz and Sidbury (1974) argue that caloric restriction has no untoward effects on growing children. Like Rivinus and colleagues, they add behavioral control techniques—mainly record keeping and stimulus control—to exercise advice and nutrition teaching, but they stress controlling the dietary (see Schwartz & Sidbury, 1980). In their program for children ages 3 years and up, they impose different levels of restriction for younger versus older patients: 3- to 8-year-olds get 300 kcal a day, whereas older youths get 500 kcal; adolescents get the most. For all, the diet is 18 percent carbohydrate, 41 percent fat, and 41 percent protein; children receive at least 1 g of protein per kg of ideal body weight. After a one- to two-day fast producing Ketonuria, a thorough physical evaluation (including serum cholesterol and glucose tolerance tests), and an assessment of weight, height, and body circumferences, the children began the diet. It lasted for about one-third of a year; then, calorie intake was raised gradually. For more weight loss, the diet was applied again one-half year later. Some of the participants were hospitalized for up to one month during the program; five days was usually enough, but some were outpatients from the start; body data were gathered regularly. From their studies, the report was not data bearing, Schwartz and Sidbury concluded that growth was normal. They went on to say " . . . markedly obese children are already advanced in their growth and skeletal maturation, and the argument that caloric restriction for limited periods of time might interfere with their growth is in fact a rationalization for nihilism" (p. 662).

Brook, Lloyd, and Wolff (1974) would probably disagree. They subjected 20 obese boys and girls, 1.5 to 16.5 years of age, to a very restrictive diet (350 kcal per day). Despite variable outcomes, it was clear that growth was affected. As the authors noted, only two of the participants managed to keep to even 50 percent of the expected growth velocity.

Mayer (1980) also would probably disagree. He warned about the dangers of reducing the caloric intake of obese children, especially those nearing a growth spurt; linear growth may be abridged (see also Ellis & Tallerman, 1934; Wilkins, 1950). And Filer (1978) warned about the hazards of calorie restriction during infancy " . . . this may be ill-advised if it means depriving an obese infant of essential nutrients including energy" (p. 90) (cf Gold & Byrne, 1979).

Rayner and Court (1975) added more data to the fears. They looked at growth velocity, 50th percentile for age and sex, in a sample of 26 overweight children given either 1000 kcal per day, this diet plus fenfluramine, or this diet plus amphetamine derivatives (chlorphtermine or diethylpropion). The children, between 38 and 113 percent overweight, were 10 boys under 4 years to just over 12 years of age and 16 girls under 4 to over 10. Evaluation occurred for a minimum of one year. Results showed that different children responded differently to intake restriction; variability was so pronounced that it obscured statistical differences. Nonetheless, it was evident that linear growth was curtailed in some youngsters and that the addition of drugs to the diet did not markedly alter this picture.

For adults, calorie restriction can produce weight losses that minimize lean tissue losses more easily, as the authors implied, than it can for children. Youngsters require enough calories for growth and lean body tissue gains while fat is lost. Rayner and Court warned, " . . . some children who are treated by dietary restriction may sustain a 10 percent or greater retardation of growth velocity . . . " (p. 124).

Weight-Loss Goals. The speed of weight loss, as indicated, often can be a function of the degree of calorie intake restriction, and therefore it is reasonable to ask if rapid weight loss risks height curtailment. As before, data-bearing answers disagree. So do opinions about how fast is too fast. Rapid weight reduction has been cited as something to strive for in the design of a childhood obesity control program (Merritt, 1978) and something to avoid (Brook et al., 1974). Weil (1977) recommends moderate rates of loss (less than .23 kg weekly) or maintenance as the child grows. Similarly, Neumann (1977), considering preschoolers and school-aged children, opted for modest goals; the objective, she feels, should be growth without gain, meaning weight control not weight loss. Taitz (1977a, b) likewise feels that the very young obese infants are better helped if the objective is just slowing rate of gain. Merritt (1979) and Merritt and Batrus (1980), for older, mildly overweight children, pushed the reduction goal to between .45 kg and .90 kg weekly. When outcomes are modest, whether intentionally or unintentionally, the therapist must repeatedly prove to the child and his parents that the efforts they go through are not in vain (see below).

Energy Imbalance and the Child's Progress

How might the Point C equation affect compliance with the Point B (behavior) targets? One way, involving the suddenness and degree of shift made in each energy term, is undesirable. If a child, isolated from his peers and embarrassed about his obesity, finds solace in food, then a drastic, sudden reduction in calorie intake would cause a percipitous decline in pleasure. The upshot of this decline, accompanying the loss of pies, cookies, and junk foods, could be nonadherence to prescribed behavior changes and dropping out of treatment. Therefore, gradual changes in the child's dietary, paced with his acceptance of them, are desirable.

Likewise dramatic, upward shifts in the calorie expenditure part of the negative energy equation may lead an obese and sedentary child to nag his way out of therapy; extra television for extra play instead of withdrawal of television privileges immediately and totally will be accepted by the child as less disruptive and fairer. Furthermore, the extra activity may positively affect the calorie intake term by fostering compliance with eating control prescriptions. It may do so by giving the child something fun to do that is incompatible with snacking.

It may also do so by reducing his appetite (but see Committee on Nutrition, 1981). There is a misconception about activity and appetite: to wit, that the effects of activity on appetite are best described by an increasing straight-line function— the more you exercise the more you eat. Evidence is available, however, that a U-shaped function better describes the activity to eating relationship. In the higher ranges of activity, eating increases accompany exercise increases (see Durnin & Brockway, 1959); but this is not true in the lower ranges of activity. Here, an increase in activity does not so definitely produce an increase in calorie intake, and further, a reduction in activity to a sedentary level may not produce a commensurate reduction in calorie intake. Some previously active but now sedentary and overweight men and women attest with sadness to the second of these statements.

Apropos of both, Mayer, Roy, and Mitra (1956), in a now classic account of the work and eating habits of a group of Bengalese men, provide data. Subjects were grouped according to work levels (that is, sedentary, light, medium, heavy, and extremely heavy), and their daily calorie intakes were measured (24-hour recall, food-buying survey). From the correspondences between levels of work and levels of intake, Mayer and associates plotted the U-shaped function; work category was on the abcissa, calorie consumption on the ordinate. Intake, it was found, was greatest at the two most divergent levels of activity; the sedentary ate like those doing the heaviest amount of work. The men doing light work took in substantially fewer calories. Moreover, the least active were among the most heavy, whereas the most active were among the least heavy. Therefore, in this study, the sedentary and the extremely active ate alike but did not weigh the same.

Of particular concern here is the finding of lower calorie intakes among those doing light work. Could a small rise in the calorie expenditure term promoted by a small rise in the level of activity (when small becomes too small is unknown) reduce calorie consumption? And could this be engineered for obese children? One study answers yes to both these queries. Epstein and co-workers (1978) had six obese 5- to 6-year-old children exercise three times weekly, 10 minutes each time, just prior to lunch; exercises included jogging, racing, calisthenics, and dancing. The authors found that small increases in activity decreased red, yellow, and green food consumption (see Chapters 4 and 5), and thus calorie intake declined significantly.

Possibly other advantages of increasing calorie outgo efforts in helping sustain compliance with behavioral prescriptions work through metabolic rate changes— through increases in metabolic rate following the cessation of exercise (Thompson, Jarvie, Lahey, & Cureton, 1982); through the exercise-induced attenuation of decreases in metabolic rate wrought by calorie intake reductions (Straw & Sonne, 1979). In regard to metabolic rate decreases, adults have been found to undergo adaptations to prolonged intake restrictions such that continuing to lose weight becomes progressively harder during treatment (Garrow, 1974; Wooley et al., 1979). Under such circumstances, the drive to break plateaus and adhere to behavioral directives may quickly dissipate (Stuart, Jensen, & Guire, 1979). These relationships have to be investigated in pediatric samples.

Guidelines for Devising
the Negative Energy Equation for Children

Unfortunately only general guidelines are available and disagreement exists.

Setting the Caloric Intake Term. As one might imagine, intake is the most frequently discussed part of the energy equation. Table 6.1 gives energy allowances (RDA, 1980) for children. These vary as the child grows older, taller, and heavier, but they do not vary as a function of gender until age 11. Thus, the recommended (not to be interpreted as required) caloric intake for infant boys and girls weighing on the average 6 kg and being on the average 60 cm long is 115 kcal/kg/day. After six months (growth to 9 kg and 71 cm), the recommended allowance drops to 105 kcal/kg/day; from 1 to 10 years; the recommended levels drop even further to about 80 kcal/kg/day (RDA, 1980). Also, it is important to note these advised intake levels are medians; they are based on longitudinal data collected in Boston, Denver, and Iowa City paralleling cross-sectional informa-

Table 6.1
Mean Heights and Weights and Recommended Energy Intake

Category	Age (years)	Weight (kg)	Height (cm)	Energy Needs (kcal)	Range*
Infants	0.0-0.5	6	60	kg × 115	95-145
	0.5-1.0	9	71	kg × 105	80-135
Children	1-3	13	90	1300	900-1800
	4-6	20	112	1700	1300-2300
	7-10	28	132	2400	1650-3300
Males	11-14	45	157	2700	2000-3700
	15-18	66	176	2800	2100-3900
Females	11-14	46	157	2200	1500-3000
	15-18	55	163	2100	1200-3000

Table adapted from Recommended Dietary Allowances, Ninth Edition, 1980. Food and Nutrition Board, National Research Council. Published by National Academy of Sciences.

*These values are 10th and 90th percentiles of energy intake, to indicate the range of energy consumption among children of these ages.

tion obtained from other studies—the HANES (RDA, 1980). Furthermore, the caloric intakes in parentheses are ranges (10th and 90th percentiles), showing the wide variability found among children in each age group examined.

To see how current intake aligns with these recommended allowances, one may employ ballistic bomb calorimetry using duplicate foods and amounts the child reportedly eats (for example, see Griffiths & Payne, 1976). Or, one may employ published tables of calories in various foods (Kraus, 1979; Appendix 2) after monitoring (24-hour recall, meal-by-meal records) the child's consumption. Then, the calorie intake level to be used in treatment may be set and the setting checked with the child's pediatrician or family physician.

The setting is important. The Committee on Dietary Allowances of the National Research Council in the United States (RDA, 1980) says,

Adequate energy intake is a requirement for efficient utilization of dietary protein for growth and maintenance. Many of the essential nutrients, particularly the minerals, are distributed widely and in low concentration in foods, especially in the low-cost staple commodities. It is, therefore, difficult to assure nutritional adequacy of diets that are low in energy content. . . . (p. 17)

The calorie intake term may have to be reset during the course of treatment and afterwards because the appropriateness of the initial setting changes as the child's body changes. With the above in mind, consider Table 6.2. It lists several

Table 6.2

A Sampling of Calorie Intake Recommendations for Treating Obese Youngsters

Source		Recommendation	Population*
Collipp, in Wilkinson (1980)	1.	600-800 kcal/day for children, promoting a .9 kg/wk loss.	C, 4-17
Dwyer, Blonde, Mayer (1972)	1.	Reduce intake by 200-275 kcal/day to produce .23 kg/wk loss. A reduction of 500 kcal/day should rarely be considered.	Unstated, but presumably 5 years.
Feig (1980)	1.	Reduce 250-500 kcal/day. (The reduction is from a table similar to 6.1.)	C, 5-13
Gold & Byrne (1979)	1.	Feed only formula, 92.4 kcal/kg.	Under 4 months
	2.	Feed only when no other reasons for crying. Table food less preferable than commercial baby foods.	All I
Golden (1979)	1.	Limit to 600-800 kcal/day to control gaining. Nutrition should be adequate as child outgrows his obesity.	C, below 5
	2.	Almost all children lose weight on 800-1000 kcal/day.	All C
Knittle (1972) (also Newmann, 1977)	1.	60 kcal/kg of ideal body weight. This diet ideally is 20% protein, 40% carbohydrate, 40% fat.	C under 12
Merritt (1978) Merritt & Batrus (1980)	1.	From 14.1 kcal/cm/day of child, subtract 500 kcal for .45 kg/wk reduction. Maintain protein above RDA level. Vitamin and mineral dosages met by 1200 kcal/day balanced diet. Below this amount, give vitamin and mineral supplements.	C, 7-11
	2.	Delay introduction of solid foods until after 6 months. Encourage home preparation of baby foods. Watch for excessive consumption of milk.	I

Source	Recommendation	Population*
Taitz (1977a)**	1. Provide enough energy for growth, about 110 kcal/ kg/day.	I, under 6 mo
	2. About 90 kcal/kg/day	I, 6-12 mo
Weil (1977)	1. Under one year, calorie intake restriction not advised.	I
	2. Skim milk, elimination of carbohydrate snacks, trim fat from meat, remove skin from fowl.	C, 1-5
	3. 20-25% calorie restriction limited to older children.	C, older than 5

*Age of child to which the numbered recommendation applies (*e.g.,* I = infants; C, 5-13 = children 5 to 13 years).
**Reflects earlier RDAs than listed in Table 6.1.

recommendations about setting the intake term by planning a calorie deficit from baseline, by advising a specific intake, or by advising an amount based upon ideal body weight.

Setting the Calorie Expenditure Term. There are fewer guidelines here than above, and fewer published attempts to set the expenditure term. Today, most would agree to set it somewhere, even if only doing so implicitly by teaching children to increase daily routines. Obese children, it is commonly held, will be better off if their calorie expenditure levels are upgraded. But there is no table of recommended energy outgo levels to which researchers and practitioners can refer; that is, there is no table of calorie expenditure analogous to Table 6.1.

Still, expenditure levels may be set for individual children in treatment. Baselines are obtainable by estimating (through direct calorimetry) calories expended. Oxygen consumption analyses also provide data (see for example, Waxman & Stunkard, 1980). Sharkey (1974) offers a simpler technique (suitable for adults but with modification suitable for children, too) that estimates basal energy expenditure from a table of values and adds in calories expended through recreation. In like manner, Foreyt and Goodrick (1981) approximate basal calorie outgo for children and then estimate daily calorie expenditure due to activity, figuring increases over basal from 50 to 100 percent that depend on the child's activity level; they use these calculations accompanied by determinations of calorie intake to formulate a daily calorie deficit for each child's treatment. Another approach, albeit possessing the reliablity and interpretative problems mentioned previously (see Foreyt & Goodrick, 1981), is having children record times spent in various pursuits (see Chapter 4). Time doing each action is then translated into calorie expenditure. But, if translated by checking a table of calorie outgo equivalents for brief and prolonged activities, even if calculations are adjusted for weight of subject, accuracy is questionable (Freedson, Katch, Gilliam, & MacConnie, 1981). Gross and net expenditures often are confused; this means that whatever else the patient would be doing if he were not exercising is not removed from the table's calculation (Epstein & Wing, 1980; Garrow, 1978b). More basic, direct assessments on children are few.

Nonetheless, the practices of setting calorie expenditure levels and monitoring adherence to them are encouraged. They are encouraged not only because they underscore the importance of habits that maximize fat loss and so on, but also because they give the child a dimension for evaluating and tracking his selection of healthful ways to become thinner. It is with these goals in mind Appendix C is provided.

Selecting Targets

Discussion in this section addresses Point B (behavior) on the obesity triangle. Changes in behavioral variables should benefit the child. They may do so physically, perhaps as indicated by producing Point C (energy) changes that cause Point A (body) changes. Or, they may do so psychologically, perhaps by making the child happier in his daily interactions. Or, they may do so both physically and psychologically. Moreover, changes in behavioral variables should yield a minimum of undesired side effects.

Foreyt and Goodrick's (1981) approach to choosing behavioral targets when treating obese children is instructive. They advise therapists and researchers to assess in three areas to build tailored programs: situations controlling eating and exercise (for example, cues to consume, locations at which consumption occurs, locations at which exercise occurs, availability of peers who exercise); skills the child lacks that by their absence makes reducing hard (for example, nutritional misinformation, exercise misinformation); cognitions that might interfere (cravings for food, thoughts that exercise hurts). Assessment tools they recommend are Coates' (1977) "Eating Analyses and Treatment Schedule (EATS)" (pp. 179–199) (which surveys and evaluates not only the quality and quantity of specific foods in the home but also food-serving variables and eating practices), written tests, and interviewing; furthermore, they recommend self-monitoring and monitoring by trained observers.

Rarely have children received such comprehensive and individualized care. Among the targets that have been selected are tantruming and food stealing (Application 2); sugary-food consumption; food preparation by the child; outside-of-home eating; eating urges; calorie intake monitoring; leaving food on the plate; exercising (Applications 4, 5, and 9); attending treatment sessions; completing homework; eating speed; adhering to food proscriptions; and reducing plate sizes (Applications 6, 7, 8, and 9). Among the strategies that have been used to assess these targets and track changes in them have been self-monitoring, parent-monitoring of children, and interviewing.

Brownell and Stunkard (1980a) highlight the importance of another possible target, a concomitant of eating: food preference. The behavioral eating test (Jeffrey et al., 1980) seems particularly well suited to its measurement. Children are asked to taste various edibles, and the amount that they consume is recorded. Pre- to post-treatment monitoring of food likes is possible, as the test's developers suggest. Modification of preferences is in the service of obesity prevention. For the already obese child's treatment, however, the concern is whether altering food likes will alter food consumption. The child undergoing treatment who sees his peers enjoying specific foods at a local restaurant may violate his dieting plan because he witnesses others eating, wants peer acceptance (see Chapter 2), craves the foods being eaten, or because of all three of these reasons. Where to aim intervention is an empirical problem.

Moving-More

Eating is but one, albeit major, of the large classes of behavior yielding intervention targets. Another, as Figure 6.1 displays, is activity. Mayer (1975), accounting for low-baseline levels among obese youngsters, comments that they may have problems "automatizing their motion" (p. 78); they exercise nonrhythmically, doing best in sports that do not require rhythm. Despite such analyses, moving-more is neglected in childhood obesity treatment. The remediative effects of exercise on childhood obesity are still unclear (Committee on Nutrition, 1981). Typically, when activity modification is attempted in therapy obese youngsters are enjoined to exercise more. Thus, Collipp (cited in Wilkinson, 1980) tells his young patients to walk, swim, or play tennis more often (see Lindner, 1980, p. 201 for other suggestions). Similarly, Merritt and Batrus (1980) ask their patients to walk or bike for 20 minutes each day, increasing this by 5 minutes each week. But these sorts of prescriptions are not given backing by behavior therapy even in more decidedly behavioral programs, at least not to the extent that eating modification prescriptions are.

There is reason to believe such lopsidedness is on the wane. Recent reviews of childhood obesity treatment by behavior therapy have recommended increasing the activity focus (Coates & Thoresen, 1980; Israel & Stolmaker, 1980). Foreyt and Goodrick (1981) extol aerobics (for example, swimming, jogging), whereas Brownell and Stunkard (1980b) praise daily routines as targets to be modified prior to the prolonged kinds of exercise (Beck et al., 1980; Epstein et al., 1981). Regardless of where the focus is directed, targeting activity in some form is likely to be beneficial.

Although more procedures for identifying specific activity targets and monitoring changes in them need to be developed, there are techniques available for doing so (see Chapter 4). Recall, for instance, Waxman and Stunkard's time-sampling of activities (six) in 15-second blocks during 15-minute periods. Similarly, Epstein and colleagues (1978) observed activities in sixty 10-second intervals per measurement period; they stocked a school gymnasium with toys (puzzels, bikes) to see whether sedentary activity or more physical play occurred. In like manner, Coates and Perry (1980) used 5-second intervals when observing the activities (sitting and running for example) of elementary school children. Pedometers, as mentioned, have been employed to assess activity levels throughout the day and over selected periods; the instrument is not error free (Brownell, 1981), but methods for improving reliability have recently been offered (Heiser, Epstein, & Wing, 1981).

Additional Targets Including Bickering

Among the other potential targets Figure 6.1 shows are social skills training, athletic skills training, self-statements about being fat and thin, deviations from plans, school performance, and the actions to be discussed next, subsumed under the general term bickering.

This target area deals with the parent–child relationship (see Olson, Pringle, & Schoenwetter, 1976), a relationship that may become particularly bad when the child appears to be cheating on the diet. To illustrate, I will briefly recount the trials and tribulations of one of my graduate students who attempted to treat an overweight 12-year-old girl. The child and her mother were seen together, although only the child required treatment; indeed, in her family, only she was overweight, having originally become so years previously. The mother could not stand her daughter's appearance but felt somehow guilty and responsible.

Prescriptions were given during each treatment hour. They were framed as homework assignments that would eventually lead to improvements in body shape. When weight losses, considered mainly by mother and child but also by therapist and supervisor to be the barometer of these improvements, failed to happen by the end of the week, bickering ensued . . . loudly and vehemently. The child's mother would demand admissions about transgressions responsible for failure. The child, in self-defense, would promptly deny complicity and would counterattack her mother's fallibility and imperfections. Frequently, the child's response to the barbs was crying—once she ran out of the office. Eventually, because of the intensity of the bickering episodes, sessions were terminated; previous attempts to stop the arguing had failed.

The relationship between this mother and child was bad at the start of treatment and deteriorated even further over time because the child's weight did not decrease. Mother's accusations led to the child's defending and counterattacking, and the fighting that resulted led to the cessation of treatment. Had we continued the offer of therapy—a misnomer in this case to be sure—it is likely that either the child or her mother would have refused it.

Did we kindle the bickering? I think so. One error was letting weight loss be the main sign of the child's progress. Doing this is hazardous because at the end of a week of behavior modification, even a very good week of it, developing youngsters may fail to reduce for several reasons, including lean tissue growth and fat losses masking weight losses. In brief, weight loss by itself can be a misleading yardstick of the child's efforts. Adaptive behaviors, not just changes in weight, should be stressed as reinforceable targets in order to lessen the chances of bickering. Furthermore, parent and child should be helped to pick moderate weight-related goals in order to lower the risk that unreasonable expectations will rise up and quash reasonable interventions. Also, teaching parents to be more supportive of the child's struggles should be included (see Application 5) if bickering seems, from interviews and observations of parents and children, to be likely, or if it actually occurs.

Conclusion

A range of possible targets exists. Interview and baseline observation help in selecting those to which treatment should be aimed at in the beginning, and continued interviewing and monitoring help in adjusting these targets and designating new ones. The objective is to keep the program tailored. Thus, selecting the right targets will remain an obstacle to the extent that initial assessment and monitoring practices are neglected. Multiple assessment procedures are needed due to the varying nature of the actions to be targeted and the potential for disagreement among measurements of even the same action (Jeffrey et al., 1980; Lang, 1971). Efforts to observe children in the style set down by Bijou, Peterson, and Ault (1968) and more recently by Coates (1977) are needed.

Selecting the right targets will also remain an obstacle to the extent that the amount of information gathered and reported continues to be restricted. The restriction makes it impossible to investigate and articulate the relationships among points on the obesity triangle, and thus prevents a demonstration that target behavior modification via behavioral prescriptions has or has not benefited the child. Again, weight loss is not the crowning arbiter of effective targeting. The absence of weight reduction should not be construed as the signal to alter targets, for there may be no weight loss at the end of a week or two because prescriptions for change have not been followed and target behaviors have not been modified and because of the physiological reasons noted above. On the other hand, there may well be poor targeting despite a noticeable weight loss. The loss may have little to do with the particular behaviors that change; perhaps treatment contains useless prescriptions and the child adopts unhealthy weight-reduction strategems.

Motivating Children

Difficult. Children may be motivated at the start of therapy, but after a few weeks or by the time therapy reaches the halfway mark, motivation often vanishes. The task of motivating children consists of getting them to attend therapy sessions, comply with treatment's prescriptions and proscriptions, and institute appropriate measures during follow-up when relapsing appears imminent. Success at one part of the task does not guarantee success at the others, for compliance in treatment does not ensure vigilance later on, regular attenders at therapy sessions are not always compliers at home (see, for example Hagen et al., 1976; Chapter 5), and sometimes compliers or children who seem to be compliers stop coming to sessions (see Application 3).

Motivation is bound up with reinforcement (Reynolds, 1968). What therapists and researchers try out as reinforcers and ways that they administer them have been reviewed in previous chapters. We have identified several kinds of reinforcers (primary, generalized) and illustrated the particulars that childhood obesity workers use (praise, toys, outings, for example). Also, we have indicated that food and drink, even though strong consequences, are not free of potential drawbacks, namely augmenting the calorie-intake term excessively and legitimizing edibles as outcomes for being good. Furthermore, we have noted that weight and fat losses are reinforcers too, but are, at the same time, imprecise mirrors of the actions producing them, because they are delayed—especially fat losses (Johnson & Stalonas, 1977; Stuart & Davis, 1972)—and they can be, as stated above, in conflict, as when fat losses mask weight losses. Moreover, also as just stated, exclusive or excessive reliance on weight loss may lead researchers and practitioners to unwarranted changes in the program and parents and children to argue.

Motivation is often seen as a specialty of the behaviorist; that is why many an obese child is referred to the behaviorist. But there is no tried and true technology the behaviorist can offer for motivating obese children. Only the conceptual framework for doing so exists. Thus, motivation remains an obstacle to therapy, several reasons for which are listed below:

1. The child is an unwilling participant. From the start of the program the child may not care to make the needed effort to reduce, having been forced rather than gently persuaded by his parents to enter the program. Antipathy towards treatment usually dooms it—the older the child the more accurate the foreshadowing is. Both parent and child are better served by delaying treatment until the child is more willing to undergo it. Perhaps in the interim, positive results will come from counseling parents alone to make gradual changes in the dietary, in the contradictory messages they give, and in the opportunities for enjoyable recreational outings they offer.

2. The child has everything. I recall one mildly overweight young lady, an 8-year-old, who wanted virtually nothing. She had nearly all the material things I could suggest as well as ample time with her mother and father. There was a dearth of usable positive reinforcers, unless things she already had were to be withdrawn and returned contingent upon progress—an understandably unacceptable strategy to this child and her parents. Finding reinforcers is a problem when mothers and fathers supply their overweight youngsters with innumerable toys, games, opportunities for movies, and so on. Suppliers usually are parents from the middle- and upper-classes, the parents who are especially likely to seek therapeutic assistance for their overweight children.

3. The child has to eat special foods. There are two ways that this may be a problem. First, the child may be made a dietary outcast (Mahoney & Mahoney, 1976a) in the home, constrained to eating a bill of fare the rest of the family does not share; such separation breeds failure. Second, for the child's sake, the family may be shifted to a special dietary, and they may rebel against it. Perhaps owing to a reduction in cookies, ice cream, and so on, they (particularly disgruntled siblings) tease and castigate the child for being the cause of the deprivation. Better tolerated by all are gradual alterations in the family's cuisine (Wheeler & Hess, 1976); and if the patient requires certain individual changes, substitutions rather than restrictions should be tried.

4. The child is out of place in the treatment group. If the child is put into a group of patients much older or younger or much heavier or lighter than he, he may feel uncomfortable. The discussion in the group may be unrelated to his level of control over food choices and activity. Feeling silly or even intimidated, he may leave the group as soon as possible.

5. The child receives untailored care and dislikes the fit. This pertains to the above problem but is more general, for it affects children seen in groups and also those seen individually. If the child is asked to comply with prescriptions and proscriptions he views as having little to do with his obesity, he may reject the total treatment package in the wake of disaffection with some of its seemingly impersonalized elements. He may do so particularly when progress is not readily apparent. An attempt to cut away the "useless" elements, the elements the child has come to believe are useless, should be undertaken. Or, discussion about their necessity should occur; the changing attitudes of the youngster towards treatment need to be monitored.

Sustaining Progress

The conditions of effective maintenance may well differ from those of effective treatment (Epstein et al., 1981; Stunkard & Penick, 1979). Whereas we obviously suffer from gaps in our knowledge of therapy, we are even more blatantly ignorant about maintenance. As with the obstacles discussed above, sustaining progress is difficult, intricate, and unresolved.

Maintenance may be thought of in several ways. If body variables (Point A) are the primary concern, successful maintenance would mean little or no relapse in weight or fat after treatment ends; the percents of overweight and overfat would remain constant or decrease. If these percents reach zero, successful maintenance after treatment ends could mean keeping the two terms of the negative energy equation nearly in balance; increases in body dimensions would be due to growing, not relapse. Considering maintenance in this way involves both body and energy (Points A and C) variables. If behavior variables are the primary concern, successful maintenance means that basically children continue with what they have been taught and targeted behavior stays modified; as a result, positive changes in the body remain. Also, early signs of relapse trigger efforts to remedy behaviors. Evidence of this kind of maintenance is the best justification for behavioral technology.

It is this kind of maintenance that Foreyt and Goodrick (1981) believe would further the child's long-term well-being. Cohen, Gelfand, Dodd, Jensen, and Turner (1980), in support, note that maintainers, seven boys and six girls, were likely to praise themselves for controlling weight, to monitor intake and weight, to decrease eating and increase activity in order to recover from a gain, and to exercise—maintainers were likely to control themselves.

But there are few clues as to how to foster this kind of maintenance. Should there be booster sessions planned for the after-treatment period? After-care meetings incorporating some portion or all of the methods used during treatment have been tried for adults, but results have been mixed (Ashby & Wilson, 1977; Domke, Lando, & Robinson, 1978; Kingsley & Wilson, 1977; Stuart & Guire, 1978). Should there be extended monitoring? Foreyt and Goodrick (1981) advise therapists to check periodically, from one to two years, on the child's actions. Should there be significant others, deployed in the child's environment, taught to bring successful maintenance to fruition?

Helpers

Parents are logical candidates for the maintenance helpers' job, for it is they who readily provide the child with television, transportation, and food. Regarding parents as feeders, Waxman and Stunkard (1980) point out that mothers oversupply their obese sons and not their thinner sons; mothers, in this study, accept a size-of-child/amount-of-food relationship. As helpers, parents are frequently in a position to encourage children to follow through with the directives of intervention, assisting in reapplication when it is called for.

Epstein and co-worker's (1981) study of overweight children, 6 to 12 years, suggests that this role as helper is possible and that directing treatment at parents is perhaps a useful way to initiate it. All the youngsters reducing enough after eight months (14 sessions) of therapy (environment alteration with nutrition and exercise teachings) to fall beneath a benchmark of 20 percent overweight maintained this progress 13 months later, if their parent(s) were treated, too. In comparison, significantly fewer youngsters given the same package but without their parent(s) formally receiving the adult version of it managed this feat. The view held by many practitioners is that parental cooperation is valuable (Collipp, 1980d; Jones, 1972; Mitchell & Fiser, 1978); parents may contribute to the persistence of their child's obesity (Olson et al., 1976). The applications reviewed in Chapter 5, by and large, echo this view; at least they imply that including parents is important (see, for example, Applications 2 through 9).

To repeat, many practitioners and researchers presume that by teaching parents to help their child the probability of long-term, extensive progress is augmented (Chapter 4). How much help they give, though, may be a critical variable. Cohen and colleagues (1980) indicate (see also Woody & Constanzo, 1981) that regainers have parents who run the weight-control programs (cf. Bleidt, 1979). As Cohen and associates note, however, parental control may be the consequence as much as the cause of regaining; the youth's failure may cue parents to take over. Which children prosper and which do not when their weight-control practices are regulated by parents and how much management is best for whom? The child's degree of control over his food supply and his opportunities for exercise is perhaps a major variable in the answer. That is, perhaps juveniles having much control compared with those having little influence respond more poorly during maintenance when parents regulate.

An even more basic question is, what should parents be taught (see Janzen & Doleys, 1981)? In our program, we give parents the lessons their children receive at the time their children receive them. The objective is to have mothers and fathers become allies and supporters, not just directors. But because the techniques parents learn during intervention may not be what they practice during maintenance, we monitor their actions during this later phase (as indicated in Application 9). In addition to teaching mothers and fathers the behavioral, nutritional, and exercise information their children learn, it may be valuable to attempt to build in flexibility—to teach parents to think behaviorally. Thus, they might be taught to observe, record, and alter where needed the types, frequencies, consequences, and antecedents of their childrens' behaviors. Furthermore, they might be taught to evaluate their own behaviors that contribute to the problems their children demonstrate; mothers who overfeed could learn to recognize and change this.

How might parents be taught such things? Lectures, discussion, practice— perhaps in self-applying obesity reduction principles (see Epstein et al., 1981; Application 8)—and feedback are major tools. Parents have been brought into the treatment process for the immediate and enduring benefit of their children in various ways: teaching parents without teaching children directly (see Application 5); teaching parents and children separately (Applications 6 and 8); teaching parents and children in individual parent–child sessions (Applications 3 and 9); teaching parents and children in group parent–child sessions (Application 7).

The comparative effectiveness of several of these permutations has been tested (see Geronilla, 1981). Kingsley and Shapiro (1977), for example, evaluated a multifaceted behavioral intervention, adapted from Stuart and Davis (1972), applied in three ways to aid overweight 10-year-olds: Either the boys and girls were seen without their parents (mothers) or with them, or only their mothers were seen (see Harris, Kirschenbaum, & Tomarken, 1981). The therapy package was evaluated after eight weekly sessions and at two follow-ups, weeks 14 and 28. Treatment groups showed weight losses by treatment's end, but differences among them were not significant, although in combination they outdid a wait-list control (see Epstein, Wing, Ossip, & Andrasik, 1981). Mothers taught alone lost the most weight for a time, compared with the other mothers; but most important to the present discussion, it made little difference at the conclusion of treatment or at follow-up how (if) they were included in the child's therapy.

Kelman and colleagues (1979 cited in Brownell & Stunkard, 1980a) reached different conclusions not by evaluating follow-up data (follow-up was unreported), but by comparing post-treatment results for pre-adolescents and adolescents. Replicating two of Kingsley and Shapiro's conditions—child-alone and mother and child seen together—and adding a third to replace the mother-alone condition, they investigated the parent-involvement variable; the new condition was teaching mother and child separately. After about a four month multi-component therapy, the authors could conclude that bringing in parents had advantages for the child. Both of the groups including mothers posted better results than the child-alone condition; the best results were from the mother-child-taught-separately group (see also Brownell, Kelman, & Stunkard, in press). More investigations incorporating different behavioral packages are needed.

Conceptualizing helpers (for example, parents, grandparents, siblings, peers) that impact on the child during maintenance as members of a community of reinforcement (Baer & Wolf, 1967, Chapter 4) reveals a potential difficulty that may interfere with the child's progress: Sometimes the community fails to act as it should. Can the child remedy this difficulty by helping the community behave better? In other words, can the child foster the persistence and continuation of his own successes by enlivening significant others in his environment to support his obesity-controlling actions? Coles (1982) has worked out a way to attempt an answer. Extrapolating from the works of Seymour and Stokes (1976) and Stokes, Fowler, and Baer (1978), he intends to teach his young obese patients, by instruction, modeling, and practice, to solicit praise from significant others in their environments. Following the conclusion of treatment involving deviation analyses (see Application 9), Coles' patients are to solicit praise from parents and siblings after completing a prescribed obesity management action. Coles divides the soliciting response into six steps: planning the praiseworthy action (for example, foregoing a snack); accomplishing the feat; evaluating whether or not to solicit praise (that is, asking oneself if the significant other is too busy to praise); naming the praiseworthy action to the potential praisegiver; waiting for praise and if it is not forthcoming saying (prompting), "That's pretty good! Don't you think so?"

(p.65); allowing the ensuing conversation to end naturally. Timing and delivery are considered important and, therefore, dealt with.

As a maintenance strategy, the soliciting tactic is interesting. The data, however, have yet to be gathered showing its applicability to the obese child. Its value possibly will be helping to keep the patient vigilant after formal treatment. Furthermore, perhaps its value will be even greater if the tactic can be extended to managing other potential agents of reinforcement in the child's environment and by so doing help him to bring a global, total environment effort to bear on the obstacle of sustaining progress.

CHAPTER 7

Adolescents

Prevalence, Connections, and Concomitants of Obesity

More than the overweight child, the overweight adolescent may be headed for the status of overweight—likely obese—adult. Stunkard and Burt (1967), as indicated in Chapter 2, noted that adolescence is a particularly risky time to be overweight. Analyzing Abraham and Nordsieck's (1960) data, they concluded that if reduction has not occurred by the teenage years, the chances the adolescent can avoid becoming an overweight adult may be over 28 to 1 (Stunkard, 1976).

How many overweight (obese) adolescents are there? Estimates are in the millions (Schwartz, 1979); considering United States teenagers alone, Powers (1980) suggests that there are three million. Discussing the influence of family as well as socioeconomic status, sex, and age on these estimates, Garn and Clark (1975) note that by the time adolescents reach their 17th year (TSNS data), those with obese parents are three times fatter (triceps skinfolds) than those with lean parents. Before adolescence wealthier girls are fatter than are poorer girls (Chapter 2), but during and after adolescence the poorer are fatter.

Using a weight-for-height index and defining obesity as 20 percent overweight, Court, Dunlop, Reynolds, Russell, and Griffiths (1976) also find, in their cross-sectional study, that demographic variables affect the prevalence of obesity. Gender affects it. In their sample of more than 5300 Australian youths, they discovered that the percentages of obese males compared to females were consistently lower at each of the ages surveyed. Thus, at ages 14, 15, and 16 years there were 4.3, 4.5, and 6.3 percent of the males labeled as obese, whereas at these same ages there were 7.9, 7.8, and 8.9 percent of the females labeled as obese (cf., Huenemann, et al., 1974 on Northern California adolescents). Defining obesity as 10 percent overweight, that is lowering criterion, Court and associates still detected greater percentages of overweight girls at every age; in fact differences between sexes were even larger.

On the whole, findings from the studies on the prevalence of adolescent obesity vary (for example, Colley, 1974; Garn & Clark, 1975; Hathaway & Sargent, 1962; Lauer et al., 1975; Richardson & Wadvalla, 1977). Disagreements arise because, as in the studies of childhood obesity, different authors apply different measures and criteria of obesity. And disagreements arise because different authors sample adolescents, who, from one study to the next and sometimes even in the same study, differ in socioeconomic status, ancestry, sex, country of birth, and in whether and to what degree their parents are obese.

Are weight and fatness excesses of childhood connected with those of adolescence? Johnston and Mack (1978) attempt to answer. They studied teenage youths in the Philadelphia area and compared those who had been light infants with those who had been heavy. More of the obese (triceps skinfold) adolescents had histories of having been heavy infants. Under 9 percent (6 out of 69) of the fat adolescent males, ages 13 to 15, were light as infants; for obese females, the corresponding figure was under 14 percent (10 out of 72). In contrast, again for ages 13 to 15, almost 36 percent (24 out of 67) of the fat adolescent males and over 22 percent (19 out of 85) of the fat adolescent females were heavy as infants; similar trends were revealed using an overweight measure (see also Johnston & Mack, 1980; Mack & Johnston, 1979).

Employing a briefer $time_1$ to $time_2$ interval, Zack, Harlan, Leaverton, and Coroni-Huntley (1979) disclose that fat children, ages 6 to 11 years, are quite likely to become fat teenagers. They reported on 2,177 subjects tested in the United States Health Examination Surveys at two times separated by two to five, usually three to four, years. Measuring skinfold thickness at three sites, Zack and co-workers learned that obesity (above the 80th percentile in skinfold thickness), remained in approximately 75 percent of their sample; the $time_1$ to $time_2$ correlation was significant. Hence, this study of childhood obesity definitely predicts adolescent obesity among male and female Blacks as well as among male and female Whites (see Lloyd et al., 1961).

Durnin and McKillop (1978), in a longitudinal investigation covering 14 years, were less certain of the connections. They started with 400 subjects but were only able to report on 102, finding different relationships for males and females. Initially they applied weight-for-height indices to categorize their sample (infants) as underweight, normal weight, overweight, or obese. Then, at follow-up (during adolescence), they assessed four skinfolds in order to gauge percent body fat. For the females, judging retrospectively, percent fat in adolescence was highly correlated with heaviness during infancy ($r = .88$), but not for the males ($r = .17$). Evaluating prospectively, infancy to adolescence, they found essentially the same poor correlation for the boys ($r = .14$). And this time for the girls the correlation was also low; the strong relationship shown previously in the retrospective account was absent. In brief, the prospective inquiry failed to indicate that early excesses strongly predicted later ones (see Committee on Nutrition, 1978).

As with the topic of prevalence, conclusions about the obesity connection of childhood with adolescence are not yet possible. And, as with the prevalence topic, answers to the connection question vary because different researchers employ different definitions and measures of obesity as well as different strategies of inquiry, and because they sample adolescents having different backgrounds.

Disease and Despair for Some

What are the physical and social–psychological concomitants of adolescent obesity? As in obese children, enduring ponderosity likely produces the same if not worse discomforts in obese adolescents. Moreover, as indicated from a retrospective inquiry, prolonged heaviness during the teenage years may be associated with the development of endometrial carcinoma. Blitzer, Blitzer, and Rimm (1976) questioned over 56,000 adult women, members of Take Off Pounds Sensibly (TOPS), to obtain information on their weight and health backgrounds. Compared with unaffected women (no cancer), those having histories of endometrial carcinoma reported significantly higher degrees of heaviness to have been present during adolescence; weight excesses in these earlier years appeared to predispose. In other words, sustained obesity is, according to these authors, a probable risk factor in the ontogenesis of endometrial carcinoma.

Physical concomitants of adolescent obesity, such as hyperinsulinism (Drash, 1973), also have been uncovered. Blood lipid abnormalities, to name another (see Chapter 2), likewise have been discussed (Clarke, Merrow, Morse, & Keyser, 1970; Walker, Bhamjee, Walker, & Martin, 1979). But they do not seem to be as marked as yet a third concomitant, blood pressure irregularities. deCastro and associates (1976b), for instance, detect a sizable difference between the percentages of overweight (9.1 percent) and nonoverweight (3 percent) hypertensive high schoolers they examined. Similarly, in a more ambitious undertaking involving over 13,000 10th graders, Miller and Shekelle (1976) obtained significant, positive correlations between measures of obesity and blood pressure. Skinfold thickness and body mass indices, body mass more so, were associated with blood-pressure elevations in 15- to 16-year-old male and female Whites as well as in male and female Blacks; correlations with systolic pressure readings were largest (see Ellison, Sosenko, Harper, Gibbons, Pratter, & Miettinen, 1980; Swartz & Leitch, 1975). Weight loss attenuates cardiovascular risk factors in some overweight teenagers (Coates et al., 1982; Dershewitz, Kahn, & Solomon, 1981).

Among the social–psychological correlates of adolescent obesity there may be self-condemnation (Cahnman, 1968) which is capable of leading teenagers toward bizarre weight-change practices having ruinous consequences (see for example, Mallick, 1980). Relatedly, there may be psychosexual and body-image problems (Dwyer, 1973; Hammar, Campbell, & Woolley, 1972; Hendry & Gillies, 1978), and there may be feelings of unacceptability in a world dominated by thins (Monello & Mayer, 1963). Victims of these undermining sequelae appear, in particular, to be teenage girls (Allon, 1980), some of whom, because they are large, see themselves as obese when in reality they are not (Beaven, 1981; Crisp, 1977; Dwyer & Mayer, 1975; Guggenheim, Poznanski, & Kaufmann, 1973; Wooley & Wooley, 1980).

Allon (1976) documented the perceptions overweight teenage girls had about how their body shapes affected their interactions with the nonoverweight. For seven months she observed 25 youths, 9 kg to 23 kg overweight, enrolled in a high school supported slimnastics class; she interviewed them and analyzed their discussions with one another. These 14- to 17-year-old girls perceived that their physiques were the foci of their interactions with agemates and others who were not obese—shape is so visible. They also perceived that their shapes caused others mixed emotions. Further, they believed their looks created a negative halo. Finally, they felt that their obvious corpulence confused thins into misjudging their physical and social skills, and by doing so limited the invitations they received to participate in various activities. In brief, these overweight girls believed, quite strongly, that being obese had a decidedly unfavorable social impact.

It remains to be seen just how ubiquitous this concern is among overweight adolescents. Potential contributors to it, condemnation of obesity by teenagers and by adults, however, do exist. Illustrating denigration by teenagers, Lerner and Korn (1972) asked 14- to 15-year-old males to describe, using 56 possible descriptors, drawings of thin, muscular, and fat adolescents. They found that these young men disparaged the fat teenager. Even those who resembled the fellow depicted in the drawing had bad things to say. More recently, Worsely (1981 a, b) evaluated the perceptions of 138 adolescents, 16-years-old, toward the obese and nonobese. Figures of fatter and thinner males and females were rated on nearly 30 semantic differential scales. Again, regardless of sex and ethnic background, the obese were viewed with disfavor (see also De Jong, 1980; Meyer & Neumann, 1977).

In regard to antipathy by elders, Hendry and Gillies (1978) demonstrated that physical education teachers regard the overweight (compared with the average weight) as having less athletic ability and (for females) being less attractive. Similarly, Canning and Mayer (1966), in a much quoted study, found what they suspect to be discrimination toward obese adolescents applying to prestigious colleges, such as the Ivy League and Seven Sister institutions. Prevalence of obesity (ponderal index), especially the prevalence of obese females, was greater in high school than in college, yet body size did not affect rates of application. Generally, less obese males and females went on to university after graduating from high school; in particular, obese compared with nonobese girls joined the labor force. But the obese were as suited as were their nonobese peers to advanced education, were as ready academically. Canning and Mayer suggest that they simply had more difficulty being accepted into outstanding places; as noted in the study, perhaps high school teachers unwittingly wrote them poorer letters of recommendation or college interviewers unwittingly judged them more negatively, or perhaps both (cf., Pargman, 1969).

Numbers of corpulent teenagers believe, mistakenly, that the solutions to all their problems await the alterations they can make in their physiques; the hoped-for, magical outcome may well lead them on the search for the magical solution—the quick cure. But even when dramatic weight losses occur they may not produce the social changes desired as Steele (1980) illustrates in her three case histories. Nor is there positive proof that adolescents who successfully alter their physiques significantly improve their self-concepts (Giotto, 1980). Some studies, however, do suggest that changes in weight can bring improvements in other untargeted areas. Stanley and co-workers (1970), for instance, recorded that adolescents responding well to weight-reduction therapy in a hospital improved at follow-up (out of hospital) scholastically. Likewise, Heyden, DeMaria, Barbee, and Morris (1973) indicate that overweight adolescents given individual care reported having more energy and demonstrated having either equal or better school grades following treatment.

Chapters 1 and 5 presented several approaches to therapy that children have received—strategies for creating the negative energy equation. Adolescents also have received these approaches; they are reviewed here.

Dieting

Practitioners and researchers offer overweight teenagers diets of varying calorie restrictions, and conduct programs in hospitals as well as in outpatient settings. Stanley and colleagues (1970), for example, imposed a 1200 kcal regimen in their six-week, hospital-based intervention; 11 adolescents, averaging about 14 years of age who were between 49 and 138 percent overweight (mean = 79 percent), received it. Losses were from 3.6 kg to 10.9 kg. During follow-up, 15 months, two furthered their reductions, one to 26.3 kg and the second to nearly 30 kg. Nine others fared more poorly, being 1.8 kg lighter and between 2.3 kg and 22.2 kg heavier than before treatment; approximately 55 percent remained close to their pre-treatment weights or extended their progress during follow-up.

Hammar, Campbell, and Wolley (1971) also investigated long-term consequences of dieting. Sixty-five overweight adolescent outpatients, mean age 14.8 years, participated in their study for about six months to a year-and-a-half. Forty-two had a low-calorie diet, not of starvation proportions, but "low" (exact figure unspecified). Twenty-three others had counselling, but neither dieted nor received nutritional advice. Teenagers who dieted did the best; nearly half lost 4.5 kg or more, whereas only 39 percent of those counselled did this well. Follow-up, averaging four years after treatment started, revealed (questionnaire data) that 24 percent of the dieted subjects maintained their successes; only about 9 percent of the counselled subjects did.

Heyden and co-workers (1973) applied a 700 kcal bill-of-fare coupled with intermittent fasting to 42 individuals, most of whom were between 13 and 17 years of age. Eight of them were seen individually accompanied by their mothers. They obtained the 700 kcal/day diet, ensuring 90 g/day of protein (more than sufficient), and, additionally, fasted one or two days each week. Results were impressive. After a mean of 5.6 months, weight losses among these very heavy youths, average weight starting 96.6 kg, were as much as 33.6 kg (mean = 18.3 kg); one girl lost and regained 11.4 kg within six months, and is, therefore, counted as not having reduced at all; six lost 4.5 kg or more, two shedding over 27 kg. Then, using Heyden and colleagues' method, half of the participants served as helpers (group leaders) to 27 other overweight juveniles they recruited. Results for this paraprofessionally run group supervised by physicians, were far less impressive. Later, seven more teenagers began the individual strategy, losing an average of 9.7 kg in from one to five months (see Asher, 1980; Brown, Forbes, Klish, Gordon, & Campbell, 1981; Dietz & Schoeller, 1982; Merritt et al., 1980; Pencharz, Motil, Parsons, & Duffy, 1980; Chapter 1).

Sometimes with adolescents, zero-calorie dieting is tried (see, for example, Nathan & Pisula, 1970). But as said in Chapter 1, one of the dangers of doing so, is loss of lean tissue, and the disappointment is transitory improvement; over 73 percent of Nathan and Pisula's subjects relapsed to or exceeded their starting weights 8 to 24 months following the starvation.

Furthermore, drugs are sometimes prescribed for adolescents, less objectionably than for children under 12 (Grollman, 1980; Chapter 1), as adjuncts to dieting. But data clarifying their advantages in this capacity are scarce. Nonprescription, over-the-counter drugs are also resorted to by desperate teenagers . . . to little avail. Moreover, unpleasant side effects (for example, nausea, insomnia) have been associated with using diet drugs (Mallick, 1980). More desirable, physical activity is sometimes added to dieting treatment for adolescents (see Heyden et al. 1973; Stanley et al., 1970); only infrequently is activity the main or exclusive intervention.

Exercising

Christakis, Sajecki, Hillman, Miller, Blumenthal, and Archer (1966) combined activity therapy with nutrition teaching; calorie restriction to promote weight loss was not emphasized. Fifty-five overweight boys, 13- to 14-years-old, received the package; 35 others—controls who were almost as overweight—received the usual gym classes their high schools offered. Nutrition education for the 55 experimentals was comprised of lectures on foods and calories, films on obesity, and opportunities to discuss specific problems. Activity therapy for them was comprised of regular gym plus teachings on body-building, weight-lifting, and physical conditioning. They exercised regularly at school and at home, progressively increasing the time they spent doing callesthenics (for example, jumping-jacks, running in place).

By the end of treatment (18 months), two controls and six experimentals dropped out. A comparison of those who remained in each group revealed that experimentals had sustained uniformly superior changes in fitness and less weight gain—means of 2.6 kg as opposed to 6.6 kg for controls. Linear growth in each group was equal, on the average 7 cm. In terms of mean reductions in overweight, experimentals were 11 percent less, controls 2 percent less; paralleling these alterations, mean triceps skinfold thicknesses decreased somewhat—.22 mm for experimentals and .04 mm for controls. Looking at upper extremes of the two conditions, 30 percent or more overweight, the authors showed that the largest group differences lay here. Teenagers this heavy in the experimental group, moreover, outdid their lighter counterparts in that group. So, the program had some value in modifying Point A (body) components of overweight male adolescents (see Moody, Wilmore, Girandola, & Royce, 1972 for Point A changes in overweight female adolescents).

Jetté, Barry, and Pearlman (1977) also focused their activity therapy for obese teenagers on evaluating Point A changes. But the changes they found in this more exclusively exercise treatment, did not involve weight or fatness variables. Twenty-one obese boys, averaging approximately 15 years of age, participated in their high school's program of physical education. Eleven, in addition, played lacrosse twice weekly, 45 minutes each time, for five months. For most Point A and B (behavior) alterations, the pre–post differences were insignificant. Those playing lacrosse regularly, however, did improve in work capacity—resting heart rate decreased significantly (12 beats per minute), exercise heart rate decreased significantly at the greatest work load (16 beats per minute) and predicted max VO_2 (maximal rate of oxygen consumption) increased.

Surgery

As stated in Chapter 1, surgery is drastic treatment. It is a last resort option for the severely obese (see Blackburn & Bistrian, 1980), the effects of which as yet (for example, effects on skeletal growth) are not entirely understood (Powers, 1980). Nearly ten years ago, Randolph and co-workers (1974) performed jujunoileal bypasses on four extremely obese juveniles, of whom three (all girls) were on the average 15.3-years-old (see Rigg, 1975). Criteria for surgery were freedom from obesity-influencing and surgery-threatening diseases, freedom from incapacitating psychological problems, willingness of parent and teenager to heed prescriptions given before and after surgery, failure at dieting (one year minimum), and being 100 percent overweight (two-year minimum). Approximate mean preoperative weight was 175 kg; the heaviest girl weighed over 198 kg. One year following surgery she weighed just over 117 kg, having lost about 81 kg. Her two peers averaged a loss of 50.8 kg. Other than diarrhea, no postoperative complications were reported (cf. Faber, Randolph, Robbins, & Smith, 1978; White, Cheek, & Haller, 1974).

More recently, Anderson and colleagues (1980) scrutinized the progress of 41 surgically treated obese individuals; 11 (Prader-Willi children) were discussed in Chapter 1; they showed a 55 percent reduction in overweight five years postoperatively. The 30 others, 15 males and 15 females of normal intelligence, average age 17 and average degree of overweight 238 percent, managed a similar improvement. Criteria for surgery, as stated in Chapter 1, were health, capacity for normal activity, and 100 percent overweight. Twenty-three received gastric bypasses, seven gastroplasties. Three years later, the mean overweight reduction was 67 percent, and two years after that it was 51 percent. Height changes during follow-up were said to be normal and no liver or other difficulties that could affect growth were found. Complications subsequent to the operation (such as infection), however, were identified for some. Worst of all, there were two deaths; one of them, a 15-year-old boy, died three days following surgery; the other, age and sex unspecified in the report, died three years following surgery.

Behavior Therapy

Studies in this section only sample those available. They are categorized as were those in Chapter 5: The focus on weight loss is separated from that on environment alteration, and this second grouping divides further into reports integrating and reports not integrating nutrition or activity advice, or both. The behavioral control of adolescent obesity, like that of childhood obesity, applies the methods and illustrates the approaches named earlier. Indeed, technologically much is the same in the treatment of adolescents and children. Recognizing this, reviewers usually discuss the two populations as if they were one. This practice, however, is unwise (Edelstein, 1981; Israel & Stolmaker, 1980). It may blur differences that need to be articulated in order for treatment to be tailored; one difference, as noted, involves the degree of control over food and activity. To date, the age variable has not received just due (Israel & Stolmaker, 1980).

Focusing on Weight Loss

The application below illustrates main features of the weight-loss-focus approach. Contingencies are placed on losing weight. Behaviors are untargeted, but behavioral procedures, such as positive reinforcement, are employed. In other words, independent variables capable of producing Point B (behavior) changes are applied to Point A (body) variables—weight; and measurements remain there. The abuse potential of the weight-loss-focus approach is partly a function of the strength of the consequences contingent on losing or not losing weight and the degree of control over the environment the adolescent has. The teenager in the application below probably had less opportunity than an adolescent living under more usual circumstances would have to do unwholesome things to herself so as to receive her weight-loss reinforcer; abuses are undisclosed.

Application 1: Consequating a Retarded Teenager's
Weight Losses

The girl in this report by Foxx (1972) was 14-years-old, retarded, and a resident of an institution. Her height and weight before treatment were listed as 160 cm and 108.5 kg. Six months of dieting prior to behavior modification resulted in a 10.4

kg loss. To increase progress, Foxx implemented a three-phase program: social reinforcement for losing weight, removal of social reinforcement, and reinstitution of reinforcement.

The program, therefore, used a single-subject design to evaluate a relatively simple strategy: positively reinforcing weight reduction. To reinforce weight reduction, an act which presumably makes the behaviors that produce it more probable, Foxx had to find a powerful, positive consequence. And he had to devise a formula for giving the consequence that would maximize its potency. From observation he learned that time with the experimenter overcame the first hurdle, and from operant-conditioning logic he knew that delivering the reinforcer as soon as possible after the event to be strengthened overcame the second hurdle. Therefore, the contingency was that if the girl reduced sufficiently by at least .68 kg weekly, she and the experimenter went together to the institution's canteen and talked; they would do so during the afternoon, once a week, soon after the weekly weight check.

The teenager knew the rules of the game from its start, but how she managed to win is unstated. Mainly, she decided whether and what to eat. Foxx correctly reasoned that the many precursors setting the occasion for his patient's acts of consumption would be unchanged had she been confined and forced to diet; she would lose weight, but in all likelihood would regain quickly. His plan, accordingly, was to keep her in the situations that compelled her to eat excessively, while he gave her reasons not to eat excessively—to wit, receiving social reinforcement for reducing. Thus, he did not teach her ways to modify actions leading to weight gain or inhibiting weight loss. She had to develop the ways herself.

Probably, she did. During 15 weeks of the first social reinforcement phase, she lost 19.5 kg—1.3 kg. every seven days. During the reversal, also 15 weeks, she lost an additional 3.4 kg—.23 kg weekly. And during the third phase, 10 weeks, her weight fell another 12.9 kg—1.3 kg weekly. Comparing the seven-day rates of loss, Foxx showed the effects of therapy: each treatment more than quintupled the losses of the intervening reversal. By the end of the program, the girl's weight reached 72.6 kg, an almost 36 kg reduction from the start, and a short time later (length unmentioned) it dropped to nearly 70.4 kg; unfortunately, height changes over this greater-than-10-month interval are unreported, and long-term follow-up data are unavailable.

Focusing on Environment Alteration

As said, this approach also seeks to alter the shape of the body, but when trying to do so, it usually applies more intricate packages of antecedent- and consequent-change methods than the weight-loss-focus approach does. And more than that approach, environment alteration targets behavioral (Point B) variables in order to bring about the Point A (body) alterations; nonetheless, unhappily, evaluation is frequently accomplished by measuring only weight or percent overweight differences.

Furthermore, as said, a distinction may be drawn between environment alteration that informs the patient about nutrition and activity principles or both and environment alteration that does not or that does little of this informing. The reports that follow vary in amount that they tell the patient. Again if I have erred in my categorizations, I apologize.

Environment Alteration:
Nutrition and/or Activity Advice Not Integrated

Two applications ensue. The first illustrates this approach with emotionally disturbed, hospitalized adolescents, the second with retarded teenagers living at home and attending a high school. The approach has also been tried with normally intelligent adolescents free of psychiatric disturbances (see Wang & Watson, 1978).

Application 2: Treating Overweight Adolescents
Hospitalized for Psychiatric Difficulties

Di Scipio, Paul, and Byers (1976) described their treatment of six severely disturbed 13- to 16-year-old girls, each of whom was grossly overweight and hospitalized, some for as long as three years. Heights were unlisted. Starting weights were from a low of 74.7 kg to a high of 94.2 kg, and magnitude of overweight was from 20.7 kg to 38.4 kg. Since admission to the hospital, all these patients had gained; one girl, in fact, had put on almost 43 kg.

Therapy for obesity was voluntary, lasting as long as four months for those wishing it; not all the girls participated for that length of time. Sensitive to creating dietary outcasts teased for being different, the authors avoided special menus. Instead they asked for reductions in extras at meals and throughout the day. The program, involving as it did a team approach, permitted continuous monitoring of the girls' efforts toward this end.

Several behavioral procedures were applied. First, there was positive reinforcement (money) for weight loss. Each .45 kg loss for the initial 2.3 kg resulted in the payment of $1.00; thereafter, payoffs for .45 kg reductions were 50¢. This downward sliding scale of monetary reinforcement is curious. Usually, losing weight is easier and motivation higher earlier in therapy, and continuing the initial rate of loss becomes progressively harder. Therefore, paying more later—paying more for harder to come by weight losses in order to make them more rewarding— may be better strategy (Chapter 2). Comparing early versus later reductions, that is week-one to week-twelve losses, the authors did indeed see the expected decline—a 1.5 kg loss to a .23 kg gain.

Next, there was response-cost; this was applied to food transgressions. Each teenager forfeited 50¢ each time she had seconds at meals or had candy, cake, or high-calorie soft drinks during other times. Girls had bankbooks assigned to them so that up-to-date records of the money transactions were available.

Third, there was social learning. Actually, as the authors illustrate, social learning in this study was a collection of tactics: praise for losing weight, praise for comments that losing weight was worthwhile, and modeling of desirable weights by group leaders. Social learning was implemented during weekly, 40 to 50 minute, group-therapy meetings.

Results, expressed in terms of weight change and comments about food transgressions, showed that response-costing illicit eating had no impact on weight loss; yet, the most successful patient was fined infrequently. She reduced 11.8 kg. Her least successful peer gained .23 kg. Because this second girl was putting on weight at about the time treatment began, the authors suggested that therapy had possibly attenuated her rate of gaining. Between the results for these two girls were those for the others, ranging from .23 kg to 5.9 kg losses.

Helping seriously disturbed teenagers reduce is difficult, to say the least; the outcome of this investigation must be considered in this light. The study is demonstrational, not experimental, and important data are missing (for example behavioral information, percent of overweight change, height change, fatness change). Notwithstanding these deficiencies, the report is provocative. Programs for treating psychotic, hospitalized adolescents are needed, especially if, as the authors imply, hospitalization breeds gaining weight. Some of the recommendations they give for initiating such programs are to seek administrative support, to finance if possible without burdening the institution, and to answer program-related questions willingly at all times.

Application 3: Treating Overweight Retarded Adolescents

Rotatori, Fox, and Switzky (1979) offered a weight-control program for six Down's Syndrome teenagers (4 girls, 2 boys) living at home, average age over 17 years and average IQ 42. Academically, the patients were approximately second-graders.

The program proceeded through four phases. Baseline, lasting about three months, entailed biweekly checks on weight; subjects gained a mean of 1.2 kg. Treatment, the second phase, was nearly identical to that of Application 4, Chapter 5, the main exception being that the regimen discussed here was 14 weeks. Through lecturing, demonstration, opportunity to practice, and feedback paced according to mastery, adolescents learned stimulus control, eating-rate reduction, self-monitoring of weight and intake, and so on. The classroom teacher gave the lessons. Teacher and parents were taught about them and about assisting the patients. Also, with parental help, teenagers rated their own compliance with the prescriptions. They obtained activity reinforcers from previously arranged reinforcer menus contingent on adherence—better adherence, better reinforcers. And they obtained them for losing weight—at least .45 kg per week.

Two meetings during five weeks comprised phase three, maintenance. The first reviewed the behavioral methods applied; the second, the homework assigned. Follow-up, the last phase, entailed weighing the boys and girls six months after the second maintenance session and then again after one year.

Results suggest that the program created the Point A (weight) changes found. But results, as is typical, are incomplete and thus tell next to nothing about behavioral outcomes, Point C (energy) variables, and other Point A components. Treatment seemed to reverse the upward trend of baseline, adolescents losing significantly; average loss was 4.7 kg, ranging from .45 kg to 7.8 kg, and everyone continued to reduce during maintenance, about 1.8 kg on the average.

Follow-up, post-maintenance to six months, revealed some regaining (two subjects), but, by and large, small reductions continued. At the year checkup, one teenager could no longer be evaluated, having graduated. Of the five remaining, three were still losing. The best was, at this time, about 10.8 kg lighter than before baseline and the worst was 1.8 kg lighter than this reference point; subtracting from post-baseline improves the picture.

Rotatori and Fox (1980) replicated much of this program with 12 moderately retarded adolescents. Another 12 retarded teenagers, in addition, received "social nutrition treatment"—dietary and exercise advice, weight-loss goal-setting, and related topics. Behavior therapy participants significantly outperformed the others, and they outdid six retarded adolescents in a wait-list control as well (see also Rotatori & Switzky, 1979).

Environment Alteration:
Nutrition and/or Activity Advice Integrated

Four applications are included here. Most of the literature on the behavioral control of adolescent obesity uses this approach.

Application 4: Group Treatment for Overweight Adolescents

Zakus, Chin, Keowm, Herbert and Held (1979), in a anecdotal account, put forth a multi-element treatment package that they applied to five adolescent girls, who averaged 16 years of age and 88.1 percent overweight (see also Botvin, Cantlon, Carter, & Williams, 1979; Brandt, Maschhoff, & Chandler, 1980; Zakus, Chin, Cooper, Makovsky & Merrill, 1981). Ten started the program, but five dropped out early. It lasted for about six months and included weekly, 90-minute group meetings (see Gross et al., 1976) conducted by a social worker and a nutritionist.

Behavioral procedures involved self-monitoring of eating, stimulus control, eating-speed reduction, reinforcing other behavior (behavior incompatible with eating), and various personalized tactics to handle individual problems. The nutrition component had tailored diets that required the regulation of meat, dairy, fruit, starch, fat, sugar, and vegetable consumption. Further, breakfast was encouraged. Computer analyses of the girls dietaries were undertaken before and during therapy. Inadequate intakes of several minerals and vitamins were uncovered and these practices corrected. Compliance with the behavioral and nutrition parts of this regimen was, as the authors report (no data), variable. Zakus and associates also had a significant-other group in their program; it was comprised of nine individuals (parents, siblings, and friends) chosen by several of the teenagers. Participants learned about eating behavior, but evidently some had difficulty applying this knowledge.

Results are dispiriting. Three girls, those having the lowest internal–external scores after treatment, lost between 2.5 kg and 5 kg. Two gained; one put on 1.1 kg, the second 5.4 kg; prior to therapy these girls, though treated by other procedures, had added substantial amounts of weight, indicating that perhaps the present program functioned as a brake on their rate of gain (see also Geller, 1978). During treatment, the worst patient, gaining the most overall, fluctuated about 19 kg, putting on 12.2 kg and taking off 6.8 kg. The best patient also fluctuated about 19 kg, yet she increased 7 kg and decreased 12 kg.

Application 5: Assessing and Treating Groups of Overweight Adolescents

Unlike Zakus and colleagues, Harris, Sutton, Kaufman, and Carmichael (1980) take many measures of outcome, but results are much the same: in a word, discouraging. The authors ran two groups of primarily adolescent-aged girls, 21 subjects in one group and 15 in the second. At the start, ages ranged from 12 to 23 years, and degree overweight from 20 to 154 percent. For the group of 21 patients, treatment lasted one year; for the other group, it lasted seven months, beginning five months later.

Harris and co-workers assessed and evaluated changes on dependent variables covering the three points of the obesity triangle. Of concern, to name some, were weight, percent overweight, medical history, nutrition, energy, attitudes, perceptions, eating, exercising, and food preference. Photographs of the patients also were taken to rate body-shape changes.

Sixty-minute group meetings originally scheduled weekly, became biweekly two months before the project ended. Sessions, conducted most often by the graduate student member of the treatment team with a physician in attendance— other team members included a psychologist and a nutritionist—embraced various topics. Some were general, such as stimulus control, nutrition, and exercise;

others were specific, being requested for special problems the group members themselves revealed. Moreover, three times within several months, significant others met, as in the previous Application. They learned about the program and how to be helpful to the patients; parents and friends of 11 of them, however, evidently elected not to participate.

As stated, results were discouraging. Dropouts were many—53 percent. Finishers, some of whom weighed well over 100 kg at the start, did not do all that well; mean loss was under 8 kg; the change is statistically significant but its clinical significance is dubious. Percent overweight reduction, 13 percent, paralleled the weight changes. And ratings of attractiveness, pre–post evaluations by independent judges on one-third of the sample (some photographs were lost), stayed about the same. On the other hand, as a group, the patients positively changed their attitudes about obesity.

This upward shift in attitudes correlated with weight loss. Not many other correlates, however, were seen, so the authors could not say much about who dropouts and reducers were likely to be. Of the few relationships they did find, one is particularly disheartening: Younger patients tended to do poorly. Older females, those in the experiment who were over 18.5 years, did better. They were the ones more likely to stay in the program and to reduce over 4.5 kg—the authors' benchmark for separating losers and nonlosers.

Height changes of the younger patients, however, need to be known in order to interpret their smaller losses; also, compliance and fatness tabulations would be of help in deciphering the effects of the package. Nonetheless, that the authors seem to be disappointed about its results is easily understood. For a protracted time they gave, as they write, "a wealth of nutritional and behavioral information . . . on eating and exercise," but bore witness to very few salutary outcomes.

Application 6: Comparing Individually Administered Treatments for Overweight Adolescents

Unlike the two preceding applications, this one (Weiss, 1977a) delivered treatment to individuals not to groups. Also dissimilar, this application attempted to systematically compare diet and behavior therapies. Furthermore, Weiss made no effort to include significant others in treatment; in fact, he asked the premier group, parents, not to interfere. His injunction possibly alerted well-meaning mothers and fathers, who may have been disrupting the weight-control efforts of their sons and daughters, (see Cohen et al., 1980), to stop aggravating the problem. If his message did this, it may have been, in and of itself, therapeutic.

Be that as it may, his concern was not to test the parent-impact variable, but rather to apply treatment. His objective was to compare the immediate and long-range effects of four interventions given to overweight teenagers, who varied per condition in average age from just over 13 years to just over 14 years; a few were as young as 9.5, others were as old as 18. Well over forty individuals, mostly females, started the program, some at weights in excess of 110 kg—mean percent overweight 42.6 percent. Seven were controls, having no contact with Weiss until treatment ended. Twelve received the standard stimulus-control package of directives. Twenty-eight received the Stuart and Davis (1972) exchange diet (see Chapter 4): Nine of these had the diet with nonredeemable points for adherence; ten others had the same diet with the points backed up by self-administered consequences; nine more had the diet with the reinforcement as well as the stimulus-control package. During the three-month intervention, all were seen individually once weekly for 10 to 15 minutes at a time, and in addition all were encouraged to exercise; instructions and ploys used to foster activity were undisclosed in the report.

Results focused on Point A (weight), percent of overweight, and, to a lesser extent, height. Overall, therapy was better than no therapy. On the weight-loss measure, all four treatment conditions were significantly superior to the control, whereas on the percent-overweight-lost measure three of the four were—the diet-only group being the exception. Likewise, on both measures of weight change, within-group differences were significant for all but the diet-only group; also, within-group differences were significant for all except the stimulus-control-only group, but just on the weight-loss variable. The combined stimulus-control and diet group, furthermore, evidenced a significant linear trend in reducing. As Weiss expressed it, almost any intervention may be productive in the short run; indeed, the results of his four treatments were equivalent.

It was at follow-up, however, that a clearer separation emerged, both stimulus-control interventions revealing their worth statistically. At that time, almost a year after the beginning of the program, each group of patients had grown about equally in height. And although some patients had maintained their weight-loss successes, others had not. (Data on individuals are available from Weiss.) Most important, greater numbers of the reducers were in the two stimulus-control conditions, and these conditions were significantly superior to the diet ones in percent overweight lost. Comparing group means, Weiss revealed that patients given stimulus control, with and without diet, regained only a fraction of what those in the diet groups combined regained. And in contrast to these diet groups, who increased in percent overweight, they decreased nearly 10 percent in overweight. Thus, stimulus-control instructions seem to have had an impact. Does adding diet advice to them strengthen it? Weiss answered yes, even though he could find no statistical difference between the two stimulus-control conditions. He argued that the combined stimulus-control group, considering weight measures and linear growth, was the best one at the 12-week evaluation; also, he argued that it better met the needs and expectations of adolescents. Teenagers, he felt, were well-served by having nutritional knowledge made available to them. They look for it.

Application 7: An Intensive Strategy for Investigating
the Treatment of Overweight Adolescents

Like Weiss, the author of this application treated overweight adolescents by seeing them individually. Coates (1977), however, provided a finer-grain analysis of outcome. His study ranks as a very thorough effort to decipher the impact of behavioral control procedures on adolescents. Also, it modeled a strategy of inquiry for understanding the treatment by patient interaction that is greatly responsible for the pronounced within-treatment variability of results found in most behavioral programs (Brownell & Stunkard, 1980a).

Essentially, Coates applied a multicomponent package and evaluated it by using a multiple-baseline design. Intervention over two months long followed a baseline lasting approximately one month. Participants were three teenage girls. One began the program about 128 percent overweight, 130 kg, 166 cm, and 16-years-old. Another began about 70 percent overweight, 88 kg, 157 cm, and 16-years-old. The third began nearly 73 percent overweight, 98 kg, 168 cm, and 15-years-old. The first two received the behavioral package, one girl one week after the other, and the third adolescent received a placebo form of treatment that included counselling on nutrition and dieting. The third teenager also was given the same lessons as her agemates at about the same time, but hers were in written form only. She did not get the application training her peers got. Because she received attention, contact, and information, however, she served as a control for the effects of these variables (Coates, 1977).

The multi-element behavioral package had more than ten components, among which were nutrition teaching, problem solving, exercise, eating-rate reduction, stimulus control, cognitive control, and food-portion reduction. Hourly meetings were held twice weekly, during which demonstrations of, practice with, and lectures about techniques occurred. For the first five weeks, some of the meetings were in the patients' homes with everyone in the family asked to attend; parents were part of the program. Besides these contacts, nonparticipant observers visited the homes at the dinner hour, four times a week for 12 weeks; observers assessed the types of food stored there, how they were served and prepared, and how the patients ate (for example, sips per minute, bites). During the program, the girls were weighed regularly and their behaviors monitored. Also, height and pre–post triceps skinfold measurements were taken.

Results detailed modifications in behavior and weight. Behaviorally treated subjects enjoyed clinically significant body changes (Coates & Thoresen, in press). For example, the originally heaviest teenager lost 9.5 kg, a 16.9 percent reduction in overweight; sixteen months following intervention, she was 45.8 kg lighter (Coates & Thoresen, 1981). Her colleague lost 5.2 kg, a 10.8 percent overweight reduction, but eventually without continuing treatment reverted back to her baseline weight (Coates and Thoresen, 1981). The control subject, howev-

er, gained during intervention. She began putting on weight by the fourth treatment week. All told she gained 2.3 kg, becoming 4 percent more overweight by its
end.

Behavior changes correlated with weight losses; in addition, the critical behavior modifications relating to the Point A (body) changes differed between the
two behaviorally treated youths, and the differences were in areas that each girl
had initially experienced difficulties (Coates & Thoresen, 1980). For instance, the
heaviest adolescent had had many rich foods readily available in her home; during
the program, she altered this situation. Also, before intervention she had consumed food frequently in various places; both problems—frequency and place—
abated over treatment. On the other hand, she experienced no eating-rate changes.
Her lighter peer, however, did. Other differences emerged as well. The implica-
tion is clear, and Coates' last comments mirror it: efficient treatment must be
tailored to the patient's needs.

Conclusions

In general, the literature on the control of adolescent obesity by behavior modification and by other strategies suffers from the same methodological and reporting
shortcomings as does the literature on childhood obesity. There are, for example:
too few follow-ups; too few demonstrations of clinical significance; too few
demonstrations that teenagers comply with prescriptions in order to change; too
few attempts to gather fatness data and elucidate the presence and effects of other
body changes as well as energy equation changes; too little assessment; and too
little monitoring. These deficiencies need to be eradicated. Also, more intensive
studies of behavioral, dietary, and exercise combinations need to be done; when
doing so, researchers should attempt to identify the interdigitations of these
combinations with the prominent characteristics (economic, social, racial, behavioral) of those adolescents receiving them.

Obstacles

Selecting the best target behaviors (see Gracianette, Williamson, Hardin, Konidoff, & Young 1980; Figure 6.1) is a major obstacle. Fodor (1980) recently
advised behavior therapists to target patient self-acceptance in their weight-loss
programs. She is concerned about the lackluster results of behaviorally based
weight-control regimes directed at adults, fearing that patients leave them with
low, perhaps even lower than when they started, self-esteem. Among the procedures her therapy strategy involved were consciousness raising to identify prejudi-
cial actions toward the obese, scrutiny of the patient's belief system related to body
shape, and cognitive restructuring. Her methods were aimed at adult women who
failed or who were likely to fail at weight control. But with modification, some of
her methods (for example, consciousness raising) seem to be appropriate for

teenagers who have yet to try to reduce or, because they request it, wish to try again. They seem to be especially appropriate for adolescent girls whose disparaging self-statements and self-perceptions help perpetuate the rejection they feel and the weight-control failures they experience.

Other major obstacles are initiating and maintaining motivation as well as sustaining progress once formal treatment ends. Apropos of the latter concern, the possible roles and variable effects of parents during and after intervention continues to be a topic of inquiry (Coates & Perry, 1980; Coates, Killen, & Slinkard, 1982; Coché, Levitz, & Jordan, 1979; Cohen et al., 1980; Kelman et al., 1979).

In addition, the obstacle of devising a negative energy equation that promotes changes in the Point A (body) variables desirable to change remains. In an attempt to pinpoint which of the two terms of this equation is most awry, some studies conclude that obese adolescents are not consuming excessively (Durnin, Lonergan, Good, & Ewan, 1974; Hampton, Huenemann, Shapiro, & Mitchell, 1967; Huenemann, 1972; Johnson, Burke, & Mayer, 1956; Stephanik, Heald, & Mayer, 1959). They find instead, that the obese are less active (Johnson et al., 1956; Stephanik et al., 1959). One of the best known of these researches, Bullen, Reed, and Mayer (1964), objectively documented this inactivity in a sample of 109 overweight adolescent girls. The authors compared the activity profiles of these teenagers to 72 others of normal weight. All the adolescents, ages 13 to 17, attended summer camps, one expressly for the heavy.

The primary method of uncovering activity differences—differences later converted to calorie expenditure estimates—was motion-picture time-sampling. At selected intervals during any of three activities, including swimming, volleyball, and tennis, the girls were filmed; then, three-second frames of these activities were analyzed and rated. A wealth of observations, 27,211, resulted.

The less overweight were the more active. For instance, when scrutinizing pictures of the swim periods, the authors found that a mean of 55 percent of the nonoverweight subjects were swimming; but only a mean of 9 percent of the overweight girls were. Calorie expenditure estimates paralleled these results. The overweight, more than their lighter peers, were rated as expending fewer calories. Yet, upon being questioned, heavy girls commended exercise just as much as did other girls; it was fun and a good opportunity to socialize.

Bradfield, Paulos, and Grossman's (1971) results conflict with those of Bullen and associates. Employing different techniques in a different setting, they found no significant energy outgo differences between small groups of obese and nonobese high school girls of similar ages—almost 17—and of similar heights— almost 166 cm. Weight for the obese cohort (N = 4) averaged 74 kg and for the nonobese (N = 6), 51 kg. Triceps skinfolds also separated the groups, averaging 24 mm for the obese and 14 mm for the nonobese.

To estimate calorie intake, Bradfield and colleagues had the girls keep three-day dietary records. To estimate calorie outgo, the authors measured heart rate. Its relationship to energy expenditure was fixed through individually determined regression lines. These were established by assessing each subject's heart rate and oxygen consumption at the same time, while she was resting or moving about. Activity level was estimated by having the girls keep three-day records of what they did and how long they did it. Also, activity level during physical education was estimated by the students' gym teacher.

Results showed that the thinner girls took in more calories than did the fatter girls. But they (the thinner) expended neither sizably more nor sizably less calories than did their corpulent peers. Energy expenditure did not discriminate. Further, there were no remarkable activity differences, neither those evident from teacher ratings nor those from three-day records. Indeed, both groups of teenagers were noticeably sedentary; much of the time they were sleeping or engaged in light to very light activity. Variability, intra-individual and intra-group, however, was higher than variability between groups. Therefore, whether a specific teenager takes in too many calories or expends too few is knowable only by assessing that teenager, and to alter the status quo for any teen, a negative energy equation has to be set down. Guidelines for adjusting the magnitudes of its two quantities, however, are in short supply. The recommended energy intakes for males and females up to 18 years of age found in Table 6.1 are of help. Nineteen-year-olds need about the same as do 18-year-olds; males averaging 70 kg and 177 cm require about 2900 kcal/day, the range being 2500 kcal to 3300 kcal; females averaging 55 kg and 163 cm require about 2100 kcal/day—range 1700 kcal to 2500 kcal (RDA, 1980). As indicated in Chapter 6, the levels advised are those believed to promote good health. They are means. A major goal is altering physique without impeding linear growth.

This objective is furthered by augmenting the calorie-outgo half of the equation, but as also indicated in Chapter 6, a list of recommendations comparable to the intake listing is unavailable. Increasing calorie expenditure is most practically accomplished by increasing physical activity. The advantages of doing so are, like those named for children, less need to rely on intake restriction when creating the therapeutic negative energy equation; maximization of fat loss; and minimization of lean body weight loss (e.g., Moody et al., 1972). More research with adolescents is necessary to uncover the effect of activity on appetite, on increasing post-exercise metabolic rate, and on attenuating dietary-induced metabolic rate drops. In sum, it appears that the concerns surrounding the task of building a safe and meaningful therapy program that exist for overweight children exist also for overweight adolescents. Future work with teenagers will tell us what other concerns there are and how to meet them.

CHAPTER 8

Current Questions, Future Directions: Concluding Comments

How may behavior therapy be of better service to obese children? There are no easy answers. To begin to find them researchers and practitioners must, at the very least, completely detail the treatment approaches offered so that these approaches are replicable. Data need to be gathered that permit different approaches to be rigorously evaluated in both the short- and long-run. In addition, enough data must be taken to permit comparisons among studies. Using the obesity triangle (see Table 6.1) as a present-day source of dependent variables pertaining to body, behavior, and energy will help researchers and practitioners to remain aware of what could be collected before, during, and after formal treatment.

Documenting the interrelationships of variables from points on the triangle is called for, so that the comprehensive impact of treatment on the child is more interpretable. The meaningfulness of treatment—its clinical significance—is more definable as more of its outcomes are made known. For instance, stating the effects of behavioral strategies on blood pressure, percent overweight, and fatness changes, and the interrelationships of these characteristics with targeted behavior classes (for example, activity) affords health-care providers greater insight into what treatment does for the child currently receiving it. Further, by knowing more about its present impact they are taking a step toward becoming more skillful in designing the next child's treatment.

Today, more questions than answers exist about therapy for obese children. My goal in this last chapter is to state many of these questions. Some have been asked already in earlier chapters; these have grown out of discussions on the contributors and concomitants of childhood obesity and the issues and obstacles involved in treating it. I'll try not to be too repetitive. Some, however, have not been addressed as yet. My hope is that the questions put forth here and those suggested earlier germinate ideas in researchers and practitioners that will be developed for future study.

Questions about the Population
of Obese Children

As noted in Chapter 2, there are a number of queries and disagreements about the incidence and natural history of childhood obesity as well as about the long-term physical consequences of the physical sequelae that are present with some obese children. Uniform sets of measures and uniform criteria of obesity are needed to answer questions and to generalize conclusions. They are also needed to understand more about the social–psychological consequences of being an obese child, and why it is that many obese youngsters remain untouched. What shields them and not others from despair? Other questions follow:

1. How do socioeconomic and racial variables interrelate with family-feeding practices and what effect do these interrelationships appear to have on numbers and sizes of fat cells in early, middle, and late childhood? Are there demonstrable patterns?
   a. Do the patterns, if found, predict response to treatment? Accordingly, are obese children of low-income Black families poor candidates for behavior modification? If so, why? (cf., Application 7, Chapter 5; Weisenberg & Fray, 1974)
   b. Which combinations of behavioral components coupled with other methods of treatment are better suited to obese children exhibiting which patterns?
   c. Which patterns predict linkages between early (time 1) and later (time 2) weight as well as fatness excesses? How does predictive accuracy change as the $time_1$ to $time_2$ interval changes?
2. What variables underlie the eating and activity behaviors of obese children (see Coché et al., 1979)?
   a. Do parents overfeed their obese children (for example, Waxman & Stunkard, 1980)?
   b. Do parents, by their own styles of eating, set an eating style for their children that contributes significantly to obesity?
   c. Is plate-cleaning enforced in the homes of obese children more than it is in the homes of nonobese ones?
   d. Is dieting modeled in the homes of obese children more than it is in the homes of nonobese ones?
3. What are the calorie-intake and calorie-expenditure differences of obese and nonobese children (Waxman & Stunkard, 1980)?
   a. How does age affect the comparisons?
   b. Does degree of obesity affect them?
   c. Does sex of child affect them?
4. Is the thermic response of food lower for obese compared with nonobese children?

    a.   What effect does dieting have on the thermic response of food?

    b.   What effect does exercise have on the thermic response of food among obese versus nonobese children?

5.   What are the activity frequency, intensity, duration, and type differences shown by obese and nonobese children?

    a.   What effects do differing amounts of activity have on appetite, calorie intake, and metabolic rate in obese and nonobese children of various ages and current histories (baselines) of activity (see Epstein et al., 1978; Chapter 6)?

6.   How general is the relationship of contradictory messages (Chapter 2) with the presence and refractoriness of childhood obesity?

    a.   Which contradictory messages are most often found?

    b.   What variables (religious, racial, economic) affect the types and numbers of contradictory messages found?

Questions about the Process and Outcome of Treating Obese Children with Behavior Therapy

Reliable and valid assessment tools are essential for measuring the components of the obesity triangle (see Brownell, 1981). Where such tools fail to exist, the imperative is to construct them; for, to the extent that precision measurements are lacking, the design, monitoring, tailoring, and evaluation of behavior therapy is limited. Questions in this section address technology of change, foci of change, delivery systems for producing change, and change itself.

1.   What role might classical conditioning have on altering the strength of modifiable food-related metabolic responses (Booth, 1980; Rodin, 1979a)?

2.   Is it valuable to attach consequences for complying with stimulus-control directives (see Mahoney et al., 1973), and does age of child interact with the use of consequences?

3.   Is cognitive restructuring valuable in working with obese children? How are ages and maturity levels involved?

4.   If food preferences can be altered through behavioral strategies to produce therapeutic effects, how may this be done least intrusively?

5.   Which behavioral strategies least intrusively alter food-getting and eating behaviors to therapeutic levels?

6.   Which behavioral strategies least intrusively alter calorie-outgo practices to therapeutic levels?

7.   What combinations of questions 4, 5, and 6 above are most effective for younger versus older children; more generally, who should get what?

    a.   How may these strategies be tailored?

8. What are the effects of targeting social skills (including assertiveness) on the body and behavioral changes of obese youths?

9. Are degree and length of contact important variables in treating obese children (see Coates et al., 1982 on adolescents)?

10. What are the most cost-effective ways to provide children of differing ages and levels of intelligence with behavioral lessons: individually or in groups? combining lecturing with demonstration, practice, and feedback (see Application 4, Chapter 5)? using programmed texts?

11. What prompts for compliance with prescriptions are effective?

12. What attrition–reduction procedures are effective?
   a. Are the effective ones correlated with noncompliance (see Hagen et al., 1976; Chapter 5)?

13. What are the positive and negative by-products of effective as well as ineffective behaviorally based programs?
   a. Which programs are more likely to have undesirable by-products for which children?

14. Are there ages when it is an especially favorable time to intervene (see Wheeler & Hess, 1977)? When, why?
   a. Are there ages when it is an especially unfavorable time to intervene? When, why?

15. What are the effects of combining behavior therapy with potent dietary and activity regimens on outcomes measured by body changes and social validation procedures?

16. In what ways (for example, contracting for maintenance, making the treatment family centered, teaching to solicit praise) can enduring treatment effects be programmed into formal treatment?
   a. As regards family-based treatments, under what circumstances are they most likely to be helpful (Coates & Thoresen, 1980) or harmful?

17. Which maintenance and continuance techniques are most cost-effective (for example, continued care, booster sessions)?

18. What is the cost-effectiveness of teaching successfully treated children to be teachers of other children (see Heyden et al., 1973 on adolescents)?

Questions about Treatment's Settings and Agents

There are several sites and combinations of sites for behavior therapy programs directed at obese youngsters, and there are various professionals and paraprofessionals to run them. Thus, in addition to university-based clinics, hospital-based inpatient and outpatient settings for health-plan subscribers, there are camps, schools, and patients' homes where all or some portion of therapy may be conducted. And in addition to dietitians, nutritionists, pediatricians, social workers, physical educators, nurses, family physicians, psychiatrists, psychologists, there are camp counselors, teachers and other school personnel, parents, siblings, and peers who may be involved.

Regarding camps as intervention sites, Brandt and associates (1980) demonstrated that these settings have potential. For five days, the authors treated 35 teenagers, residents of a camp for overweight adolescents, by applying environment alteration with diet and exercise teachings. The mean age of the participants, mostly girls, was over 14. (Replicating their program in a similar setting with obese children could prove to be worthwhile.) The youths seen were taught various lessons including how to keep records, how to target behaviors, and how to relax. They also learned about daily exercise, calorie expenditure, calorie intake, food preparation, and basic nutrition; teaching plans are available from the authors.

Changes in obesity-triangle components were evaluated, some immediately following treatment and others after three and six months. For example, average six-month weight loss was 1.5 kg., ranging from -15.4 kg. to +7.7 kg. Average three-month skinfold thickness reduction was 3.6 mm; mean height increase, determined at the longer follow-up, was 1.52 cm. Self-perceptions, moreover, improved over time, and places of eating decreased in number.

As indicated (Application 1, Chapter 5), for camp to be most meaningful as the site of intervention, follow-through to the home environment is necessary. Modifications in the setting wherein control over eating and activity is maximal may dissipate rapidly in the one wherein control over them is far less; training and hoping is often insufficient.

Weight-reduction camps provide researchers and practitioners with settings to program comprehensively and daily, as do the schools; as Brownell and Kaye (1982) theorize, these may be excellent treatment milieus; numbers of youngsters could be helped there.

For years, dietary and activity regimens have been designed for and conducted in schools (see for example Huse, Branes, Colligan, Nelson, & Palumbo, 1982: Huse, Palumbo, Nelson, & Hick, 1978; Seltzer & Mayer, 1970). Behavior therapy additions to them have usually been more recent. Botvin and co-workers (1979), for instance, evaluated changes in weight and fatness among more than 100 overweight 7th and 8th graders, numbers of whom were treated for 10 weeks with environment alteration tactics (such as stimulus control) joined by nutrition education and exercise teachings. Significantly more of those who were so treated (70 percent) compared with those who were not (43 percent) reduced their triceps skinfold thicknesses. Likewise, significantly more of the treated (51 percent) versus controls (16 percent) lost weight.

Also using a school setting and also applying a 10-week program of environment alteration integrating nutrition and activity teachings, Brownell and Kaye (1982) reported Point A (weight) changes. But their findings were more encouraging than those of Botvin and colleagues. Brownell and Kaye taught behavioral contracting, intake monitoring, stimulus-control of eating, speed-control of eating, reinforcement control of eating, as well as exercise and attitude change to 63, 5- to 12-year-old children who were 10 percent or more overweight. Further, they taught them about obesity, nutrition, aerobics, routine activities, and so forth. Written booklets were used to present information; very young children had the information presented orally. What's more, not only the children but also their parents, teachers, and the school administrators were taught.

The objective of all this teaching, as the authors say, was supporting the children's efforts by capitalizing on the social forces in their environments. Hence, besides these agents, Brownell and Kaye also included peers, food-service personnel and the school's physical education instructor. The coordinator for the project was a nurse's aide who weighed the youngsters weekly, graphed their progress, and praised their triumphs. Furthermore, she marshalled public acclaim for them by arranging a school assembly, during which certificates of participation were distributed (see Application 6, Chapter 5).

Results showed that compared with 14 nonrandomly selected youngsters, five from the therapy setting and nine from another school, significantly more of the treated children reduced weight (95.2 percent versus 21.4 percent). They lost significantly more weight, too (means of 4.4 kg decrease versus 1.2 kg gain for controls). And they sustained a greater reduction in percent overweight (means of 15.4 percent loss versus 2.8 percent gain for controls). Nineteen percent of the youths treated shed at least 6.8 kg and more than 6 percent shed over 9 kg. Evaluating against a three-year retrospective weight baseline taken on the 63 children, Brownell and Kaye revealed that weight gain was not only stopped but reversed. Unfortunately, however, readers know little of how the children brought about these clinical benefits or of how long they managed to keep them.

Another intervention setting is the home. Therapists treating there may instruct obese children, siblings of these children, and parents about modifications to make both in home and away from it. Giving prescriptions and evaluating compliance may be aided by home observations on selected targets (see Coates, 1977 on adolescents). Much of the child's treatment, therefore, may occur in the child's home. The literature, however, reflects no trend towards home-based treatment. Nor does it reflect a trend toward making comparative feasibility studies of the various possible treatment sites. For the most part, single-setting or multiple-setting demonstrations that rely on showing Point A (weight) changes exist. These programs treat without determining if there are specific effects traceable to specific settings.

Evaluative studies to correct this insufficiency would be welcome. One eventual product of regimens that combine for example office, school, and home-based programs for obese children, while probing for setting-specific effects, will be comprehensive plans that seek and predict multiple changes. In order to bring about these multiple changes, these comprehensive plans may enlist multiple agents of change, the significant individuals, with whom, as Brownell and Kaye indicate, the obese child associates. They are brothers, sisters, and classmates who are taught to help him follow specific prescriptions and who are taught to stop denigrating obesity with words and deeds, to stop promoting the vicious circle (see Chapter 2). They are also teachers who learn to deliver and monitor components of behavioral programs. And they are parents, grandparents, aunts, and uncles who learn to support the child's efforts, perhaps by praise, by ceasing to bicker, and by stopping contradictory messages. They are a number of persons who are given parts to play in mounting a total offensive on the obese child's behalf; future research will uncover what these parts should be, who should be given what part, and how best to teach.

About parents and their roles, various questions follow:

1. How much and what kinds of parent involvement (such as interveners, as supporters of therapist-run programs) for which children (for example, different ages, different degrees of control over food acquisition) furthers or interferes with the goals of treatment?
2. How much and what kinds of parent involvement for which children furthers or interferes with the goals of maintenance (see Cohen et al., 1980)?
3. What skills should parents be taught for treatment and for maintenance? Is teaching problem-solving skills an efficient way to reduce the need for renewed professional intervention?
   a. What is the value of programmed texts with video and audio supplementation in teaching parents?
   b. Should parents be taught by becoming patients themselves or by remaining untreated partners with the therapist (see Epstein et al., 1981; Applications 8 and 9, Chapter 5).
4. What pre-treatment practices of parents in relation to their children affect how they should be included in therapy and what they should be taught?

Questions about Prevention

Can childhood obesity be prevented? What value is there in preventing it? If it is valuable to prevent it, when is the optimal time to take preventive steps? What should these steps be? Today, prevention is an arguable topic (Coates & Thoresen, 1980). There are many who advise that it be tackled (for example, Bray, 1979; Court, 1979; Golden, 1979; Lloyd, 1977; Lloyd & Wolf, 1980; Myres & Yeung, 1979; Weil, 1977). And there are a few who have risen to the challenge.

For example, though cognizant of the large amount of disagreement that one can find on the subject, Pisacano, Lichter, Ritter, and Siegal (1978) are nonetheless supportive of attempting preventive efforts. In their discussion, they suggest that modifying an infant's taste preferences, by modifying his diet, will alter the development of subsequent obesity and perhaps, by so doing, affect his later well-being. They report that teaching mothers of 80 three-month-old infants to use Prudent Diet principles in feeding the babies lowered the numbers of these infants who were overweight; they were compared with 50 other babies, seen earlier, fed a more traditional bill-of-fare. At age three, greater than 25 percent of the traditionally fed were still overweight—change in prevalence of overweight from three months to three years had been about a 9 percent decrease. Change in overweight prevalence for the Prudent Diet group had been far more dramatic—from 25 percent of them being overweight at three months to about 1.3 percent of them at three years.

As an aspect of prevention, conditioning food preferences (acceptances) is in its early stages. Brownell and Stunkard (1980a), like Pisacano and colleagues, highlight its potential; they cite studies that attempt to modify food likes among the very young and nonobese. In one Brownell and Stunkard discuss, the food acceptances of toddlers are manipulated. Herbert-Jackson and Risley (1977), its authors, showed that they could increase the supply of protein and calcium preschoolers and toddlers received without substantially adding to the caloric content of the youngsters's diets. Twenty-one children at a day care center were subjects in this investigation; they ranged in age from 1 to 2.5 years. While at the center, the children had snacks and lunch daily. Briefly, Herbert-Jackson and Risley looked at the willingness of these children to sample recipes with and without the addition of meat, textured vegetable protein (TVP), or nonfat dry milk solids. They found that whereas preferences for particular foods existed, the preferences were unaffected by the presence or absence of the supplements. Also which supplements were used had no major impact. Notably, compared to meat, TVP and nonfat dry milk solids are inexpensive, easy to store, nutritional, and low in calories (see also Herbert-Jackson & Risely, 1975, 1976; Herbert-Jackson, Cross, & Risley, 1977).

In a less controlled study, Hofacker and Brenner (1976) report a simple maneuver for getting hospitalized children to consume more vegetables. Essentially, the authors associated the act of eating these foods with growing "strong and beautiful." Thirteen dieticians dressed themselves in costumes depicting vegetables and, after being introduced to the youngsters in the audience, paraded— "Vegetable parade"—in front of them. A party of vegetable eating followed. This low-cost, award-winning strategy for reducing neophobia (Rozin, 1976) led to sampling vegetables and throwing less of them away; follow-up was, unfortunately, brief (see also, Madsen, Madsen, & Thompson, 1974).

Focusing on not only food choices but also eating and activity behaviors, Smiciklas-Wright and D'Augelli (1978) described (no outcome data presented) their obesity prevention effort. This study recognized and capitalized on the family's impact on the child's diet, ingestion, and activity (see Hertzler, 1981).

The authors taught parents, small groups of them at one time, to assess family patterns in these areas, to modify them, and to evaluate the modifications accomplished. The five-week program they offer is interdisciplinary; for example, nutritionists and behaviorists head it. In addition to dealing with calorie intake and expenditure, the program also taught parents to handle new problems almost certain to arise afterwards. In short, it attempted to foster preparedness. Mothers and fathers were taught the behavior modification process (see Chapter 3) of assessment, intervention, and evaluation.

The worth in relation to price of such an effort remains to be seen. What to teach families and the immediate as well as long-term effects of the teachings greatly need study:

1. Which youngsters (for example, both parents obese) are most likely to profit from obesity prevention attempts? What characteristics do they manifest?
2. What nutritional, activity, and behavioral teachings should be directed at families with children designated as candidates for obesity-prevention programs? For example, will and when will sustained exercise increments forestall adipose hypercellularity and diminish the probability of refractory adult obesity (see Thompson et al., 1982)?
3. How valuable will programmed texts about preventing obesity be in well-baby clinics?
4. What impact, positive and negative effects and side effects, have childhood obesity prevention programs on the physical, social, and psychological well-being of youngsters as they grow into adolescence and adulthood (see Coates & Thoresen, 1980)?

Conclusions

Doubtless, there are a multitude of other questions for behavioral researchers and practitioners to ask about behavior therapy for the obese child. To be of greatest service, to substantially change the picture of treatment painted in Chapter 1, behavior therapy will have to grow: It will have to target more comprehensively; it will have to evaluate its immediate and long-term effects more completely; it will have to develop its methods and measurements more stringently. Such growth, coupled with efforts to ascertain what procedures work best for whom will help it to better meet the needs of obese children who differ in age, background, and need.

Relatedly, behavior therapy will have to examine policies for lowering its costs and raising its benefits: It will have to cultivate practices in new therapy settings and ways to deploy the potentially signficant agents of change already in them.

Further, behavior therapy will have to wade into the muddy waters of prevention: It is here, ultimately, that it may do the most good for children.

Finally, behavior therapy will more and more have to accept a component role in and be accepted as a vital component of child health care and child health research: It will have to increasingly become one of the tools of programs for obesity control and one of those for prevention that various professionals (for example, dieticians, pediatricians, physical educators) jointly orchestrate. Indeed, it will have to play such an interdisciplinary part if it is ever to improve its chances against narrow outcomes, outcomes that are at best only statistically not clinically significant.

Much remains to be done.

Appendixes

Appendix A
Recommended Dietary Allowances

FOOD AND NUTRITION BOARD, NATIONAL ACADEMY OF SCIENCES-NATIONAL RESEARCH COUNCIL
RECOMMENDED DAILY DIETARY ALLOWANCES,[a] Revised 1980

Designed for the maintenance of good nutrition of practically all healthy people in the U.S.A.

Age (years)	Weight (kg)	Weight (lb)	Height (cm)	Height (in)	Protein (g)	Vita-min A (µg RE)[b]	Vita-min D (µg)[c]	Vita-min E (mg α-TE)[d]	Vita-min C (mg)	Thia-min (mg)	Ribo-flavin (mg)	Niacin (mg NE)[e]	Vita-min B-6 (mg)	Fola-cin (µg)[f]	Vitamin B-12 (µg)	Cal-cium (mg)	Phos-phorus (mg)	Mag-nesium (mg)	Iron (mg)	Zinc (mg)	Iodine (µg)
Infants																					
0.0-0.5	6	13	60	24	kg × 2.2	420	10	3	35	0.3	0.4	6	0.3	30	0.5[g]	360	240	50	10	3	40
0.5-1.0	9	20	71	28	kg × 2.0	400	10	4	35	0.5	0.6	8	0.6	45	1.5	540	360	70	15	5	50
Children																					
1-3	13	29	90	35	23	400	10	5	45	0.7	0.8	9	0.9	100	2.0	800	800	150	15	10	70
4-6	20	44	112	44	30	500	10	6	45	0.9	1.0	11	1.3	200	2.5	800	800	200	10	10	90
7-10	28	62	132	52	34	700	10	7	45	1.2	1.4	16	1.6	300	3.0	800	800	250	10	10	120
Males																					
11-14	45	99	157	62	45	1000	10	8	50	1.4	1.6	18	1.8	400	3.0	1200	1200	350	18	15	150
15-18	66	145	176	69	56	1000	10	10	60	1.4	1.7	18	2.0	400	3.0	1200	1200	400	18	15	150
19-22	70	154	177	70	56	1000	7.5	10	60	1.5	1.7	19	2.2	400	3.0	800	800	350	10	15	150
23-50	70	154	178	70	56	1000	5	10	60	1.4	1.6	18	2.2	400	3.0	800	800	350	10	15	150
51+	70	154	178	70	56	1000	5	10	60	1.2	1.4	16	2.2	400	3.0	800	800	350	10	15	150
Females																					
11-14	46	101	157	62	46	800	10	8	50	1.1	1.3	15	1.8	400	3.0	1200	1200	300	18	15	150
15-18	55	120	163	64	46	800	10	8	60	1.1	1.3	14	2.0	400	3.0	1200	1200	300	18	15	150
19-22	55	120	163	64	44	800	7.5	8	60	1.1	1.3	14	2.0	400	3.0	800	800	300	18	15	150
23-50	55	120	163	64	44	800	5	8	60	1.0	1.2	13	2.0	400	3.0	800	800	300	18	15	150
51+	55	120	163	64	44	800	5	8	60	1.0	1.2	13	2.0	400	3.0	800	800	300	10	15	150
Pregnant					+30	+200	+5	+2	+20	+0.4	+0.3	+2	+0.6	+400	+1.0	+400	+400	+150	h	+5	+25
Lactating					+20	+400	+5	+3	+40	+0.5	+0.5	+5	+0.5	+100	+1.0	+400	+400	+150	h	+10	+50

[a] The allowances are intended to provide for individual variations among most normal persons as they live in the United States under usual environmental stresses. Diets should be based on a variety of common foods in order to provide other nutrients for which human requirements have been less well defined.

[b] Retinol equivalents. 1 retinol equivalent = 1 µg retinol or 6 µg β carotene.

[c] As cholecalciferol. 10 µg cholecalciferol = 400 IU of vitamin D.

[d] α-tocopherol equivalents. 1 mg d-α tocopherol = 1 α-TE.

[e] 1 NE (niacin equivalent) is equal to 1 mg of niacin or 60 mg of dietary tryptophan.

[f] The folacin allowances refer to dietary sources as determined by *Lactobacillus casei* assay after treatment with enzymes (conjugases) to make polyglutamyl forms of the vitamin available to the test organism.

[g] The recommended dietary allowance for vitamin B-12 in infants is based on average concentration of the vitamin in human milk. The allowances after weaning are based on energy intake (as recommended by the American Academy of Pediatrics) and consideration of other factors, such as intestinal absorption.

[g] The increased requirement during pregnancy cannot be met by the iron content of habitual American diets nor by the existing iron stores of many women; therefore the use of 30-60 mg of supplemental iron is recommended. Iron needs during lactation are not substantially different from those of nonpregnant women, but continued supplementation of the mother for 2-3 months after parturition is advisable in order to replenish stores depleted by pregnancy.

189

Food	Calories by Weight or Portion (Kcal)
Apple (raw)	16/28 g
Artichoke (boiled)	13/28 g
Asparagus (whole spears)	6/28 g
Bacon (fried, drained)	
Canadian	2.8/1 g
Strips	6/1 g
Bananas (raw with skin)	17/28 g
Beans	
Green (boiled)	7/28 g
Kidney (cooked)	33/28 g
Lima (cooked)	39/28 g
Bologna	3/1 g
Bread	
White	65/one slice
Wheat	57/one slice
Broccoli (boiled, drained)	8/28 g
Butter	34/1 tsp
Cake	
Angel food	2.8/1 g
Chocolate layer	3.3/1 g
Gingerbread	2.8/1 g
Pound cake	4.1/1 g
Candy	
Caramel (plain)	4/1 g
Chocolate peanuts	5.6/1 g
Milk chocolate (Hershey)	5.4/1 g
Granola bar	5/1 g
Cantaloupe (raw with skin)	4/28 g
Carrots (raw)	12/28 g
Cashews (shelled, roasted)	5.7/1 g
Catsup	1.1/1 g
Cauliflower (fresh)	3/28 g
Celery	4/28 g
Cereals (ready to eat)	
Sugar first ingredient	3.9/1 g
Sugar second ingredient	2.5/1 g
Granola (with raisins & almonds)	4.3/1 g
Cheese	
American (processed)	3.8/1 g
Cheddar	4/1 g
Cottage (creamed)	1/1 g

Food	Calories by Weight or Portion (Kcal)
Cheese (Continued)	
Cottage (uncreamed)	.9/1 g
Monterey jack	3.6/1 g
Swiss (processed)	3.6/1 g
Cheese spread (processed)	2.8/1 g
Cherries (raw)	13/28 g
Chewing gum	
Regular	9/1 stick
Sugarless	8/1 stick
Bubble gum (large)	85/1 piece
Chicken	
Broiled meat	1.4/1 g
Pot pie	9.9/1 g
Cookies (plain)	5/1 g
Corn on cob (raw, no husks)	15/28 g
Corned Beef (cooked)	3.8/1 g
Crab (steamed without shell)	.9/1 g
Crackers	
Graham	3.8/1 g
Saltines	4.3/1 g
Cucumber (raw, with skin)	3.9/28 g
Cupcakes (plain)	3.7/1 g
Doughnuts	
Cake (plain)	3.9/1 g
Jelly	3.5/1 g
Powdered	4.9/1 g
Eggs	
Fried	86/1 medium
Scrambled (milk added)	97/1 medium
Flounder (baked)	2/1 g
Frankfurters (cooked)	3/1 g
Grapefruit (raw, pulp)	11.5/28 g
Grapes (raw with seeds & stems)	12/28 g
Gumdrops	3.5/1 g
Halibut (broiled fillets)	1.7/1 g
Ham (cooked, roasted)	
Lean and fat	3.5/1 g
Lean only	2.1/1 g
Hamburger	
Ground beef (lean, cooked)	2.2/1 g
Ground round (lean, cooked)	1.9/1 g

Food	Calories by Weight or Portion (Kcal)
Honey	3/1 g
Ice Cream	
12% fat	2/1 g
16% fat	2.2/1 g
Ice milk	1.5/1 g
Jelly beans	2.4/1 g
Lamb	
Chops (loin, lean, cooked)	1.9/1 g
Shoulder (roasted, no bone)	3.4/1 g
Lettuce (raw)	2.9/28 g
Liver (beef, fried)	2.3/1 g
Lobster (cooked meat)	.96/1 g
Luncheon meat	
Boiled ham	2.3/1 g
Salami	3.1/1 g
Macaroni	
Cooked (10 min)	1.5/1 g
Cooked (15 min)	1.1/1 g
Margarine (reg.)	23/1 tsp
Meat Loaf	2/1 g
Milk (cup approx. 245 g)	
Whole	160/1 cup
2%	145/1 cup
Skim	88/1 cup
M & M's (regular)	5/1 g
Mushrooms (raw, whole, untrimmed)	7.8/28 g
Mustard	1.1/1 g
Noodles (egg)	
Uncooked	3.8/1 g
Cooked	1.2/1 g
Oranges (raw, peeled)	14/28 g
Peach (raw)	11/28 g
Peanuts (roasted)	
With skins	5.8/1 g
Without skins	5.8/1 g
Peanut butter	6/1 g
Pears (raw)	17/28 g
Plum (Damson, without pits)	18/28 g
Pop (see Soft drinks)	
Popcorn (popped)	
In oil, no butter	4.6/1 g
Plain	3.9/1 g

Food	Calories by Weight or Portion (Kcal)
Pork Chops (lean, broiled)	2.8/1 g
Pork Sausage (cooked)	4.8/1 g
Potatoes (cooked)	
Baked in skin	.9/1 g
Boiled in skin	.8/1 g
French-fried	2.7/1 g
Mashed (with milk)	.7/1 g
Raisins	2.9/1 g
Rice (cooked, long grain)	1/1 g
Roasts	
Rib (lean, cooked)	2.4/1 g
Rump (lean, cooked)	2.1/1 g
Salmon (meat)	
Canned (red, sockeye)	1.7/1 g
Fresh (broiled)	1.2/1 g
Scallops (cooked)	1.1/1 g
Shrimp (fried with bread crumbs, batter)	2.3/1 g
Soft Drinks	
Colas	146/360 ml
Gingerale	130/360 ml
Root Beer	155/360 ml
Seven-Up	146/360 ml
Soup	
Chicken consomme	44/one cup
Cream of chicken	115/one cup
Split pea	130/one cup
Vegetable	75/one cup
Sour cream	9/1 tsp
Spaghetti	
Cooked (10 min)	1.5/1 g
Cooked (15 min)	1.1/1 g
Spareribs (pork, cooked)	
fatty	4.7/1 g
thin	4.1/1 g
Spinach (raw, untrimmed)	7.4/28 g
Steak (beef, broiled, lean)	
Club	4.5/1 g
Porterhouse	4.6/1 g
T-bone	4.7/1 g
Sirloin	3.9/1 g
Strawberries (raw, trimmed)	10.5/28 g

Food	Calories by Weight or Portion (Kcal)
Tomato (raw, unpeeled)	6.3/28 g
Tuna (canned)	
In oil (drained)	1.9/1 g
In water	1.2/1 g
Turkey (roasted)	
Meat and skin	2.2/1 g
Light meat only	1.8/1 g
Dark meat only	2/1 g
Veal chop (medium fat, loin, cooked)	2.4/1 g
Watermelon	3.5/28 g
Yogurt	
Fruit	1-1.2/1 g
Plain (partially skimmed)	.5-.6/1 g

Sources: Kraus, B., *Calories and Carbohydrates*. New York: Grosset and Dunlap, 1979; Chaback, E., *The Complete Calorie Counter*. New York: Dell, 1979; Netzer, C., and Chaback, E. *Brand-Name Calorie Counter* (abridged). New York: Dell, 1979; Pennington, J. A. T., and Church, H. Nichols, *Food Values of Portions Commonly Used* (13 Edition). New York: Harper & Row, 1980; Watt, B. K., and Merrill, A. L. *Composition of Foods* (Agriculture Handbook No. 8, U.S. Department of Agriculture). Washington, D.C.: U.S. Government Printing Office, 1975.

Listing is alphabetical and calorie values are approximations.

Appendix C
Calorie Outgo Levels
for Prolonged Activities

Prolonged Activity	Approximate Calories Expended per Minute for 41 kg Person
Badminton	
Playing moderately	3.4
Playing strenuously	5.8
Biking	
Slowly (5 mph)	3
Fast (13 mph)	6.4
Running (Jogging)	
Take your time jog (5 mph)	6
Faster pace (7.5 mph)	9
Really moving (10 mph)	12
Skating	3-9
Skiing (Cross-country)	
Leisurely pace (3 mph)	5+
Moderate pace (5 mph)	7
Soccer	5.4
Swimming (Crawl)	
Slow	2.8
Fast	6.4
Tennis	4+
Walking	
Stroll (2 mph)	2+
Fair clip (3 mph+)	3+

Sources: Fitness Finders, *A Unique Approach to Personal Fitness*. Pennsylvania: Fitness Finders, 1969; Jordan, H. A., Levitz, L. S., and Kimbrell, G. M. *Eating is Okay*. New York: Rawson Associates, 1976; Sharkey, B. J. *Physiological Fitness and Weight Control*. Missoula: Mountain Press Publishing Co., 1974.

Calorie levels are approximations for a 41 kg person. Add 10 percent for each 7 kg above 41 kg and subtract 10 percent for each 7 kg under 41 kg. The table is to be used only as a guide for increasing prolonged activities (see Chapter 6).

Appendix D
Growth Charts (Height, Weight, Age)

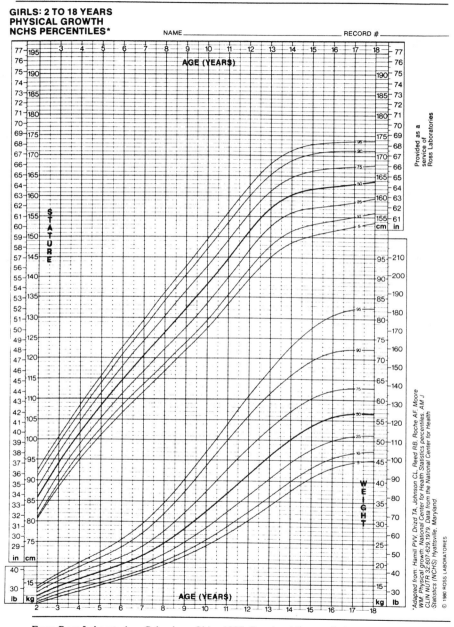

**GIRLS: 2 TO 18 YEARS
PHYSICAL GROWTH
NCHS PERCENTILES***

NAME _____ RECORD # _____

From Ross Laboratories, Columbus, Ohio, 1980. Reprinted by permission.

The weight objective may be set by first determining the percentile rank of the patient's height for age (upper curves) and then finding his or her weight at the same percentile rank and age (lower curves).

196

Appendix D (continued)
Growth Charts (Height, Weight, Age)

BOYS: 2 TO 18 YEARS
PHYSICAL GROWTH
NCHS PERCENTILES*

NAME_____ RECORD #_____

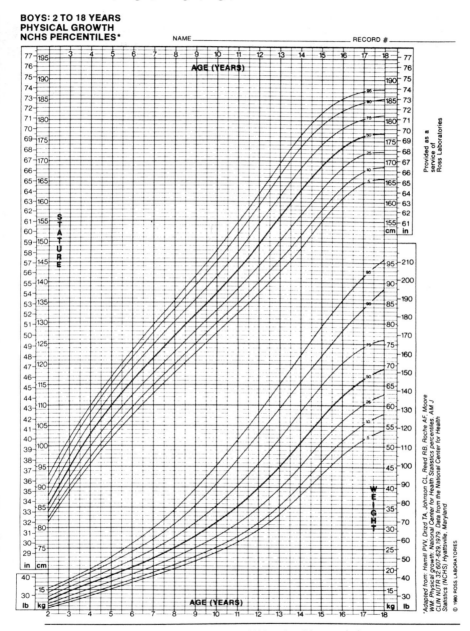

From Ross Laboratories, Columbus, Ohio, 1980. Reprinted by permission.

The weight objective may be set by first determining the percentile rank of the patient's height for age (upper curves) and then finding his or her weight at the same percentile rank and age (lower curves).

Appendix E
Triceps Skinfold Percentiles—Smoothed percentiles of triceps skinfold for boys
2–18 years, by age: United States, 1963–65, 1966–70, and 1971–74

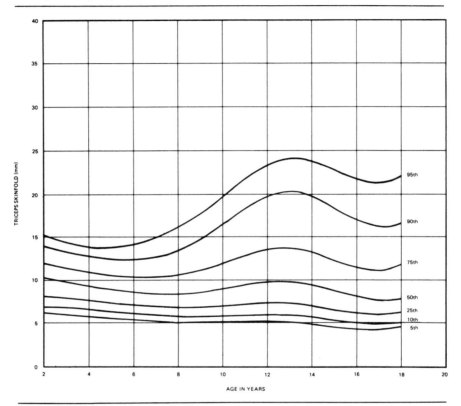

Source: Johnson, C. L., Fulwood, R., Abraham, S., and Bryner, J. D. *Basic Data on Anthro-*
pometric Measurements and Angular Measurements of the Hip and Knee Joints for Selected Age
Groups 1–74 Years of Age. (Vital and Health Statistics: Series 11; no.219, D.H.H.S. Publication
No., PHS 81–1669). Hyattsville, Maryland: US Department of Health and Human Resources,
1981.

These values are not to be considered "ideals" (Owen, 1982).

Appendix E (continued)
Triceps Skinfold Percentiles—Smoothed percentiles of triceps skinfold for girls ages 2–18, by age: United States, 1963–65, 1966–70, and 1971–74

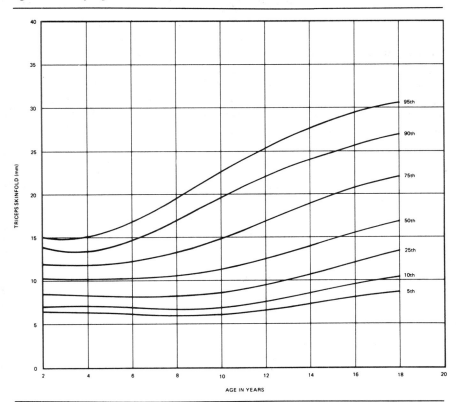

Source: Johnson, C. L., Fulwood, R., Abraham, S., and Bryner, J. D. *Basic Data on Anthropometric Measurements and Angular Measurements of the Hip and Knee Joints for Selected Age Groups 1–74 Years of Age.* (Vital and Health Statistics: Series 11; no.219, D.H.H.S. Publication No., PHS 81–1669). Hyattsville, Maryland: US Department of Health and Human Resources, 1981.

These values are not to be considered "ideals" (Owen, 1982).

Physician Consent Form

I am aware that my patient, _____,
is participating in a behavioral control program for obesity at the

_____ .
According to my knowledge, there is no medical reason that would prevent
_____ from participating in this
program. The calorie intake level assigned to this patient will not likely be
lower than _____ .

Physician's signature _____
Date _____

Appendix G
Interview with Contradictory Message Listing

Name: _____

Birthdate: _____   Address_____

Height: _____ in. _____ cm.   Phone no. _____

Weight: _____ lb. _____ kg

Right arm skinfold _____

Waist size: _____

Number of years of school completed: Mother: _____ years
                                                                              Father: _____ years

Occupation: Mother: _____ Father: _____

Ethnic origin: Mother: _____ Father: _____

Approximate annual family income: _____

Child's Obesity History

Age of obesity onset (when was it first noticed?) _____

Are any other family members or close relatives overweight?

Yes _____ No _____

    If yes, who? (relation to child) _____

      how much overweight?   _____ lb _____ lb _____ lb

      age of obesity onset ? _____

Is the child currently in a period of: (check one)

    weight gain _____

    weight loss _____

    constant weight _____

Has the child engaged in any dieting attempts?   Yes _____   No _____

If yes, how many attempts within the past 12 months? _____

    Who initiated the last dieting attempt ? _____

    What was the child's reaction to the last dieting attempt?

    _____

    Was the last dieting attempt successful or unsuccessful?

    _____

    What was the reason for terminating the last diet?

    _____

    On the average, how long does a dieting attempt last?

    _____

Is the child presently taking any medications? Yes_____   No_____
If yes, are they parent- or physician-prescribed? _____
What is the child's past medical history of:
  illness? _____
  operations?_____
  accompanying medications?_____
Were there any accompanying weight changes?   Yes_____ No_____

Eating Practices

How many formal (sit-down) meals does the child have per day?_____
Does the whole family eat at the same time for each meal?
  Yes_____   No_____
  If not, with whom does the child eat:
    Breakfast?_____
    Lunch? _____
    Dinner? _____

Does the child eat snacks between meals?   Yes_____ No_____
If yes, what do these snacks usually consist of?_____
What time(s) of day does snacking occur?_____
What is the child doing while snacking? _____
Are snacks readily available to the child? Yes_____No_____
Who else in the family snacks between meals? _____
What time(s) of day does snacking occur?_____
What activities are usually accompanied by snacking?_____
When eating a meal, is the child served portions of food?
  Yes_____ No_____
  If yes, who generally serves the food? _____
Is the child encouraged to "clean up" the food on his/her plate?
  Yes_____ No_____
Is it common to reward the child with food for being good?
  Yes_____ No_____
Is the child's eating ever restricted as a form of punishment?
  Yes_____ No_____
Does the child eat lunch at school? Yes_____ No_____
Must the child spend lunch time in the school cafeteria?
  Yes_____ No_____
  If no, where may the students go for lunch? _____
When the child and friends are together, is it common for the group to buy
snacks? Yes_____ No_____
When going to a movie, is the child given money for treats?
  Yes_____ No_____
When out shopping, do you usually stop for snacks? Yes_____ No_____

Activity Practices

Does the child engage in any regular sports activities?
  Yes _____ No _____
  If yes, what kind?_____
Do other family members engage in regular sports activities?
  Yes _____ No _____
  If yes, who? _____
  What kind? _____
How many hours per day does the child spend watching TV?
  _____ hrs/day
How many hours per day does the child spend reading? _____ hrs/day
Does the child know how to:
  Ride a bike?   Yes _____   No _____
  Swim?   Yes _____   No _____
  Roller-skate?   Yes _____   No _____
  Ice skate?   Yes _____   No _____
How close is the nearest playground or gymnasium? _____
  How frequently does the child go there? _____ (times per month)
When the child gets together with friends, what kind of activity does the
group usually engage in?_____
What is the child's general means of transportation to and from
school? _____
  How far away is school? _____

Attitude Questionnaire

Is the child's obesity a problem? Yes _____ No _____
  If yes, in what way is it a problem?_____
  If no, do you think it might become a problem in the future?
  Yes _____No_____
  If yes, in what way? _____
Do you think it is healthier for a child to be overweight than it is for a
child to be underweight? Yes _____ No _____
Do family members ever tease the child about being overweight?
  Yes _____No _____
What do you think is the major cause of the child's overweight condition?
_____
Is this major cause controllable? Yes_____ No_____
  If yes, how? _____
  If no, why not? _____
Do you think that society is biased against obese children?

Yes _____ No _____
If yes, in what way? _____
Do you think that society is biased against obese adults?
Yes _____ No _____
If yes, in what way? _____

Social Skills (For interviewer to estimate)

Self Perception

Body image
Athletic prowess
Physical attractiveness

Contradictory Messages (See Ch. 2)

Message Surveyed: Clean your plate if you want dessert, but you're getting too
fat from eating too many sweets.
At dinnertime, are you ever told that food is costly and you shouldn't
waste it? Yes ( ) No ( )
*How often during the week are you told at dinnertime that food is very
costly and you shouldn't waste it? _____ .
At dinnertime, are you ever told to think of those who are starving—those
who aren't as lucky as you?
Yes ( ) No ( )
*How often at dinnertime during the week are you told to think about people
who are starving? _____ .
How often each week are you told that eating sweet things like pie, ice
cream, cookies and cake makes people heavy? _____ .
Who tells you, if anyone, that eating sweet things like pie, ice cream, and
cake makes people heavy? _____ .
Do your parents ever tell you that you do not eat enough at dinner?
Yes ( ) No ( )
Do your parents ever tell you that you eat too much at dinner?
Yes ( ) No ( )
Do your parents ever tell you that you eat too many sweets?
Yes ( ) No ( )
To eat dessert, do you have to finish your dinner?
Yes ( ) No ( )
Who, if anyone, ever tells you that to get dessert you should eat all
your dinner? _____ .
How often each week are you told to finish your dinner?
_____ .

Message Surveyed: Food is splendor, but fat is ugly.
   Do your parents ever say that it is bad for someone to be overweight?
   Yes (   )   No (   )
  * How many times last week did your parents say that?
   _____

   Do your brothers or sisters ever say that being overweight is bad?
   Yes (   ) No (   )   *How often?_____
   What does a fancy dinner at your house consist of?
   _____

   _____

   How many times last month did you have fancy dinners?
   _____

   Typically, what is served for dinner?
   _____

Message Surveyed: Eat to be friendly, but best friends aren't fat.
   How many times a week do you go with your friends somewhere to
   buy food? _____ .
   How many times a week do you go somewhere with your friends to eat
   something (e.g., ice cream, candy)? _____ .
   Do friends at school ever give you things to eat?
   Yes (   )   No (   )
   Do kids in school ever tease other kids for being overweight?
   Yes (   )   No (   )
   Are some of your good friends overweight?
   Yes (   )   No (   )
   Who are your best friends?   (Names) _____

   _____

   _____

Message Surveyed: Play with us to be one of us, but we don't like fatsos.
   Do you like sports? Yes (   )   No (   )
   Do kids at school or on your block nearby or ever choose you to play on
   a team? Yes (   )   No (   )
   Do teachers at school ever ask you to play on a team?
   Yes (   )   No (   )
   Are overweight people ever good at team sports?
   Yes (   )   No (   )
   [If the answer is no to the above question, ask] :   Does a person have to
   be thin or muscular to be good at team sports? Yes (   )   No (   )

Do you play team sports after school?
Yes ( )   No ( )
Do you play team sports at recess?
Yes ( )   No ( )

When possible, information is to be obtained from patient.

*Ask only if preceding question is answered "Yes."

From Rallo, 1982. Also from Michael D. LeBow, *Weight Control: The Behavioural Strategies* (Chichester: John Wiley & Sons, Ltd.,1981, pp. 300–302). Copyright © 1981 by John Wiley & Sons, Ltd. Reprinted by permission of the publisher.

References

Abraham, S., Collins, G., & Nordsieck, M. Relationship of childhood weight status to morbidity in adults. *Public Health Reports,* 1971, 86, 273–284.

Abraham, S. & Nordsieck, M. Relationship of excess weight in children and adults. *Public Health Reports,* 1960, 25, 263–273.

Abrahms, J. L. & Allen, G. J. Comparative effectiveness of situational programming, financial payoffs, and group pressures in weight reduction. *Behavior Therapy,* 1974, 5, 391–400.

Abramson, E. E. & Jones, D. Reducing junk food palatibility and consumption by aversive conditioning. *Addictive Behaviors,* 1981, 6, 145–148.

Adams, N., Ferguson, J., Stunkard, A. J., & Agras, S. The eating behavior of obese and nonobese women. *Behaviour Research and Therapy,* 1978, 16, 225–232.

Addison, R. M. & Homme, L. The reinforcing event (RE) menu. *NSPI Journal,* 1966, 5, 8–9.

Alley, R. A., Narduzzi, J. V., Robbins, T. J., Weir, T. F., Sabeh, G., & Danowski, T. S. Measuring success in the reduction of obesity in childhood. *Clinical Pediatrics,* 1968, 7, 112–118.

Allon, N. Tensions in interactions of overweight adolescent girls. *Women Health,* 1976, 1, 14–23.

Allon, N. Sociological aspects of overweight youth. In P. J. Collipp (Ed.), *Childhood obesity* (2nd ed.). Littleton, Massachusetts: PSG Publishing, 1980.

Altman, K., Bondy, A., & Hirsch, G. Behavioral treatment of obesity in patients with Prader-Willi syndrome. *Journal of Behavioral Medicine,* 1978, 1, 403–412.

Anderson, A. E., Soper, R. T., Scott, D. H. Gastric bypass for morbid obesity in children and adolescents. *Journal of Pediatric Surgery,* 1980, 15, 876–881.

Andres, R. Influence of obesity on longevity in the aged. *Advances in Pathobiology,* 1980, 7, 238–246.

Apfelbaum, M., Fumeron, F., Dunica, S., Magnet, M., Brigant, L., Boulange, A., & Hors, J. Genetic approach to family obesity: Study of HLA antigens in 10 families and 86 unrelated obese subjects. *Biomedicine,* 1980, 33, 98–100.

Aragona, J., Cassady, J., & Drabman, R. Treating overweight children through parental training and contingency contracting. *Journal of Applied Behavior Analysis*, 1975, 8, 269–278.

Arteaga, H. P., DosSantos, J. E., Dutra de Oliviera, J. E. Obesity among school children of different socioeconomic levels in a developing country. *International Journal of Obesity*, 1982, 6, 291–297.

Ashby, W. A. & Wilson, G. T. Behavior therapy for obesity: Booster sessions and long-term maintenance of weight loss. *Behaviour Research and Therapy*, 1977, 15, 451–464.

Asher, P. Fat babies and fat children: The prognosis of obesity in the very young. *Archives of Diseases in Childhood*, 1966, 41, 672–673.

Asher, W. L. Obese teenagers. In P. J. Collipp (Ed.), *Childhood obesity* (2nd ed.). Littleton, Massachusetts: PSG Publishing, 1980.

Ashwell, M., Priest, P., & Bondoux, M. Adipose tissue cellularity in obese women. In A. Howard (Ed.), *Recent advances in obesity research: I*. London: Newman Publishing, 1975.

Ayllon, T. Intensive treatment of psychotic behavior by stimulus satiation and food reinforcement. *Behaviour Research and Therapy*, 1963, 1, 53–61.

Ayllon, T. & Azrin, N. H. *The token economy: A motivational system for therapy and rehabilitation*. New York: Appleton-Century-Crofts, 1968.

Bacon, G. E. & Lowrey, G. H. A clinical trial of fenfluramine in obese children. *Current Therapy Research*, 1967, 9, 626–634.

Baer, D. M. A note on the absence of Santa Claus in any known ecosystem: A rejoinder to Willems. *Journal of Applied Behavior Analysis*, 1974, 7, 167–169.

Baer, D. M. & Wolf, M. M. *The entry into natural communities of reinforcement*. Paper presented at the Meeting of the American Psychological Association, Washington, D. C., 1967.

Baer, D. M. Wolf, M. M., & Risley, T. R. Some current dimensions of applied behavior analysis, *Journal of Applied Behavior Analysis*, 1968, 1, 91–97.

Ballard, B. B., Gipson, M. T, Guttenberg, W., & Ramsey, K. Palatibility of food as a factor influencing obese and normal-weight childrens' eating habits. *Behaviour Research and Therapy*, 1980, 18, 598–600.

Bandura, A. *Principles of behavior modification*. New York: Holt, Rinehart & Winston, 1969.

Bandura, A. & Simon, K. M. The role of proximal intentions in self-regulation of refractory behavior. *Cognitive Therapy and Research*, 1977, 1, 177–194.

Baritussio, A., Enzi, G., Rigon, G., Molinori, M., Fnelmen, E. M., Crebaldi, G. Effect of anorexiant drugs on growth hormone secretion in obese children. *Pharmacological Research Communications*, 1978, 10, 529–540.

Barker, V. C. J. The angle of obesity: A simple measurement for body typing. *New Zealand Medical Journal*, 1976, 84, 437–439.

Beaven, S. J. Attitudes to appearance in adolescence. *Journal of Human Nutrition*, 1981, 35, 335–338.

Beck, S. Epstein, L. H., Wing, R. R., & Ossip, D. J. *The effects of lifestyle and programmed exercise on weight loss in obese children.* Poster presented at the meeting of Association for Advancement of Behavior Therapy, New York, 1980.

Bellack, A. S. Behavior therapy for weight reduction. *Addictive Behaviors,* 1975, 1, 73–82.

Bellack, A. S., Glanz, L. M., & Simon, R. Self-reinforcement style and covert imagery in the treatment of obesity. *Journal of Consulting and Clinical Psychology,* 1976, 44, 490–491.

Bellack, A. S. & Rozensky, R. H. The selection of dependent variables for weight reduction studies. *Journal of Behavior Therapy and Experimental Psychiatry,* 1975, 6, 83–84.

Bellack, A. S. & Schwartz, J. Assessment for self-control programs. In M. Hersen & A. S. Bellack (Eds.), *Behavioral assessment: A practical handbook.* New York: Pergamon Press, 1976.

Berchtold, P., Jorgens, V., Finke, C., & Berger, M. Epidemiology of obesity and hypertension. *International Journal of Obesity,* 1981, 5(Suppl. 1), 1–7.

Berendez, H. W. Effect of maternal acetonuria on I.Q. of offspring. In H. S. Cole (Ed.), *Early diabetes in early life.* New York: Academic Press, 1975.

Berenson, G. S. Risk factors in children—the early natural history of atherosclerosis. In G. Schettler, Y. Goto, & G. Klose (Eds.), *Atherosclerosis IV.* Heidelberg, Germany: Springer-Verlag, 1977.

Berenson, G.S., Foster, M.S., Frank, G.C., Frerichs, R. R., Srinivasan, S. R., Voors, A. W., & Webber, L. S. Cardiovascular disease risk factor variables at the preschool age—The Bogalusa Heart Study. *Circulation,* 1978, 57, 603–612.

Bernfeld, J. & Lesieur, G. Eating habits of the obese child and its family. *Information Retrieval* (IRL), 1976, 2(No. 2500), 196.

Bijou, S. W., Peterson, R. F., & Ault, M. H. A method to integrate descriptive and experimental field studies at the level of data and empirical concepts. *Journal of Applied Behavior Analysis,* 1968, 1, 175–191.

Birch, L. L., Marlin, D. W., Kramer, L., Peyer, C. Mother–child interaction patterns and the degree of fatness in children. *Journal of Nutrition Education,* 1981, 13, 17–21.

Biron, P., Mongeau, J. G., & Bertrand, D. Familial resemblences of body weight and weight/height in 374 homes with adopted children. *Journal of Pediatrics,* 1977, 91, 555–558.

Bistrian, B. R. & Sherman, M. Results of the treatment of obesity with a protein-sparing modified fast. *International Journal of Obesity,* 1978, 2, 143–148.

Blackburn, G. L. The liquid protein controversy—a closer look at the facts. *Obesity and Bariatric Medicine,* 1978, 7, 25–28.

Blackburn, G. L. & Bistrian, B. R. Surgical techniques in the treatment of adolescent obesity. In P. J. Collipp (Ed.), *Childhood obesity* (2nd ed.). Littleton, Massachusetts: PSG Publishing, 1980.

Blackburn, G. L. & Greenberg, I. Multidisciplinary approach to adult obesity therapy. *International Journal of Obesity,* 1978, 2, 133–142.

Bleidt, B. B. A comparison of two behavioral approaches to the treatment of obesity in children. *Dissertation Abstracts International,* 1979, 40, 440–B.

Blitzer, P. W., Blitzer, E. C., Rimm, A. A. Association between teenage obesity and cancer. *Preventive Medicine,* 1976, 5, 20–31.

Bonato, D. & Boland, F. J. *Response inhibition deficits and obesity in children: A disconfirmation.* Manuscript submitted for publication, 1982.

Booth, D. A. First steps toward an integrated quantitative approach to human feeding and obesity with some implications for research into treatment. In G. H. Bray (Ed.), *Recent advances in obesity research: II.* London: Newman Publishing, 1978.

Booth, D. A. Acquired behavior controlling energy intake and output. In A. J. Stunkard (Ed.), *Obesity.* Philadelphia: W. B. Saunders, 1980.

Börjeson, M. Overweight children. *Acta Paediatrica Scandinavia,* 1962, 51(Suppl 132).

Börjeson, M. The aetiology of obesity in children: A study of 101 twin pairs. *Acta Paediatrica Scandinavia,* 1976, 65, 279–287.

Börjeson, M. The etiology of obesity in children. In P. J. Collipp (Ed.), *Childhood obesity* (2nd ed.). Littleton, Massachusetts: PSG Publishing, 1980.

Botvin, G. J., Cantlon, A., Carter, B. J., & Williams, C. L. Reducing adolescent obesity through a school health program. *The Journal of Pediatrics,* 1979, 95, 1060–1062.

Bowerman, W. J., Harris, W. E. & Shea, J. M. *Jogging.* New York: Grosset and Dunlap, 1978.

Bradfield, R., Paulos, J., & Grossman, H. Energy expenditure and heart rate of obese high school girls. *American Journal of Clinical Nutrition,* 1971, 24, 1482–1488.

Brandt, G., Maschhoff, T., & Chandler, N. S. A residential camp experience as an approach to adolescent weight management. *Adolescence,* 1980, 15, 807–822.

Bray, G. A. *The obese patient.* Toronto: W. B. Saunders Company, 1976.

Bray, G. A. Obesity in America. *International Journal of Obesity,* 1979, 3, 363–375.

Bray, G. A., Greenway, F. L., Molitch, M. E., Dahms, W. T., Atkinson, R. L., & Hamilton, K. Use of anthropometric measures to assess weight loss. *The American Journal of Clinical Nutrition,* 1978, 31, 769–773.

Bridgewater, C. A., Walsh, J. A., Jeffrey, D. B., Ballard, B., & Peterson, P. *The behavioral assessment of children's food preferences.* Paper presented at the meeting of the Association for Advancement of Behavior Therapy, Toronto, November, 1981.

Brook, C. G. D. Obesity: The fat child. *British Journal of Hospital Medicine,* 1980, 24, 517–522.

Brook, C. G. D., Huntley, R. M. C., & Slack, J. Influence of heredity and environment in the determination of skinfold thickness in children. *British Medical Journal,* 1975, 2, 719–721.

Brook, C. G. D., Lloyd, J. K., & Wolff, D. H. Relation between age of onset of obesity and size and number of adipose cells. *British Medical Journal,* 1972, 2, 25–27.

Brook, C. G. D., Lloyd, J. K., & Wolff, O. H. Rapid weight loss in children. *British Medical Journal,* 1974, 3, 44.

Brown, M. R., Forbes, G. B., Klish, W. J., Gordon, A., & Campbell, M. A. Protein-sparing modified fast in obese adolescents: Long-term effect on lean body mass. *Pediatric Research,* 1981, 15, Abstract 519, 527.

Brownell, K. D. Assessment of eating disorders. In D. H. Barlow (Ed.), *Assessment of adult disorders.* New York: Guilford, 1981.

Brownell, K. D., Heckerman, C. L., & Westlake, R. J. *Therapist and group contact as variables in the behavioral treatment of obesity.* Paper presented at the meeting of the Association for the Advancement of Behavior Therapy, New York, December 1976. (Also in *Journal of Consulting and Clinical Psychology,* 1978, 46, 593–594)

Brownell, K. D., Heckerman, C. L., Westlake, R. J., Hayes, S. C., & Monti, P. M. The effect of couples training and partner cooperativeness in the behavioral treatment of obesity. *Behaviour Research and Therapy,* 1978, 16, 323–333. (Also, paper presented at the Association for Advancement of Behavior Therapy, Atlanta, 1977)

Brownell, K. D. & Kaye, F. S. A school-based behavior modification, nutrition education and physical activity program for obese children. *American Journal of Clinical Nutrition,* 1982, 35, 277–283.

Brownell, K. D., Kelman, J. H., & Stunkard, A. J. Treatment of obese children with and without their mothers: Changes in weight and blood pressure. *Pediatrics,* in press.

Brownell, K. D. & Stunkard, A. J. Behavior therapy and behavior change: Uncertainties in programs for weight control. *Behaviour Research and Therapy,* 1978, 16, 301.

Brownell, K. D. & Stunkard, A. J. Behavioral treatment for obese children and adolescents. In A. J. Stunkard (Ed.), *Obesity.* Philadelphia: W. B. Saunders, 1980a.

Brownell, K. D. & Stunkard, A. J. Physical activity in the development and control of obesity. In A. J. Stunkard (Ed.), *Obesity.* Philadelphia: W. B. Saunders, 1980b.

Brownell, K. D. & Stunkard, A. J. Couples training, pharmacotherapy, and behavior therapy in the treatment of obesity. *Archives of General Psychiatry,* 1981a, 38, 1224–1229.

Brownell, K. D. & Stunkard, A. J. Differential changes in plasma high-density lipoprotein-cholesterol levels of obese men and women during weight reduction. *Archives of Internal Medicine,* 1981b, 141, 1142–1146.

Brozek, J., Grande, F., Anderson, J. T., & Keys, A. Densitometric analysis of body composition: Revision of some quantitative assumptions. *Annals of the New York Academy of Science,* 1963, 110, 113–140.

Bruch, H. Obesity in childhood IV: Energy expenditure of obese children. *American Journal of Diseases of Children,* 1940, 60, 1082–1109.

Bruch, H. Hunger and instinct. *Journal of Nervous and Mental Disease,* 1969, 149, 91–114.

Bruch, H. Juvenile obesity: Its courses and outcome. In C. V. Rowlan (Ed.), *Anorexia and obesity.* Boston: Little, Brown, 1970.

Bruch, H. *Eating disorders.* New York: Basic Books, 1973.

Bruch, H. The importance of overweight. In P. J. Collipp (Ed.), *Childhood obesity.* Littleton, Massachusetts: PSG Publishing, 1975.

Bruch, H. Developmental considerations of anorexia nervosa and obesity. *Canadian Journal of Psychiatry,* 1981, 26, 212–217.

Buchberger, J. The problem of obesity in children in mountain areas and in cities. *Information Retrieval* (IRL), 1977, 2, 106.

Bullen, B., Reed, R. B., & Mayer, J. Physical activity of obese and nonobese adolescent girls appraised by motion picture sampling. *American Journal of Clinical Nutrition,* 1964, 14, 211–223.

Buskirk, E. R. Obesity: A brief overview with an emphasis on exercise. *Federation Proceedings,* 1974, 33, 1948–1951.

Cahn, A. Growth and caloric intake of heavy and tall children. *Journal of the American Dietetic Association,* 1968, 53, 476–480.

Cahnman, W. J. The stigma of obesity. *Sociological Quarterly,* 1968, 9, 283–299.

Canadian Paediatric Society, Breast-feeding: What is left besides the poetry? *Canadian Journal of Public Health,* 1978, 69, 13–20.

Canning, H. & Mayer, J. Obesity: Its possible effect on college acceptance. *New England Journal of Medicine,* 1966, 275, 1172–1174.

Capell, J. & Martin, J. *Obesity: Multidisciplinary study, treatment and prevention in the adult and pediatric rehabilitation program.* Poster presented at the meeting of the Association for the Advancement of Behavior Therapy, San Francisco, 1975.

Carman, D. D. Infant and childhood obesity. *Pediatric Nursing,* 1976, Nov/Dec, 33–38.

Carroll, C., Miller, D., and Nash, J. C. *Health: The science of human adaptation.* Dubuque, Iowa: Wm. C. Brown, 1976.

Carroll, L. J. & Yates, B. T. Further evidence for the role of stimulus control training in facilitating weight reduction after behavioral therapy. *Behavior Therapy,* 1981, 12, 287–291.

Carroll, L. J., Yates, B. T., & Gray, J. J. Predicting obesity reduction in behavioral and non-behavioral therapy from client characteristics: The self-evaluation measure. *Behavior Therapy,* 1980, 11, 189–197.

Cautela, J. R. Treatment of compulsive behavior by covert sensitization. *Psychological Record,* 1966, 16, 33–41.

Cautela, J. R. Covert sensitization. *Psychological Reports,* 1967, 20, 459–468.

Cautela, J. R. The treatment of overeating by covert conditioning. *Psychotherapy: Theory, Research, and Practice,* 1972, 9, 211–216.

Cautela, Jr. R. & Baron, M. G. Covert conditioning: A theoretical analysis. *Behavior Modification,* 1977, 1, 351–367.

Cautela, J. R. & Kastenbaum, R. A reinforcement survey schedule for use in therapy, training and research. *Psychological Reports,* 1967, 20, 115–130.

Chaback, E. *The Complete Calorie Counter.* New York: Dell, 1979.

Charney, E., Goodman, H. C., McBride, M., Lyon, B., & Pratt, R. Childhood antecedents of adult obesity. Do chubby infants become obese adults? *The New England Journal of Medicine,* 1976, 295, 6–9.

Chiumello, G., Guercio, M. J., Carnelutti, M., & Bidone, G. Relationship between obesity, chemical diabetes, and beta pancreatic function in children. *Diabetes,* 1969, 18, 238–243.

Christakis, G., Sajecki, S., Hillman, R. W., Miller, E., Blumenthal, S., & Archer, M. Effect of a combined nutrition education and physical fitness program on the weight status of obese high school boys. *Federation Proceedings,* 1966, 25, 15–19.

Christensen, A. & Barrios, E. *Partners, payoffs and pounds.* Paper presented at the meeting of the Western Psychological Association, Sacramento, June 1975.

Churchill, J. A. & Berendez, H. W. Intelligence of children whose mother had acetonuria during pregnancy. In Pan American Organization Committee on Medical Research, *Perinatal factors affecting human development.* Washington, D. C.: Pan American Sanitary Bureau (Science Publication No. 185:30–35), 1969.

Clarke, R. P., Merrow, S. B., Morse, E. H., & Keyser, D. E. Interrelationships between plasma lipids, physical measurements, and body fatness of adolescents in Burlington, Vermont. *The American Journal of Clinical Nutrition,* 1970, 23, 754–763.

Coates, T. J. The efficacy of a multicomponent self-control program in modifying the eating habits and weight of three obese adolescents (Doctoral dissertation, Stanford University, 1977). *Dissertation Abstracts International,* 1977–1978, 38, 1295–1296. (University order no. 77–18, 204)

Coates, T. J., Jeffery, R. N., Slinkard, L. A., Killen, J. D., & Danaher, B. G. Frequency of contact and monetary reward in weight loss, lipid change, and blood pressure reduction with adolescents. *Behavior Therapy,* 1982, 13, 175–185.

Coates, T. J., Killen, J. D., & Slinkard, L. A. Parent participation in a treatment program for overweight adolescents. *International Journal of Eating Disorders,* 1982, 1, 37–48.

Coates, T. J. & Perry, C. Multifactorial risk reduction with children and adolescents: Taking care of the heart in behavior group therapy. In D. Upper & S. M. Ross (Eds.), *Behavior group therapy: An annual review.* Champaign, Illinois: Research Press, 1980.

Coates, T. & Thoresen, C. Treating obesity in children and adolescents: A public health problem. *American Journal of Public Health,* 1978, 68, 143–151.

Coates, T. J. & Thoresen, C. E. Obesity among children and adolescents: The problem belongs to everyone. In B. Lahey & A. Kazdin (Eds.), *Advances in clinical child psychology* (Vol. 3). New York: Plenum, 1980.

Coates, T. J. & Thoresen, C. E. Behavior and weight changes in three obese adolescents. *Behavior Therapy,* 1981, 12, 383–399.

Coates, T. J. & Thoresen, C. E. Treating obesity in adolescents: A behavioral approach. In J. M. Ferguson & C. B. Taylor (Eds.), *Advances in behavioral medicine.* Englewood Cliffs, New Jersey: Prentice-Hall, in press.

Coché, J., Levitz, L. S., & Jordan, H. A. Behavioral group psychotherapy for overweight children and adolescents. In D. Upper & S. M. Ross (Eds.), *Behavioral group therapy 1979.* Champaign, Illinois: Research Press, 1979.

Cohen, F., Gelfand, D. M., Dodd, D. K., Jensen, J., & Turner, C. Self-control practices associated with weight loss maintenance in children and adolescents. *Behavior Therapy,* 1980, 1, 26–37.

Cole, T. J., Donnet, M. L., & Stanfield, J. P. Weight-for-height indices to assess nutritional status—a new index on a slide-rule. *The American Journal of Clinical Nutrition,* 1981, 34, 1935–1943.

Coles, R. *Behavioral treatment of obese children.* Unpublished doctoral dissertation in preparation. University of Manitoba, 1982.

Colletti, G., Savrin, E. & Stern, L. *An applied behavior analysis approach to follow-up intervention for weight control of six obese children and their mothers.* Paper presented at the meeting of the Association for Advancement of Behavior therapy, San Francisco, December 1979.

Colley, J. R. T. Obesity in school children. *British Journal of Preventative and Social Medicine,* 1974, 28, 221–225.

Collipp, P. J. (Ed.), *Childhood obesity* (2nd ed.). Littleton, Massachusetts: PSG Publishing, 1980a.

Collipp, P. J. Differential diagnosis of childhood obesity. In P. J. Collipp (Ed.), *Childhood obesity* (2nd ed.). Littleton, Massachusetts: PSG Publishing, 1980b.

Collipp, P. J. Long Island child life program. In P. J. Collipp (Ed.), *Childhood obesity* (2nd ed.). Littleton, Massachusetts: PSG Publishing, 1980c.

Collipp, P. J. Suggestions for leaders of childhood obesity groups. In P. J. Collipp

(Ed.), *Childhood obesity* (2nd ed.). Littleton, Massachusetts: PSG Publishing, 1980d.

Committee on Nutrition. Fetal and infant nutrition and susceptibility to obesity. *Nutrition Reviews,* 1978, 36, 122–126.

Committee on Nutrition. Nutritional aspects of obesity in infancy and childhood. *Pediatrics,* 1981, 68, 880–883.

Coplin, S. S., Hine, J., & Gormican, A. Outpatient dietary management in the Prader-Willi syndrome. *Journal of the American Dietetic Association,* 1976, 68, 330–334.

Corbin, C. B. & Pletcher, P. Diet and physical activity patterns of obese and nonobese elementary school children. *The Research Quarterly,* 1968, 39, 922–928.

Costanzo, P. R. & Woody, E. Z. Externality as a function of obesity in children: Pervasive style eating-specific attribute? *Journal of Personality and Social Psychology,* 1979, 37, 2286–2296.

Court, J. M. Obesity in childhood. *Medical Journal of Australia,* 1977, 1, 888–891.

Court, J. M. The development of obesity in childhood. *Medical Journal of Australia,* 1979, 2, 248–250.

Court, J. M. & Dunlop, M. Obesity from infancy: A clinical entity. In A. Howard (Ed.), *Recent advances in obesity research: I.* London: Newman Publishing, 1975.

Court, J. M., Dunlop, M. Reynolds, M., Russell, J., & Griffiths, L. Growth and development of fat in adolescent school children in Victoria: Part I. *Australian Pediatric Journal,* 1976, 12, 296–304.

Court, J. M., Hill, G. J., Dunlop, M., & Boulton, T. J. C. Hypertension in childhood obesity. *Australian Pediatric Journal,* 1974, 10, 296–300.

Craddock, D. *Obesity and its management.* London: Churchill Livingstone, 1978.

Crisp, H. H. Some psychobiological aspects of adolescent growth and their relevance for the fat/thin syndrome (anorexia nervosa). *International Journal of Obesity,* 1977, 1, 231–238.

Crow, R. A., Fawcett, J. N., & Wright, P. Maternal behavior during breast- and bottle-feeding. *Journal of Behavioral Medicine,* 1980, 3, 259–277.

Danaher, B. C. Theoretical foundations and clinical applications of the Premack Principle: Review and critique. *Behavior Therapy,* 1974, 5, 307–324.

Davies, C. T. M., Godfrey, S., Light, M., Sargeant, A. J., & Zeidifard, E. Cardiopulmonary responses to exercise in obese girls and young women. *Journal of Applied Physiology,* 1975, 38, 373–376.

Day, L. P. The psychological adjustment of obese versus nonobese children. *Dissertation Abstracts International,* 1982, 42, 2982B.

deCastro, F. J., Biesbroeck, R., Erickson, C., Farrell, P., Leong, W., Murphy, D., & Green, R. Hypertension in adolescents. *Clinical Pediatrics,* 1976a, 15, 24–26.

deCastro, F. J., Christianson, S. & Lollar, P. Blood pressures in children. *Missouri Medicine,* 1976b, June, 263–264.

DeJong, W. The stigma of obesity: The consequences of naive assumptions concerning the causes of physical deviance. *Journal of Health and Social Behavior,* 1980, 21, 75–87.

DeLuca, R. V. *Effects of fixed-interval and fixed-ratio schedules of reinforcement on exercise with obese and nonobese boys.* Unpublished masters thesis, University of Manitoba, 1982.

Dershewitz, R. A., Kahn, H. A., & Solomon, N. The relationship of weight-loss to blood pressure in the obese, hypertensive adolescent. *Maryland State Medical Journal,* 1981, 30, 53–56.

DeSchampheleire, I., Parent, M. A., & Chatteur, C. Excessive carbohydrate intake in pregnancy and neonatal obesity: Study in Cap Bon, Tunisia. *Archives of Diseases in Childhood,* 1980, 55, 521–526.

Deschamps, I., Desjeux, J. F., Machinot, S., Rolland, F., & Lestradet, H. Effects of diet and weight loss on plasmaglucose, insulin, and free fatty acids in obese children. *Pediatric Research,* 1978, 12, 757–760.

Deutsch, R. M. *Realities of nutrition.* Palo Alto: Bull Publishing, 1976.

Diament, C. & Wilson, G. T. An experimental investigation of the effects of covert sensitization in an analogue eating situation. *Behavior Therapy,* 1975, 6, 499–509.

Dickson, B. E., Szparaga, C., Epstein, L. H., Wing, R. R., Koeske, R., & Zidansek, J. *The effects of a lifestyle exercise program on fitness and weight loss in obese children.* Paper presented at the meeting of the Association for Advancement of Behavior Therapy, Toronto, November 1981.

Dietz, W. H. & Schoeller, D. A. Optimal dietary therapy for obese adolescents: Comparison of protein plus glucose and protein plus fat. *The Journal of Pediatrics,* 1982, 100, 638–644.

Dine, M. S., Gartside, P. S., Glueck, C. J., Rheines, L., Greene, G., & Khoury, P. Where do the heaviest children come from? A prospective study of white children from birth to 5 years of age. *Pediatrics,* 1979, 63, 1–7.

Dinoff, M., Rickard, H. G., & Colwick, J. Weight reduction through successive contracts. *American Journal of Orthopsychiatry,* 1972, 42, 110–113.

Di Scipio, W. J., Paul, H., & Byers, A. C. *Applied social behavior analysis of overeating in hospitalized psychotic girls.* Paper presented at the meeting of the Association of Behavior Analysis, Chicago, May 1976.

Ditschunheit, H., Jons, E. & Englehardt, I. On the incidence of obesity in childhood. *International Journal of Obesity,* 1978, 2, 475–476.

Dodd, D. K., Birky, H. J., & Stalling, R. B. Eating behavior of obese and normal weight females in a natural setting. *Addictive Behaviors,* 1976, 1, 321–325.

Domke, J. A., Lando, H. A., & Robinson, D. C. *Efficacy of follow-up booster sessions in treating obesity.* Paper presented at the meeting of the American Psychological Association, Toronto, August 1978.

Dorner, G. Influence of early postnatal nutrition on body weight in adolescence. *Information Retrieval* (IRL), 1979, 4(2491), 67.

Dorner, G., Grychtolik, H., & Julitz, M. Overfeeding in the first three months of life as a significant risk factor for the development of obesity and resulting disorders. *Deutsche Gesundheituesen,* 1977, 32, 6–9. Cited in Grinker, J. A. Behavioral and metabolic factors in childhood obesity, in M. Lewis and L. A. Rosenblum (Eds.), *The uncommon child.* New York: Plenum Press, 1981.

Douglass, T. S. Endocrinological and other uncommon causes of obesity. In P. S. Powers, (Ed.), *Obesity: The regulation of weight.* Baltimore: Williams & Wilkins, 1980.

Drabman, R. S., Cordua, G. D., Hammer, D., Jarvie, G. J., & Horton, W. Developmental trends in eating rates of normal and overweight preschool children. *Child Development,* 1979, 50, 211–216.

Drabman, R. S., Hammer, D., & Jarvie, G. J. Eating rates of elementary school children. *Journal of Nutrition Education,* 1977a, 9, 80–82.

Drabman, R. S., Hammer, D., & Jarvie, G. J. Eating styles of obese and nonobese black and white children in a naturalistic setting. *Addictive Behaviors,* 1977b, 2, 83–86.

Drash, A. Relationship between diabetes mellitus and obesity in the child. *Metabolism,* 1973, 22, 337–344.

Drenick, E. J. The prognosis of conventional treatment in severe obesity. In P. Bjorntorp, M. Cairella, & A. N. Howard, (Eds.), *Recent advances in obesity research: III.* London: John Libbey, 1981.

Drenick, E. J. & Johnson, D. Weight reduction by fasting and semistarvation in morbid obesity: Long-term follow-up. *International Journal of Obesity,* 1978, 2, 123–132.

Dressendorfer, R. Lean body mass increase with exercise. *Obesity and Bariatric Medicine,* 1975, 4, 188–190.

Dubois, S., Hill, D. E., & Beaton, G. H. An examination of factors believed to be associated with infantile obesity. *The American Journal of Clinical Nutrition,* 1979, 32, 1997–2004.

Dugdale, A. E. & Lovell, S. Measuring childhood obesity. *The Lancet,* 1981, 11, 1224.

DuRant, R. H. & Linder, C. W. An evaluation of five indexes of relative body weight for use with children. *Journal of the American Dietetic Association,* 1981, 78, 35–41.

DuRant, R. H., Martin, D. S., Linder, C. W., & Weston, W. The prevalence of obesity and thinness in children from a lower socioeconomic population receiving comprehensive health care. *The American Journal of Clinical Nutrition,* 1980, 33, 2002–2007.

Durnin, J. V. G. A. & Brockway, J. M. Determination of total energy expenditures in man by indirect calorimetry: Assessment of the accuracy of a modern technique. *British Journal of Nutrition,* 1959, 13, 41–57.

Durnin, J. V. G. A., Lonergan, M. E., Good, J., & Ewan, A. A cross-sectional nutritional and anthropometric study with an interval of 7 years, on 611 young adolescent school children. *British Journal of Nutrition,* 1974, 32, 169–179.

Durnin, J. V. G. A. & McKillop, F. M. The relationship between body build in infancy and percentage body fat in adolescence: A 14-year follow-up on 102 infants. *Proceedings of the Nutrition Society,* 1978, 37, 80A–81A.

Durnin, J. V. G. A. & Womersley, J. Body fat assessed from total body density and its estimation from skinfold thickness: Measurements on 481 men and women aged 16–72 years. *British Journal of Nutrition,* 1974, 32, 77–97.

Dwyer, J. T. Psychosexual aspects of weight control and dieting behavior in adolescence. *Medical Aspects Human Sexuality,* 1973, 7, 82–114.

Dwyer, J. Diets for children and adolescents that meet the dietary goals. *American Journal of Diseases of Children,* 1980, 134, 1073–1080.

Dwyer, J. T., Blonde, C. V., & Mayer, J. Treating obesity in growing children, Part 2. *Postgraduate Medicine,* 1972, 51, 111–115.

Dwyer, J. & Mayer, J. The dismal condition: Problems faced by obese adolescent girls in American Society. In G. R. Bray (Ed.), *Obesity in perspective,* Vol. 2, Part 2 (DHEW Publication no. 75–708, National Institute of Health). Washington, D. C.: U. S. Government Printing Office, 1975.

Dyrenforth, S. R., Freeman, D. G., & Wooley, S. C. Self-esteem, body type preference, and sociometric ratings of peers in pre-school children. Cited in S. C. Wooley, O. W. Wooley, & S. R. Dyrenforth. Theoretical, practical, and social issues in behavioral treatments of obesity. *Journal of Applied Behavior Analysis,* 1979, 12, 3–25.

Dyrenforth, S. R., Wooley, O. W., & Wooley, S. C. A woman's body in a man's world: A review of findings on body image and weight control. In J. R. Kaplan (Ed.), *A woman's conflict: The special relationship between woman and food.* Englewood Cliffs, New Jersey: Prentice-Hall, 1980.

Edelman, B. Developmental differences in the conceptualization of obesity. *Journal of the American Dietetic Association,* 1982, 80, 122–126.

Edelstein, B. Changing teenage eating behavior. *Connecticut Medicine,* 1981, 45, 496–500.

Edwards, D. W. W., Hammond, W. H., Healy, M. L. R., Tanner, T. M., & Whitehouse, R. H. Design and accuracy of calipers for measuring subcutaneous tissue thickness. *British Journal of Nutrition,* 1955, 9, 133–143.

Edwards, K. A. An index for assessing weight change in children: Weight/height ratios. *Journal of Applied Behavior Analysis,* 1978, 11, 421–429.

Edwards, L. W., Dickes, W. F., Alton, I. R., & Hakanson, E. Y. Pregnancy in the massively obese: Course, outcome, and obesity prognosis of the infant. *American Journal of Obstetrics and Gynecology,* 1978, 131, 479–483.

Eid, E. E. Follow-up study of physical growth of children who had excessive weight gain in first six months of life. *British Medical Journal*, 1970, 2, 74–76.

Ellis, R. W. B. & Tallerman, K. H. Obesity in childhood: A study of fifty cases. *Lancet*, 1934, 2, 615.

Ellison, R. C., Newburger, J. W., & Gross, D. M. Pediatric aspects of essential hypertension. *Journal of the American Dietetic Association*, 1982, 80, 21–25.

Ellison, R. C., Sosenko, J. M., Harper, G. P., Gibbons, L., Pratter, F. E., & Miettinen, O. S. Obesity, sodium intake and blood pressure in adolescents. *Hypertension*, 1980, 2(Suppl. I), 178–182.

Epstein, L. H., Masek, B. J. & Marshall, W. R. A nutritionally based school program for control of eating in obese children. *Behavior Therapy*, 1978, 9, 766–778.

Epstein, L. H., Nuss, M. M., Wing, R. R., Koeske, R., Zidansek, J., & Dickson, B. E. *The long-term effects of programmed aerobic and lifestyle exercise on weight in obese pre-adolescents.* Paper presented at the meeting of the Association for Advancement of Behavior Therapy, Toronto, November 1981.

Epstein, L. H., Parker, L., McCoy, J. F., & McGee, G. Descriptive analysis of eating regulation in obese and nonobese children. *Journal of Applied Behavior Analysis*, 1976, 9, 407–415.

Epstein, L. H., & Wing, R. R. Aerobic exercise and weight. *Addictive Behaviors*, 1980, 5, 371–388.

Epstein, L. H., Wing, R. R., Koeske, R., Andrasik, F., & Ossip, D. J. Child and parent weight loss in family-based behavior modification programs. *Journal of Consulting and Clinical Psychology*, 1981, 49, 674–685.

Epstein, L. H., Wing, R. R., Koeske, R., Ossip, D., & Beck, S. A comparison of lifestyle change and programmed aerobic exercise on weight and fitness changes in obese children. *Behavior Therapy*, 1982, 13, 651–665.

Epstein, L. H., Wing, R. R., Ossip, D. J. & Andrasik, F. Parent/child weight loss in family based behavior modification. Paper presented at the 2nd Annual Meeting of the Society of Behavioral Medicine, 1981.

Epstein, L. H., Wing, R. R., Steranchak, L., Dickson, B., & Michelson, J. Comparison of family-based behavior modification and nutrition education for childhood obesity. *Journal of Pediatric Psychology*. 1980, 5, 25–36.

Faber, J., Randolph, J. G., Robbins, S., & Smith, J. C. Zinc and copper status in young patients following jejunoileal bypass. *Journal of Surgical Research*, 1978, 24, 83–86.

Farrell, S. R., Layton, M. S., Ford, F., & Tervo, R. C. Obesity and diet in a spina bifida clinic: Associated factors and management. *Journal of the Canadian Dietetic Association*, 1981, 42, 160–166.

Feig, B. K. *The parents' guide to weight control for children ages 5 to 13 years.* Springfield, Illinois: Charles C Thomas, 1980.

Feinstein, A. R. The measurement of success in weight reduction: An analysis of methods and a new index. *Journal of Chronic Diseases,* 1959, 10, 439–456.

Ferguson, J. Slimming: New ideas on behaviour. *Community Outlook,* 1981, May 14, 171–176.

Ferris, A. G., Laus, M. J., Hosmer, D. W., & Beal, V. A. The effect of diet on weight gain in infancy. *The American Journal of Clinical Nutrition,* 1980, 33, 2635–2642.

Ferster, C. B., Culbertson, S., & Boren, M. C. P. *Behavior Principles,* 2nd ed. Englewood Cliffs, New Jersey: Prentice-Hall, 1975.

Ferster, C. B., Nurnberger, I. I., & Levitt, E. B. The control of eating. *Journal of Mathetics,* 1962, 1, 87–109.

Ferster, C. B. & Perrott, M. C. *Behavior principles.* New York: Appleton-Century-Crofts, 1968.

Ferster, C. B. & Skinner, B. F. *Schedules of reinforcement.* New York: Appleton-Century-Crofts, 1957.

Filer, L. Early nutrition: Its long-term role. *Hospital Practice,* 1978, 13, 87–95.

Fisch, R. O., Bilek, M. R., & Ulstrom, R. Obesity and leanness at birth and their relationship to body habitus in later childhood. *Pediatrics,* 1975, 56, 521–528.

Fisher, Jr., E. B., Green, L., Friedling, C. Levenkron, J. & Porter, F. L. Self-monitoring of progress in weight-reduction: A preliminary report. *Journal of Behavior Therapy and Experimental Psychiatry,* 1976, 7, 363–365.

Fitness Finders. *A unique approach to personal fitness.* Pennsylvania: Fitness Finders, 1969.

Fodor, I.G. *Behavior therapy for the overweight woman: A time for reappraisal.* Paper presented at the meeting of the International Congress of Behavior Therapy, Jerusalem, July 1980.

Follick, M. S., Henderson, O., Herbert, P., & Abrams, D. *Plasma lipoprotein changes associated with behavioral weight loss intervention.* Paper presented at the meeting of the Society of Behavioral Medicine, New York, November 1980.

Fomon, S. J. Factors influencing food consumption in the human infant. *International Journal of Obesity,* 1980, 4, 348–350.

Foreyt, J. P. & Goodrick, G. K. Childhood obesity. In E. J. Mash & L. G. Terdal (Eds.), *Behavioral assessment of childhood disorders.* New York: The Guilford Press, 1981.

Foreyt, J. P. & Hagen, R. L. Covert sensitization: Conditioning or suggestion? *Journal of Abnormal Psychology,* 1973, 82, 17–23.

Foreyt, J. P. & Parks, J. T. Behavioral controls for achieving weight loss in the severely retarded. *Journal of Behavior Therapy and Experimental Psychiatry,* 1975, 6, 27–29.

Foster, T. A., Voors, A. W., Webber, L. S., Frerichs, R. R., & Berenson, G. S. Anthropometric and maturation measurements of children ages 5 to 14 years in a biracial community—The Bogalusa Heart Study. *The American Journal of Clinical Nutrition,* 1977, 30, 582–591.

Fowler, R. S., Fordyce, W. E., Boyd, V. D., & Masock, A. The mouthful diet: A behavioral approach to overeating. *Rehabilitation Psychology,* 1972, 19, 98–106.

Foxx, R. M. Social reinforcement of weight reduction: A case report on an obese retarded adolescent. *Mental Retardation,* 1972, 10, 21–23.

Freedson, P. S., Katch, V. L., Gilliam, T. B., & MacConnie, S. Energy expenditure in prepubescent children: Influence of sex and age. *The American Journal of Clinical Nutrition,* 1981, 34, 1827–1830.

Frerichs, R. R., Webber, L. S., Srinivasan, S. R., & Berenson, G. S. Relation of serum lipids and lipoproteins to obesity and sexual maturity in white and black children. *American Journal of Epidemiology,* 1978, 108, 486–496.

Frisancho, A. R. Triceps skinfold and upperarm muscle size norms for assessment of nutritional status. *American Journal of Clinical Nutrition,* 1974, 27, 1052–1057.

Frisancho, A. R. New norms of upper limb fat and muscle areas for assessment of nutritional status. *American Journal of Clinical Nutrition,* 1981, 34, 2540–2545.

Garb, J. L., Garb, J. R., & Stunkard, A. J. Social factors and obesity in Navajo Indian Children. In A. Howard (Ed.), *Recent advances in obesity research,* Vol. 1. London, England: Newman Publishing, 1975.

Garn, S. M. & Bailey, S. M. Fatness similarities in adopted peers. *American Journal of Clinical Nutrition,* 1976, 29, 1067–1068.

Garn, S. M., Bailey, S. M., Solomon, M. A., & Hopkins, P. J. Effect of remaining family members on fatness prediction. *The American Journal of Clinical Nutrition,* 1981, 34, 148–153.

Garn, S. M. & Clark, D. C. Nutrition, growth, development, and maturation: Findings from the ten-state nutrition survey of 1968–1970. *Pediatrics,* 1975, 56, 306–319.

Garn, S.M. & Clark, D.C. Trends in fatness and the origins of obesity. *Pediatrics,* 1976, 57, 443–456.

Garn, S. M., Clark, D. D., & Guire, K. E. Growth, body composition, and development of obese and lean children. In M. Winick (Ed.), *Childhood obesity.* New York: Wiley, 1975.

Garn, S. M., Cole, P. E., & Bailey, S. M. Effect of parental fatness levels on the fatness of biological and adoptive children. *Ecology of Food and Nutrition,* 1977, 6, 91–93.

Garn, S. M., Hopkins, P. J., & Ryan, A. S. Differential fatness gain of low income boys and girls. *The American Journal of Clinical Nutrition,* 1981, 34, 1465–1468.

Garrison, R. J., Wilson, P. J., Castelli, W. P., Fenleib, M., Kannel, W. B., & McNamara, P. M. Obesity and lipoprotein cholesterol in the Framingham Offspring Study. *Metabolism,* 1980, 29, 1053–1060.

Garrow, J. S. *Energy balance and obesity in man.* New York: American Elsevier Publishing Company, 1974.

Garrow, J. S. Infant feeding and obesity of adults. *Bibliotheca Nutritoet Dieta,* Vol. 26, 29–35, Basel: Karger, 1978a.

Garrow, J. S. The regulation of energy expenditure in man. In G. A. Bray (Ed.), *Recent advances in obesity research: II.* London: Newman Publishing, 1978b.

Garrow, J. S. Overview: New approaches to body composition. *The American Journal of Clinical Nutrition,* 1982, 35(Suppl.), 1152–1158.

Gaul, D. J., Craighead, E., & Mahoney, M. J. Relationship between eating rates and obesity. *Journal of Consulting and Clinical Psychology,* 1975, 43, 123–125.

Geller, S. E. Behavioral weight control for obese adolescents: Preliminary findings and future considerations. *Psychological Reports,* 1978, 42, 1233–1234.

Geller, S. E., Keane, T. M., & Scheirer, C. J. Delay of gratification, locus of control, and eating patterns in obese and nonobese children. *Addictive Behaviors,* 1981, 6, 9–14.

Geronilla, L. S. A study of weight control in pediatric obesity using mothers as behavior modifiers. *Dissertation Abstracts International,* 1981, 42, 2027–B.

Gillum, R. F., Jeffery, R. W., Gerber, W. G., Elmer, P. J., & Prineas, R. J. *Primary prevention of hypertension through weight and dietary sodium restrictions.* Paper presented at the meeting of the Society of Behavioral Medicine, New York, November 1980.

Ginsberg-Fellner, F. Growth of adipose tissue in infants, children, and adolescents: Variations in growth disorders. *International Journal of Obesity,* 1981, 5, 605–611.

Ginsberg-Fellner, F., Jagendorf, L. A., Carmel, H., & Harris, T. Overweight and obesity in preschool children in New York City. *The American Journal of Clinical Nutrition,* 1981, 34, 2236–2241.

Ginsberg-Fellner, F. & Knittle, J. L. Weight reduction in young obese children I. Effects on adipose tissue cellularity and metabolism. *Pediatric Research,* 1981, 15, 1381–1389.

Giotto, M. I. The effect of peer support upon ideal weight attainment and the self-concept of adolescent girls involved in a multidimensional physical education program. *Dissertation Abstracts International,* 1980, 40, 4413A–4414A.

Gold, S. C. & Byrne, A. M. *Obesity in infants* (letter). *Hospital Practice,* 1979, 14, 17.

Goldblatt, P. B., Moore, M. E., & Stunkard, A. J. Social factors in obesity. *Journal of the American Medical Association,* 1965, 192, 1039–1044.

Goldbloom, R. B. Obesity in childhood. *Canadian Medical Association Journal,* 1975, 113, 139.

Golden, M. P. An approach to the management of obesity in childhood. *Pediatric Clinics of North America,* 1979, 26, 187–197.

Goldstein, J. L. & Failkow, P. J. The Alstrom syndrome: Report of 3 cases with further delineation of the clinical pathophysiological and genetic aspects of the disorder. *Medicine,* 1973, 52, 53–71.

Goodman, N., Richardson, S. A., Dornbusch, S. M., & Hastorf, A. H. Variant reactions to physical disabilities. *American Sociological Review,* 1963, 28, 429–435.

Gordon, A. & Boulton, T. J. C. Do fat children think differently about food? *Australian Paediatric Journal,* 1978, 14, 174–176.

Gormally, J., Buese-Moscati, E., Clyman, R., & Forbes, R. R. Research design issues for behavioral treatment of obesity. *JSAS Catalog of Selected Documents in Psychology,* 1977, 7, (Ms. no. 1462), 34.

Gormally, J. Rardin, D., & Black, S. Correlates of successful response to a behavioral weight control clinic. *Journal of Counseling Psychology,* in press.

Gracianette, C., Williamson, D., Hardin, B., Konidoff, C. & Young, L. *Behavioral treatment of adolescent obesity: Modification of eating habits versus exercise habits.* Paper presented at the meeting of the Association for Advancement of Behavior Therapy, New York, November, 1980.

Griffiths, M. & Payne, P. R. Energy expenditure in small children of obese and non-obese parents. *Nature,* 1976, 260, 698–700.

Grimes, W. B. & Franzini, L. R. Skinfold measurement techniques for estimating percentage body fat. *Journal of Behavior Therapy and Experimental Psychiatry,* 1977, 8, 65–69.

Grinker, J. A. Appetite control: Morphological and psychological considerations. In P. J. Collipp (Ed.), *Childhood obesity* (2nd ed.). Littleton, Massachusetts: PSG Publishing, 1980.

Grinker, J. A. Behavioral and metabolic factors in childhood obesity. In M. Lewis and L. A. Rosenblum (Eds.), *The uncommon child.* New York: Plenum, 1981.

Grinker, J. & Hirsch, J. Metabolic and behavioral correlates of obesity. In *Physiology, emotion and psychosomatic illness: A CIBA Foundation Symposium.* Amsterdam: Associated Scientific Publishers, 1972.

Grinker, J. A., Price, J. M., & Greenwood, M. R. C. Studies of taste in childhood obesity. In D. Novin, W. Wyricka, G. Bray (Eds.), *Hunger: Basic mechanisms and clinical implications.* New York: Raven Press, 1976.

Grollman, A. Drug therapy of obesity in children. In P. J. Collipp (Ed.), *Childhood obesity*. Littleton, Massachusetts: PSG Publishing, 1980.

Gross, I., Wheeler, M., & Hess, K. The treatment of obesity in adolescents using behavioral self-control: An evaluation, *Clinical Pediatrics*, 1976, 15, 920–924.

Gross, T., Sokol, R. J., & King, K. C. Obesity in pregnancy: Risks and outcome. *Obstetrics and Gynecology*, 1980, 56, 446–450.

Guggenheim, K., Poznanski, R., & Kaufmann, N. A. Body build and self-perception in 13- and 14-year-old Israeli children and their relationship to obesity. *Israel Journal of Medical Science*, 1973, 9, 120–128.

Gurney, R. Hereditary factor in obesity. *Archives of Internal Medicine*, 1936, 57, 557–561.

Gurr, M. I. & Kirtland, J. Adipose tissue cellularity—a review: I. Techniques for studying cellularity. *International Journal of Obesity*, 1978, 2, 401–427.

Guthrie, H. A. *Introductory nutrition*. St. Louis: C. V. Mosby, 1975.

Guy, R. The growth of physically handicapped children with emphasis on appetite and physical activity. *Public Health*, 1978, 92, 145–154.

Hagen, R. L. Theories of obesity: Is there any hope for order? In B. J. Williams, S. Martin, & J. P. Foreyt (Eds.), *Obesity: Behavioral approaches to dietary management*. New York: Brunner/Mazel, 1976.

Hagen, R. L., Foreyt, J. P., & Durham, T. W. The dropout problem: Reducing attrition in obesity research. *Behavior Therapy*, 1976, 7, 463–471.

Hager, A., Sjöström, L., Arvidsson, B., Björntorp, P., & Smith, U. Adipose tissue cellularity in obese school girls before and after dietary treatment. *American Journal of Clinical Nutrition*, 1978, 31, 68–75.

Hager, A. & Thorell, J. I. Insulin secretion and peripheral insulin sensitivity in obese children. Evidence of deficient glucose-stimulated early insulin release despite hyperinsulinemia. *International Journal of Obesity*, 1979, 3, 349–358.

Hamill, P. V. V., Drizd, T. A., Johnson, C. L., Reed, R. B., & Roche, A. F. *NCHS growth curves for children birth—18 years*. (Vital and Health Statistics—Series 11, No. 165. DHEW Publication No., PHS 78–1650). Washington, D. C.: US Government Printing Office, 1977.

Hamill, P. V. V., Drizd, T. A., Johnson, C. L., Reed, R. B., Roche, A. F., & Moore, W. M. Physical growth: NCHS percentiles. *American Journal of Clinical Nutrition*, 1979, 32, 607–629. Data from the National Center for Health Statistics Hyattsville, Maryland. Columbus, Ohio: Ross Laboratories, 1980.

Hammar, S. L., Campbell, M. M., Campbell, V. A., Moores, N. L., Sareen, C., Garies, F. J., & Lucas, B. An interdisciplinary study of adolescent obesity. *Journal of Pediatrics*, 1972, 80, 373–383.

Hammar, S. L., Campbell, V., & Wooley, J. Treating adolescent obesity: Long range evaluation of previous therapy. *Clinical Pediatrics*, 1972, 10, 46–52.

Hampton, M. C., Huenemann, R. L., Shapiro, L. R., & Mitchell, B. W. Caloric and nutrient intakes of teenagers. *Journal of the American Dietetic Association,* 1967, 50, 385–396.

Hancock, T. Baby food bonanza boosted by big business. *Canadian Family Physician,* 1977, 23, 8.

Harris, E. S., Kirschenbaum, D. S. & Tomarken, A. J. *Parental involvement in behavioral weight loss therapy for preadolescents.* Paper presented at the meeting of the Association for Advancement of Behavior Therapy, Toronto, November 1981.

Harris, M. B. Self-directed program for weight control: a pilot study. *Journal of Abnormal Psychology,* 1969, 74, 263–270.

Harris, M. B., Sutton, M., Kaufman, E. M., & Carmichael, C. W. Correlates of success and retention in a multi-faceted, long-term behavior modification program for obese adolescent girls. *Addictive Behaviors,* 1980, 5, 25–34.

Harrison, G. G., Udall, J. N., & Morrow, G. Maternal obesity, weight gain in pregnancy and infant birth weight. *American Journal of Obstetrics and Gynecology,* 1980, 136, 411–412.

Hathaway, M. L. & Sargent, D. W. Overweight in children. *Journal of the American Dietetic Association,* 1962, 40, 511–515.

Hawk, L. Thrusting greatness upon them. *Journal of Psychosomatic Research,* 1977, 21, 277–285.

Hawk, L. J. & Brook, C. G. D. Influence of body fatness in childhood on fatness in adult life. *British Medical Journal,* 1979, 1, 151–152.

Hayes, S. C. Single case experimental design and empirical clinical practice. *Journal of Consulting and Clinical Psychology,* 1981, 49, 193–211.

Heckerman, C. L. & Zitter, R. E. *Spouse monitoring and reinforcement in the treatment of obesity.* Paper presented at the meeting of the Association for Advancement of Behavior Therapy, San Francisco, December 1979.

Heiman, M. F. The management of obesity in the post-adolescent developmentally disabled client with Prader-Willi syndrome. *Adolescence,* 1978, 13, 291–296.

Heiser, J. R., Epstein, L. H. & Wing, R. R. Mechanical reliability of pedometers. *The Behavior Therapist,* 1981, 4, 21–22.

Hendry, L. B. & Gillies, P. Body type, body esteem, school, and leisure: A study of overweight, average, and underweight adolescents. *Journal of Youth and Adolescence,* 1978, 7, 181–195.

Herbert-Jackson, E., Cross, M. Z., & Risley, T. R. Milk types and temperature: What will young children drink? *Journal of Nutrition Education,* 1977, 9, 76–79.

Herbert–Jackson, E. & Risley, T. R. *Behavioral nutrition: Providing an empirical basis for improved child nutrition counseling.* Paper presented at the meeting of the American Psychological Association, Chicago, September 1975.

Herbert-Jackson E. & Risley, T. R. *Behavioral nutrition: Expanding applications for behavioral technology.* Paper presented at the meeting of the Association for Advancement of Behavior Therapy, New York, December 1976.

Herbert-Jackson, E. & Risley, T. R. Behavioral nutrition: Consumption of foods of the future by toddlers. *Journal of Applied Behavior Analysis,* 1977, 10, 407–413.

Hersen, M. & Barlow, D. H. *Single case experimental designs: Strategies for studying behavior change.* New York: Pergamon Press, 1976.

Hertzler, A. A. Obesity—impact of family. *Journal of the American Dietetic Association,* 1981, 79, 525–529.

Heyden, S., DeMaria, W., Barbee, S. & Morris, M. Weight reduction in adolescents. *Nutrition and metabolism,* 1973, 15, 295–304.

Hill, S. W. & McCutcheon, N. B. Eating responses of obese and non-obese humans during dinner meals. *Psychosomatic Medicine,* 1975, 37, 395–401.

Hirsch, J. Cell number and size as a determinant of subsequent obesity. In M. Winick (Ed.), *Childhood obesity.* New York: John Wiley & Sons, 1975.

Hirsch, J. & Han, R. W. Cellularity of rat adipose tissue: Effects of growth, starvation, and obesity. *Journal of Lipid Research,* 1969, 10, 77–82.

Hirsch, J. & Knittle, J. L. Cellularity of obese and nonobese human adipose tissue. *Federal Proceedings,* 1970, 29, 1516–1521.

Hofacker, R. & Brenner, N. Vegetable parade persuades children to try new foods. *Journal of Nutrition Education,* 1976, 8, 21–24.

Holm, V. A. & Pipes, P. L. Food and children with Prader-Willi syndrome. *American Journal of Diseases of Children,* 1976, 130, 1063–1067.

Homme, L. E. Control of coverants: The operants of the mind. *Psychological Record,* 1965, 15, 501–511.

Homme, L. E., deBaca, P. C., Devine, J. V., Steinhorst, R., & Rickert, E. J. Use of the Premack principle in controlling the behavior of nursery school children. *Journal of the Experimental Analysis of Behavior,* 1963, 6, 544.

Horan, D. B. Attitudes of nondisabled preschool and kindergarten students toward visibly-disabled and obese children and an investigation of an intervention to modify those attitudes: An empirical study. *Dissertation Abstracts International,* 1982, 42, 3015A–3016A.

Horan, J. J. & Johnson, R. G. Coverant conditioning through a self-management application of the Premack Principle: Its effect on weight reduction. *Journal of Behavior Therapy and Experimental Psychiatry,* 1971, 2, 243–249.

Howard, A. N., Dub, I., & McMahon, M. The incidence, cause and treatment of obesity in Leicester school children. *Practitioner,* 1971, 207, 662–668.

Huenemann, R. L. Food habits of obese and nonobese adolescents. *Postgraduate Medicine,* 1972, 51, 99–105.

Huenemann, R. L. Environmental factors associated with preschool obesity, Part I. *Journal of the American Dietetic Association,* 1974a, 64, 480–487.

Huenemann, R. L. Environmental factors associated with preschool obesity, Part II. *Journal of the American Dietetic Association,* 1974b, 64, 488–491.

Huenemann, R. L., Hampton, M. C., Behnke, A. R., Schapiro, L. R., & Mitchell, B. W. *Teenage nutrition and physique.* Springfield, Illinois: Charles C Thomas, 1974.

Huse, D. M., Branes, L. A., Colligan, R. C., Nelson, R. A., & Palumbo, P. J. The challenge of obesity in childhood I. Incidence, prevalence, and staging. *Mayo Clinic Proceedings,* 1982, 57, 279–284.

Huse, D. M., Palumbo, P. J., Nelson, R. A., & Hick, J. F. Grammar school site for identifying and treating obese children. *International Journal of Obesity,* 1978, 2, 365.

Illingsworth, R., Harvey, C. & Gin, S. T. Relation of birthweight to physical development in childhood. *Lancet,* 1949, 2, 598.

Isbitsky, J. R. & White, D. R. Externality and locus of control in obese children. *The Journal of Psychology,* 1981, 107, 163–172.

Israel, A. C. & Saccone, A. J. Follow-up effects of choice of mediator and target of reinforcement on weight loss. *Behavior Therapy,* 1979, 10, 260–265.

Israel, A. C. & Stolmaker, L. Behavioral treatment of obesity in children and adolescents. In M. Hersen, R. Eisler, & P. M. Miller (Eds.), *Progress in behavior modification,* Vol. 10. New York: Academic Press, 1980.

Israsena, T., Israngkura, M., & Srivuthana, S. Treatment of childhood obesity. *Journal of the Medical Association of Thailand,* 1980, 63, 433–437.

Jackson, J. N. & Ormiston, L. H. Diet and weight control clinic: A status report. Unpublished manuscript, Stanford University, 1977.

Jacobelli, A., Simeoni, A., Vecci, E., & Agostino, A. Outpatient treatment of juvenile obesity. *Information Retrieval Limited,* 1979, 4, 72.

Janda, L. H. & Rimm, D. G. Covert sensitization in the treatment of obesity. *Journal of Abnormal Psychology,* 1972, 80, 37–42.

Janzen, G. & Doleys, D. M. *Parental modeling and reinforcement in the treatment of childhood obesity.* Paper presented at the meeting of the Association for Advancement of Behavior Therapy, Toronto, November 1981.

Jeffery, R. W., Thompson, P. D., & Wing, R. R. Effects on weight reduction of strong monetary contracts for calorie restriction or weight loss. *Behaviour Research and Therapy,* 1978, 16, 363–369.

Jeffery, R.W., Wing, R. R., & Stunkard, A. J. Behavioral treatment of obesity: The state of the art. *Behavior Therapy,* 1978, 9, 189–199.

Jeffrey, D. B. & Katz, R. C. *Take it off and keep it off: A behavioral program for weight loss and healthy living.* Englewood Cliffs, New Jersey: Prentice-Hall, 1977.

Jeffrey, D. B., Lemnitzer, N. B., Hickey, J. S., Hess, M. J., McLellarn, R. W., & Stroud, J. M. The development of a behavioral eating test and its relationship to a self-report food preference scale. *Behavioral Assessment,* 1980, 2, 87–98.

Jelliffe, D. B. & Jelliffe, E. F. Fat babies: Prevalence, perils, prevention. *Journal of Tropical Pediatrics and Environmental Child Health,* 1975, 21, 123–159.

Jetté, M., Barry, W., & Pearlman, L. The effects of an extracurricular physical activity program on obese adolescents. *Canadian Journal of Public Health,* 1977, 68, 39–42.

Joachim, R. The use of self-monitoring to effect weight loss in a mildly retarded female. *Journal of Behavior Therapy and Experimental Psychiatry,* 1977, 8, 213–215.

Johnson, C. L., Fulwood, R., Abraham, S., & Bryner, J. D. *Basic data on anthropometric measurements and angular measurements of the hip and knee joints for selected age groups 1–74 years of age.* (Vital and Health Statistics: Series II; no. 219. DHHS Publication No., PHS 81–1660). Hyattsville, Maryland: US Department of Health and Human Resources, 1981.

Johnson, M. L., Burke, B. S., & Mayer, J. Relative importance of inactivity and overeating in the energy balance of obese high school girls. *American Journal of Clinical Nutrition,* 1956, 4, 37–44.

Johnson, R. E., Mastropaolo, J. A., & Wharton, M. A. Exercise, dietary intake, and body composition. *Journal of the American Dietetic Association,* 1972, 61, 399–403.

Johnson, R. M. Evaluating child's ideal weight. (Ask the practicing physician). *Obesity and Bariatric Medicine,* 1979, 8, 188.

Johnson, W. G., Parry, W., & Drabman, R. S. The performance of obese and normal size children on a delay of gratification task. *Addictive Behaviors,* 1978, 3, 205–208.

Johnson, W. G. & Stalonas, P. Measuring skinfold thickness—A cautionary note. *Addictive Behaviors,* 1977, 2, 105–108.

Johnson, W. G., Wildman, H. E., & O'Brien, T. The assessment of program adherence: The achilles' heel of behavioral weight reduction? *Behavioral Assessment,* 1980, 2, 297–301.

Johnston, F. E. & Mack, R. W. Obesity in urban black adolescents of high and low relative weight at 1 year of age. *American Journal of Diseases of Children,* 1978, 132, 862–864.

Johnston, F.E. & Mack, R. W. Obesity, stature, and one year relative weight of 15-year-old youths. *Human Biology,* 1980, 52, 35–41.

Jones, H. E. The fat child. *Practitioner,* 1972, 208, 212–219.

Jongmans, J. G. *Vermagerings-Therapieen.* Unpublished doctoral dissertation, Psychological Laboratory of the University of Amsterdam, 1969.

Jonides, L. Childhood obesity: A treatment approach for private practices, *Pediatric Nursing,* 1982, 8, 320–322.

Jordan, H. A. & Berland, T. *The doctor's calories-plus diet.* Chicago: Contemporary Books, 1981.

Jordan, H. A. & Levitz, L. S. Behavior modification in the treatment of childhood obesity. In M. Winick (Ed.), *Childhood obesity.* New York: Wiley, 1975.

Jordan, H. A., Levitz, L., & Kimbrell, G.M. The 24-hour activity clock. Unpublished data form, 1976a.

Jordan, H. A., Levitz, L. S., & Kimbrell, G. M. In S. Gelman (Ed.), *Eating is okay.* New York: Rawson Associates Publishers, Inc., 1976b.

Jordan, H. A. & Spiegel, T. A. Palatability and oral factors and their role in obesity. In *The Chemical senses and nutrition.* New York: Academic press, 1977.

Jordan, H. A., Stellar, E., & Duggan, S. Z. Voluntary intragastric feeding in man. *Communications in Behavioral Biology,* 1968, 1, 65–68.

Jung, R. T., Gurr, M. I., Robinson, M. P., & James, W. P. T. Does adipocyte hypercellularity in obesity exist? *British Medical Journal,* 1978, 2, 319–321.

Kahle, E. B., Walker, R. B., Eisenman, P. A., Behall, K. M., Hallfrisch, J., & Reiser, S. Moderate diet control in children: The effects on metabolic indicators that predict obesity-related degenerative diseases. *The American Journal of Clinical Nutrition,* 1982, 35, 950–957.

Kahn, E. G. Obesity in children. *Journal of Pediatrics,* 1970, 77, 771–774.

Kanfer, F. H. Self-monitoring: Methodological limitations and clinical applications. *Journal of Consulting and Clinical Psychology,* 1970, 35, 148–152.

Kanfer, F. H. The many faces of self-control, or behavior modification changes its focus. In R. B. Stuart (Ed.), *Behavioral self-management: Strategies, techniques and outcomes,* New York: Brunner/Mazel, 1977.

Kannel, W. B. & Dawber, T. R. Atherosclerosis: a pediatric problem. *Journal of Pediatrics,* 1972, 80, 544–554.

Kaoukis, G. *The two-bucket system.* Device developed by G. Kaoukis, University of Manitoba, 1980.

Kaplan, D. L. Eating style of obese and nonobese persons (Doctoral dissertation, University of Pennsylvania, 1977). *Dissertation Abstracts International,* 1977, 38, 5574B–5575B. (University Microfilms no. 7806603.)

Kappy, M. S. & Plotnick, L. Erythrocyte insulin binding in obese children and adolescents. *Journal of Clinical Endicrinology and Metabolism,* 1980, 51, 1440–1446.

Kazdin, A. E. Methodological and interpretive problems of single-case experimental designs. *Journal of Consulting and Clinical Psychology,* 1978, 46, 629–642.

Keane, T. M., Geller, S. E., & Scheirer, C. J. A parametric investigation of eating styles in obese and nonobese children. *Behavior Therapy,* 1981, 12, 280–286.

Keller, S. M., Colley, J. R. T., & Carpenter, R. G. Obesity in school children and their parents. *Annals of Human Biology,* 1979, 6, 443–455.

Kelman, S. J., Brownell, K. D., & Stunkard, A. J. The role of parental participation in the treatment of obese adolescents. Unpublished manuscript, 1979. Cited in A. J. Stunkard (Ed.), *Obesity.* Philadelphia: W. B. Saunders, 1980, 424–425 and 435.

Kessen, W. Signs of risk of obesity in newborn babies. *International Journal of Obesity*, 1980, 4, 341–347.

Keys, A. & Brozek, J. Body fat in adult man. *Physiology Review*, 1953, 33, 245–325.

Khan, M. A. Nutrition and current concepts of obesity. *CRC Critical Reviews in Food Science and Nutrition*, 1981, 14, 135–151.

Kiesler, D. J. Some myths of psychotherapy research and the search for a paradigm. *Psychological Bulletin*, 1966, 65, 110–136.

Kingsley, R. G. & Shapiro, J. A comparison of three behavioral programs for the control of obesity in children. *Behavior Therapy*, 1977, 8, 30–36.

Kingsley, R. G. & Wilson, G. T. Behavior therapy for obesity: A comparative investigation of long-term efficacy. *Journal of Consulting and Clinical Psychology*, 1977, 45, 288–298.

Kirscht, J. P., Becker, M. H., Haefner, D. P., & Maiman, L. A. Effects of threatening communications and mothers' health beliefs on weight change in obese children. *Journal of Behavioral Medicine*, 1978, 1, 147–157.

Knittle, J. L. Obesity in childhood: A problem in adipose tissue cellular development. *Journal of Pediatrics*, 1972, 6, 1048–1059.

Knittle, J. L. Basic concepts in the control of childhood obesity. In M. Winick (Ed.), *Childhood obesity*. New York: John Wiley & Sons, 1975.

Knittle, J. L., Ginsberg-Fellner, F., & Brown, R. E. Adipose tissue development in man. *American Journal of Clinical Nutrition*, 1977, 30, 762–766.

Knittle, J. L., Timmers, K., Ginsberg-Fellner, F., Brown, R. E., & Katz, D. P. The growth of adipose tissue in children and adolescents. *Journal of Clinical Investigation*, 1979, 63, 239–246.

Koh, E. T. Selected anthropometric measurements for a low-income black population in Mississippi. *Journal of the American Dietetic Association*, 1981, 79, 555–561.

Kohrs, M. B., Wang, L. L., Ekland, D., Paulsen, B., & O'Neal R. The association of obesity with socioeconomic factors in Missouri. *The American Journal of Clinical Nutrition*, 1979, 32, 2120–2128.

Kowalczyk, J. Analysis of familial, somatic and psychic aspects in children with simple obesity. *Polish Medical Sciences and History Bulletin*, 1976, 15, 65–68.

Kramer, M. S. Do breast-feeding and delayed introduction of solid foods protect against subsequent obesity. *The Journal of Pediatrics*, 1981, 98, 883–887.

Kraus, B. *Calories and carbohydrates*. New York: Grosset and Dunlap, 1979.

Laditan, A. A. O. Excessive weight gain in infancy and childhood in developing countries: Association with modern methods of infant feeding. *Journal of Human Nutrition*, 1981, 35, 139–140.

Lancet. Helping obese children. *Lancet*, 1978, 1, 1189–1190.

Lang, P. J. The mechanics of desensitization and the laboratory study of fear. In

C. M. Franks (Ed.), *Behavior therapy: Appraisal and status*. New York: McGraw-Hill, 1969.

Lang, P. J. The application of psychophysiological methods to the study of psychotherapy and behavior modification. In A. E. Bergin & S. L. Garfield (Eds.), *Handbook of psychotherapy and behavior change*. New York: Wiley, 1971.

Lansky, D. A methodological analysis of research on adherence and weight loss: Reply to Brownell and Stunkard (1978). *Behavior Therapy*, 1981, 12, 144–149.

Lasarev, S. G. Morbidity among children with excessive body weight during the first year of life. *Pediatriya*, 1978, 10, 33–36. (*Information Retrieval*, 1979, 4, no. 1328, 70.)

Lauer, R. M., Connor, W. E., Leaverton, P. E., Reiter, M. A., & Clarke, W. R. Coronary heart disease risk factors in school children: The Muscatine study. *The Journal of Pediatrics*, 1975, 86, 697–706.

Lauer, R. M. & Shekelle, R. B. (Eds.), *Childhood prevention of atherosclerosis and hypertension*. New York: Raven Press, 1980.

LeBow, M. D. *Behavior modification: A significant method in nursing practice*. Englewood Cliffs, New Jersey: Prentice-Hall, 1973.

LeBow, M. D. *Approaches to modifying patient behavior*. New York: Appleton-Century-Crofts, 1976.

LeBow, M. D. Can lighter become thinner? *Addictive Behaviors*, 1977, 2, 87–93.

LeBow, M. D. *Weight control: The behavioral strategies*. Chichester and New York: Wiley, 1981a.

LeBow, M. D. Obstacles to effectively treating obese children. *Child Behavior Therapy*, 1981b, 3, 29–39.

LeBow, M. D., Buser, M., Coles, R., Hanel, F., & Vallentyne, S. Building weight control plans in children. Unpublished manuscript, 1979.

LeBow, M. D., Chipperfield, J., & Magnusson, J. *The effects of sex, weight, and social context on cleaning-the-plate behaviour*. Paper presented at the meeting of the Association for Advancement of Behavior Therapy, Los Angeles, November 1982.

LeBow, M. D., Goldberg, P. S. & Collins, A. Eating behavior of overweight and nonoverweight persons in the natural environment. *Journal of Consulting and Clinical Psychology*, 1977, 45, 1204–1205.

LeBow, M. D. & LeBow, B. L. *Deviation analysis in the behavioral treatment of overweight adults*. Unpublished manuscript, 1981.

LeBow, M. D. & Perry, R. P. *If only I were thin*. Winnipeg, Manitoba: Prairie Publishing, 1977.

LeBow, M. D. & Skopec, M. *A behavioral weight reduction program for college students*. Unpublished manuscript, Dartmouth Medical School, 1973.

Lechowick, F. *The effect of effort and food preferability on food consumption of obese and nonobese children*. Unpublished master's thesis, University of Manitoba, 1981.

Leitenberg, H. The use of single case methodology in psychotherapy research. *Journal of Abnormal Psychology*, 1973, 82, 87–101.

Leon, G. R., Bemis, K. M., Meland, M., & Nussbaum, D. Aspects of body image perception in obese and normal weight youngsters. *Journal of Abnormal Child Psychology*, 1978, 6, 361–371.

Lerner, R. M. The development of stereotyped expectancies of body build-behavior relations. *Child Development*, 1969a, 40, 137–141.

Lerner, R. M. Some female stereotypes of male body-build-behavior relations. *Perceptual and Motor Skills*, 1969b, 28, 363–366.

Lerner, R. M. & Gellert, E. Body build identification, preference and aversion in children. *Developmental Psychology*, 1969, 456–462.

Lerner, R. M. & Korn, S. J. The development of body-build stereotypes in males. *Child Development*, 1972, 43, 908–920.

Lerner, R. M. & Pool, K. B. Body-build stereotypes: A cross cultural comparison. *Psychological Reports*, 1972, 31, 527–532.

Lerner, R. M. & Schroeder, C. Physique identification preference and aversion in kindergarten children. *Developmental Psychology*, 1971, 5, 538.

Levine, R. S., Hennekens, C. H., Rosner, B., Gourley, J., Gelband, H. & Jesse, M. S. Cardiovascular risk factors among children of men with premature myocardial infarction. *Public Health Reports*, 1981, 96, 58–69.

Levitz, L. S., Jordan, H. A., LeBow, M. D., & Coopersmith, M. L. Weight loss five years after behavioral treatment. In R. C. Hawkins (Chair). *Maintenance of weight loss in behavioral treatment programs*. Symposium presented at the meeting of the American Psychological Association, Montreal, 1980.

Lindner, P. Techniques of management for the inactive obese child. In P. J. Collipp (Ed.), *Childhood obesity* (2nd ed.). Littleton, Massachusetts: PSG Publishing, 1980.

Lloyd, J. K. Prognosis of obesity in infancy and childhood. *Postgraduate Medicine Journal*, 1977, 53, 111–115.

Lloyd, J. K. & Wolff, O. H. Overnutrition and obesity. In F. Falkner (Ed.), *Prevention in childhood of health problems in adult life*. Geneva: World Health Organization, 1980.

Lloyd, J. K., Wolff, O. H., & Whelen, W. S. Childhood obesity: A long-term study of height and weight. *British Medical Journal*, 1961, 2, 145–148.

Lohman, T. G. Skinfolds and body density and their relation to body fatness: A review. *Human Biology*, 1981, 53, 181–225.

Londe, S., Bourgoignie, J. J., Robson, A. M., & Goldring, D. Hypertension in apparently normal children. *The Journal of Pediatrics*, 1971, 78, 569–577.

Loro, A. D., Fisher, E. B., Jr., & Levenkron, J. C. Comparison of established and innovative weight reduction treatment procedures. *Journal of Applied Behavior Analysis*, 1979, 12, 141–155.

Lynds, B. G., Seyler, S. K., & Morgan, B. M. The relationship between elevated blood pressure and obesity in black children. *American Journal of Public Health,* 1980, 70, 171–173.

Mack, R. W. & Johnston, F. E. Height, skeletal maturation and adiposity in adolescents with high relative weight at one year of age. *Annals of Human Biology,* 1979, 6, 77–83.

Maddox, G. L., Back K. W., & Liederman, V. R. Overweight as social deviance and disability. *Journal of Health and Social Behavior,* 1968, 9, 287–298.

Madsen, C. H., Madsen, C. K., & Thompson, F. Increasing rural Head Start children's consumption of middle class meals. *Journal of Applied Behavior Analysis,* 1974, 7, 257–262.

Mahoney, B. K., Rogers, T., Straw, M., & Mahoney, M. J. *Results and implications of a problem solving treatment program for obesity.* Paper presented at the Meeting of the Association for Advancement of Behavior Therapy, Atlanta, December 1977.

Mahoney, M. J. Self-reward and self-monitoring techniques for weight control. *Behavior Therapy,* 1974, 5, 48–57.

Mahoney, M. J. Fat fiction. *Behavior Therapy,* 1975a, 6, 416–418.

Mahoney M. J. The obese eating: Bites, beliefs, and behavior modification. *Addictive Behaviors.* 1975b, 1, 47–54.

Mahoney, M. J. & Mahoney, K. *Permanent weight control.* New York: Norton & Company, 1976a.

Mahoney, M. J. & Mahoney, K. Treatment of obesity: A clinical exploration. In B. J. Williams, S. Martin & J. P. Foreyt (Eds.), *Obesity: Behavioral approaches to dietary management.* New York: Brunner/Mazel, 1976b.

Mahoney, M. J., Moura, N. G. M., & Wade, T. C. Relative effectiveness of self-reward, self-punishment, and self-monitoring techniques for weight loss. *Journal of Consulting and Clinical Psychology,* 1973, 40, 404–407.

Mallick, J. M. The adverse effects of weight control in teenage girls. *Dissertation Abstracts International,* 1980, 41, 895–B.

Mann, R. A. The behavior–therapeutic use of contingency contracting to control an adult behavior problem. Weight control. *Journal of Applied Behavior Analysis,* 1972, 5, 99–109.

Marshall, D. G., Elder, J., O'Basky, D., Wallace, D. J., & Liberman, R. P. Behavioral treatment of Prader-Willi syndrome. *The Behavior Therapist,* 1979, 2, 22–24.

Marston, A. R., London, P., & Cooper, L. M. A note on the eating behavior of children varying in weight. *Journal of Child Psychology and Psychiatry,* 1976, 17, 55–58.

Martin, J. E. & Sachs, D. A. The effects of a self-control weight loss program on an obese woman. *Journal of Behavior Therapy and Experimental Psychiatry,* 1973, 4, 155–159.

Martin, M. M. & Martin, A. L. A. Obesity, hyperinsulinism, and diabetes mellitus in childhood. *Journal of Pediatrics,* 1973, 82, 192–201.

Mason, E. Obesity in pet dogs. *The Veterinary Record,* 1970, 86, 612–616.

Mathews, D. K. & Fox, E. L. *The physiological basis of physical education and athletics* (2nd ed.). Philadelphia: W. B. Saunders, 1976.

Matson, J. L. Social reinforcement by the spouse in weight control: A case study. *Journal of Behavior Therapy and Experimental Psychiatry,* 1977, 8, 327–328.

Mayer, J. *Overweight: Causes, cost, and control.* Englewood Cliffs, New Jersey: Prentice-Hall, 1968.

Mayer, J. *Human nutrition.* Springfield, Illinois: Charles C Thomas, 1972.

Mayer, J. Obesity during childhood. In M. Winick (Ed.), *Childhood obesity.* New York: John Wiley & Sons, 1975.

Mayer, J. The best diet is exercise. In P. J. Collipp (Ed.), *Childhood obesity* (2nd ed.). Littleton, Massachusetts: PSG Publishing, 1980.

Mayer, J., Roy, P., & Mitra, K. P. Relation between calorie intake, body weight and physical work: Studies in an industrial male population in West Bengal. *American Journal of Clinical Nutrition,* 1956, 4, 169–175.

McFall, R. M. Parameters of self-monitoring. In R. B. Stuart (Ed.), *Behavioral self-management: Strategies, techniques and outcome.* New York: Brunner/Mazel, 1977.

McReynolds, W. T., Lutz, R. N., Paulsen, B. K., & Kohrs, M. B. Treatment manual for the food management (stimulus control) treatment. *JSAS Catalog of Selected Documents in Psychology,* 1975, 5, 286.

Mellbin, T. & Vuille, J. C. The relative importance of rapid weight gain in infancy as a precursor to childhood obesity. *Pediatric and Adolescent Endicrinology,* Vol. 1, 78–83. Basel: Karger, 1976.

Merritt, R. J. Treatment of pediatric and adolescent obesity. *International Journal of Obesity,* 1978, 2, 207–214.

Merritt, R. J. Obesity in pediatric patients. *Comprehensive Therapy,* 1979, 5, 26–34.

Merritt, R. J. & Batrus, C. The role of the dietitian in the treatment of pediatric obesity. In P. J. Collipp (Ed.), *Childhood obesity* (2nd ed.). Littleton, Massachusetts, 1980.

Merritt, R. J., Bistrian, B. R., Blackburn, G. L., & Suskind R. M. Consequences of modified fasting in obese pediatric and adolescent patients. I Protein sparing modified fast. *Journal of Pediatrics,* 1980, 96, 13–19.

Merritt, R. J., Blackburn, G. L., Bistrian, B. R., Palumbo, J., & Suskind, R. M. Consequences of modified fasting in obese pediatric and adolescent patients: Effect of a carbohydrate free diet on serum proteins. *American Journal of Clinical Nutrition,* 1981, 39, 2752–2755.

Merritt, R. J., Schlaman, C. L., Bistrian, B. R., & Suskind, R. M. Protein supplemented fasting in children. *International Journal of Obesity*, 1978, 2, 365–366.

Metropolitan Life Insurance Tables, 1959. Metropolitan Life Insurance Company. New Weight Standards for Men and Women. *Statistical Bulletin*, 1959, 40(1).

Meyer, E. E. & Neumann, C. G. Management of the obese adolescent. *Pediatric Clinics of North America*, 1977, 24, 123–132.

Meyer, V. & Crisp, A. H. Aversion therapy in two cases of obesity. *Behaviour Research and Therapy*, 1964, 2, 143–147.

Miller, P. M. & Sims, K. L. Evaluation and component analysis of a comprehensive weight control program. *International Journal of Obesity*, 1981, 5, 57–65.

Miller, R. A. & Shekelle, R. B. Blood pressure in tenth-grade students. *Circulation*, 1976, 54, 993–1000.

Milstein, R. M. Responsiveness in newborn infants of normal weight and overweight parents. *Dissertation Abstracts International*, 1978, 39, 2478B–2479B.

Mitchell, C. O. & Fiser, R. H. Exogenous childhood obesity: A promising application of a combined approach for treatment of obesity in the young child. *International Journal of Obesity*, 1978, 2, 366.

Mobbs, J. Childhood obesity. *International Journal of Nursing Studies*, 1970, 7, 3–18.

Monello, L. F. & Mayer, J. Obese adolescent girls: An unrecognized 'minority' group. *American Journal of Clinical Nutrition*, 1963, 13, 35–39.

Moody, D. L., Wilmore, J. H., Girandola, R. N., & Royce, J. P. The effects of a jogging program on the body composition of normal & obese high school girls. *Medicine and Science in Sports*, 1972, 4, 210–213.

Moore, M. E., Stunkard, A. J., & Srole, L. Obesity, social class and mental illness. *Journal of the American Medical Association*, 1962, 181, 962–966.

Morgan, J. The pre-school child: Diet, growth and obesity. *Journal of Human Nutrition*, 1980, 34, 117–130.

Morgavan, C. B. Effects of degree of children's obesity and compliant vs noncompliant behavior on adult's evaluation and reinforcement of the children. *Dissertation Abstracts International*, 1976, 37, 1919B.

Morris, R. W. & Chinn, S. Weight for height as a measure of obesity in English children five to eleven years old. *International Journal of Obesity*, 1981, 5, 367–376.

Morris, S. S., Farrier, S. C., Rogers, C. S., & Tapper, L. J. Feeding behaviors, food attitudes, and body fitness in infants. *Journal of the American Dietetic Association*, 1982, 80, 330–334.

Mossberg, N. Obesity in children: A clinical-prognostical investigation. *Acta Paediatrica*, 1948, 35, Supplement 2, 1.

Murata, M., Fujita, Y., Yamazaki, K., Hoshina, K., & Imai, M. The fatty liver in childhood obesity: Does it result in liver inflammation and fibrosis. *International Journal of Obesity,* 1978, 4, 486.

Murphy, J. K., Williamson, D. A., Buxton, A., Moody, S. C., Absher, N., & Warner, M. *The effects of spouse involvement and contingency contracting upon weight loss.* Paper presented at the meeting of the Association for Advancement of Behavior Therapy, New York, November 1980.

Myres, A. & Yeung, D. L. Obesity in infants: Significance aetiology and prevention. *Canadian Journal of Public Health,* 1979, 70, 113–119.

Naiman, D. J. Effect of prior exposure to food and nonfood slides upon the reward ratings and selections by obese and nonobese school-age children. *Dissertation Abstracts International,* 1978, 38, 7235A–7236A.

Nathan, S. Body image in chronically obese children as reflected in figure drawings. *School Psychology Digest,* 1976, 5, 456–463.

Nathan, S. L. & Pisula, D. Psychological observations of obese adolescents during starvation treatment. *Journal of the American Academy of Child Psychiatry,* 1970, 9, 722–740.

Netzer, C. & Chaback, E. *Brand-name calorie counter* (abridged). New York: Dell, 1979.

Neumann, C. & Alpaugh, M. Birth weight doubling time: A fresh look. *Pediatrics,* 1976, 57, 469–473.

Neumann, C. G. Obesity in pediatric practice: Obesity in the preschool and school-age child. *Pediatric Clinics of North America,* 1977, 24, 117–122.

New, M. I. & Rauh, W. Childhood obesity and hypertension. In P. J. Collipp (Ed.), *Childhood obesity* (2nd ed.). Littleton, Massachusetts: PSG Publishing, 1980.

Newman, H. H., Freeman, F. N., & Holzinger, K. N. *Twins: A study of heredity and environment.* Chicago: University of Chicago Press, 1937.

Neyzi, O., Saner, G., Binyildiz, P., Yazicioglu, S., Emre, S., & Gurson, C. Relationship between body weight in infancy and weight in later childhood and adolescence. In Z. Laron (Ed.), *Pediatric and adolescent endicrinology* Vol. 1: *The adipose Child.* Basel: Karger, 1976.

Nisbett, R. E. Hunger, obesity, and the ventromedial hypothalamus. *Psychological Review,* 1972, 79, 433–453.

Nisbett, R. E. Starvation and the behavior of the obese. In G. A. Bray & J. E. Bethune (Eds.), *Treatment and management of obesity.* New York: Harper & Row, 1974.

Niswander, K. & Jackson, E. C. Physical characteristics of the gravida and their association with birth weight and perinatal death. *American Journal of Obstetrics and Gynecology,* 1974, 119, 306–313.

Noppa, H., Bengtsson, C., Isaksson, B., & Smith, U. Adipose tissue cellularity in adulthood and its relation to childhood obesity. *International Journal of Obesity,* 1980, 4, 253–263.

Nutt, H. H. Infant nutrition and obesity. *Nursing Forum,* 1979, 18, 131–157.

Olson, C. M., Pringle, D. J., & Schoenwetter, C. D. Parent child interaction: Its relation to growth and weight. *Journal of Nutrition Education,* 1976, 8, 67–70.

O'Neil, P. M., Currey, H. S., Hirsch, A. A., Riddle, E. E., Taylor, C. I., Malcolm, R. J., & Sexauer, J. D. Spouse effect in behavioral obesity therapy. *Addictive Behaviors,* 1979, 4, 167–177.

Orenstein, D. M., Boat, T. F., Owens, R. P., Horowitz, J. G., Primiano, F. P., Germann, K., & Doershuk, C. F. The obesity hypoventilation syndrome in children with Prader-Willi syndrome: A possible role for familial decreased response to carbon dioxide. *The Journal of Pediatrics,* 1980, 97, 765–767.

Osborne, J. G. Free-time as a reinforcer in the management of classroom behavior. *Journal of Applied Behavior Analysis,* 1969, 2, 113–118.

Oscai, L. B. & Williams, B. T. Effect of exercise on overweight middle-aged males. *Journal of the American Geriatric Society,* 1968, 16, 794–797.

Ounsted, M. & Sleigh, G. The infant's self-regulation of food intake and weight gain. *Lancet,* 1975, 2, 1393–1397.

Owen, G. M. Measurement, recording, and assessment of skinfold thickness in childhood and adolescence: Report of a small meeting. *The American Journal of Clinical Nutrition,* 1982, 35, 629–638.

Pargman, D. The incidence of obesity among college students. *The Journal of School Health,* 1969, 29, 621–627.

Pařizková, J. Body composition and exercise during growth and development. In G. L. Rarick (Ed.), *Physical activity: Human growth and development.* New York: Academic Press, 1973.

Pařizková, J. *Body fatness and physical fitness.* The Hague, The Netherlands: Martinus Nijhoff b.v., Publishers, 1977.

Patterson, G. R. & Gullion, M. E. *Living with children.* Champaign, Illinois: Research Press, 1971.

Pavlov, I. P. *Conditioned reflexes.* London: Oxford University Press, 1927. Republished in 1960, New York: Dover Publications, Inc. Translated by G. V. Anrep.

Pearce, J., LeBow, M. D., & Orchard, J. Role of spouse involvement in the behavioral treatment of overweight women. *Journal of Consulting and Clinical Psychology,* 1981, 49, 236–244.

Peckham, C. H. & Christianson, R. E. The relationship between pre-pregnancy weight and certain obstetric factors. *American Journal of Obstetrics and Gynecology,* 1971, 111, 1–7.

Peña, M., Barta, L., Regöly-Mérel, A., & Tichy, M. The influence of physical exercise upon the body composition of obese children. *Acta Paediatrica Academiae Scientiarum Hungaricae,* 1980, 21, 9–14.

Pencharz, P. B., Motil, K. J., Parsons, H. G., & Duffy, D. J. The effect of an energy-restricted diet on the protein metabolism of obese adolescents: Ni-

'trogen-balance and whole-body nitrogen turnover. *Clinical Science,* 1980, 59, 13–18.

Penick, S. B., Filion, R., Fox, S., & Stunkard, A. J. Behavior modification in the treatment of obesity. *Psychosomatic Medicine,* 1971, 33, 46–55.

Pennington, J. A. T. & Nichols-Church, H. *Food Values of Portions Commonly Used,* 13th Edition. New York: Harper & Row, 1980.

Perri, M. G., Twentyman, C., Stalonas, P. M., Toro, P. A., & Zastowny, T. R. *Evaluation of social support systems in the behavioral treatment of obesity.* Paper presented at the meeting of the American Psychological Association, Montreal, September 1980.

Perry, R. P., LeBow, M. D., & Buser, M. M. An exploration of observational learning in modifying selected eating responses of obese children. *International Journal of Obesity,* 1979, 3, 193–199.

Petrash, S. P. Some indices of the state of health of obese school children. *Pediatriya,* 1977, 9, 34–35. [*Information Retrieval,* 1978, 3(1310), 73.]

Phillips, D., Fischer, S. C., & Singh, R. A children's reinforcement survey schedule. *Journal of Behavior Therapy and Experimental Psychiatry,* 1977, 8, 131–134.

Pipes, P. & Holm, V. Weight control of children with Prader-Willi syndrome. *Journal of the American Dietetic Association,* 1973, 62, 520–524.

Pisacano, J. C., Lichter, H., Ritter, J. & Siegal, A. P. An attempt at prevention of obesity in infancy. *Pediatrics,* 1978, 61, 360–364.

Pleas, J. *A test of the helper therapy principle in weight management.* Paper presented at the meeting of the International Congress on Obesity, Washington, D.C., October 1977.

Polich, J. J., Stauter, J., Kirkpatrick, P. T., & Larson, M. Childhood obesity. *The Journal of Family Practice,* 1978, 7, 849–855.

Polished Apple. *Nutrition filmstrips for children.* Malibu, California: The Polished Apple, 1976.

Pollack, M. L., Cureton, T. K., & Greniger, L. Effects of frequency of training on working capacity, cardiovascular function, and body composition in adult men. *Medical Science in Sports,* 1969, 1, 70–74.

Pollitt, E. & Wirtz, S. Mother–infant feeding interaction and weight gain in the first month of life. *Journal of the American Dietetic Association,* 1981, 78, 596–601.

Poskitt, E. M. E. Overfeeding and overweight in infancy and their relation to body size in early childhood. *Nutrition and Metabolism,* 1977, 21(Suppl. 1), 54–55.

Poskitt, E. M. E. & Cole, T. J. Do fat babies stay fat? *British Medical Journal,* 1977, 1, 7–9.

Poskitt, E. M. E. & Cole, T. J. Nature, nurture, and childhood overweight. *British Medical Journal,* 1978, 1, 603–605.

Powers, P. S. *Obesity: The regulation of weight*. Baltimore: Williams & Wilkins, 1980.

Premack, D. Reinforcement theory. In D. Levine (Ed.), *Nebraska Symposium on Motivation: 1965*. Lincoln: University of Nebraska Press, 1965, 123–180.

Rallo, J. *An exploration of the effects of parental modeling on the acquisition of eating behaviours by obese children*. Unpublished master's thesis, University of Manitoba, 1982.

Ramirez, M. E. & Mueller, W. H. The development of obesity and fat patterning on Tokelau children. *Human Biology*, 1980, 52, 675–687.

Randolph J. Discussion on Anderson et al., 1980. *Journal of Pediatric Surgery*, 1980, 15, 881.

Randolph, J. G., Weintraub, W. H., & Rigg, A. Jejunoileal bypass for morbid obesity in adolescents. *Journal of Pediatric Surgery*, 1974, 9, 341–345.

Rappoport, S. Obesity and the pediatrician. *American Journal of Diseases of Children*, 1974, 12, 597.

Ravelli, G. P. & Belmont, L. Obesity in nineteen-year-old men: Family size and birth order associations. *American Journal of Epidemiology*, 1979, 109, 66–69.

Ravelli, G. P., Stein, Z. A., & Susser, M. W. Obesity in young men after famine exposure in utero and early infancy. *New England Journal of Medicine*, 1976, 295, 349–353.

Ravitch, M. Discussion on Anderson et al, 1980. *Journal of Pediatric Surgery*, 1980, 15, 881.

Rayner, P. H. W. & Court, J. M. The effect of dietary restriction and anorectic drugs on linear growth velocity in childhood obesity. *Postgraduate Medical Journal*, 1975, 51, 120–125.

RDA. *Recommended Dietary Allowances* (9th ed.). Washington, D.C.: National Academy of Sciences, 1980.

Reynolds, G. S. *A primer of operant conditioning*. Glenview, Illinois: Scott, Foresman & Company, 1968.

Richardson, B. D. & Wadvalla, M. The bearing of height, weight, and skinfold thickness on obesity in four South African ethnic groups of school pupils of 17 years. *Tropical and Geographical Medicines*, 1977, 29, 82–90. In *Information Retrieval* (IRL), 1978, 3, No. 302, 59–60.

Richardson, S. A., Goodman, N., Hastorf, A. H. & Dornbusch, S. M. Cultural uniformity in reaction to physical disabilities. *American Sociological Review*, 1961, 26, 241–247.

Rigg, C. A. Jejunoileal bypass for morbidly obese adolescent. *Acta Paediatrica Scandinavia*, 1975, 256, 62–63.

Rimm, I. J. & Rimm, A. A. Association between juvenile onset obesity and severe adult obesity in 73,532 women. *American Journal of Public Health*, 1976, 6, 479–481.

Rimm, I. J., Rimm, A. A, & Hartz, A. Comments on obesity study. *American Journal of Public Health,* 1976, 66, 906–907.

Rivinus, T. M., Drummond, T., & Combrinck-Graham, L. A group-behavior treatment program for overweight children: Results of a pilot study. In *The adipose child pediatric adolescence endocrinology,* Vol. 1. Basel: Karger, 1976, 212–218.

Rivlin, R. S. The use of hormones in the treatment of obesity. In M. Winick (Ed.), *Childhood obesity.* New York: Wiley, 1975.

Roche, A. F. The adipocyte-number hypothesis. *Child Development,* 1981, 52, 31–43.

Rodin, J. Effects of obesity and set point on taste responsiveness and ingestion in humans. *Journal of Comparative and Physiological Psychology,* 1975, 89, 1003–1009.

Rodin, J. Bidirectional influences of emotionality, stimulus responsivity, and metabolic events in obesity. In J. D. Maser and M. E. P. Seligman (Eds.), *Psychopathology: Experimental Models.* San Francisco: W. H. Freeman and Company, 1977.

Rodin, J. *Obesity theory and behavior therapy: An uneasy couple.* Paper presented at the meeting of the Association for Advancement of Behavior Therapy, San Francisco, December 1979a.

Rodin, J. Obesity: Why the losing battle? *JSAS Catalog of Selected Documents in Psychology,* 1979b, 9, 17.

Rodin, J. The externality theory today. In A. J. Stunkard (Ed.), *Obesity.* Philadelphia. W. B. Saunders, 1980.

Rodin, J. Psychological factors in obesity, In P. Bjorntorp, M. Cairella, A. N. Howard (Eds.), *Recent advances in obesity research: III.* London: John Libbey, 1981.

Rodin, J. & Slochower, J. Externality in the nonobese: Effects of environmental responsiveness on weight. *Journal of Personality and Social Psychology,* 1976, 33, 338–344.

Romanczyk, R. G., Tracy, D. A., Wilson, G. T., & Thorpe, G. L. Behavioral techniques in the treatment of obesity: A comparative analysis. *Behaviour Research and Therapy,* 1973, 11, 629–640.

Rona, R. J. & Chinn, S. National study of health and growth: social and family factors and obesity in primary school children. *Annals of Human Biology,* 1982, 9, 131–145.

Rony, H. R. *Obesity and leaness.* Philadelphia: Lea & Febiger, 1940.

Rose, H. E. & Mayer, J. Activity, caloric intake, fat storage, and energy balance of infants. *Pediatrics,* 1968, 41, 18–29.

Rosenbaum, M. S., Faris, A. W., Shriner, J. F., Blankenship, V. H., & Suskind, M. Managing overweight children: Effects of a protein sparing modified fast (PSMF) diet, exercise, and behavior modification. *American Journal of Clinical Nutrition,* 1982, 35, 856.

Rosenbaum, M. S., Faris, A. W., Shriner, J. F., & Suskind, R. M. Weight reduction and physical fitness in overweight children. *Pediatric Research,* 1981, 15, 455.

Rosenthal, B. S., Allen, G. J., & Winter, C. Husband involvement in the behavioral treatment of overweight women: Initial effects and long-term follow-up. *International Journal of Obesity,* 1980, 4, 165–173.

Rosenthal, B. S. & Marx, R. D. Differences in eating patterns of successful and unsuccessful dieters, untreated overweight and normal weight individuals. *Addictive Behaviors,* 1978, 3, 129–134.

Ross, K. E., Daniels, L., & Douglas, H. M. The obese child: Observations in the gymnasium of the Adelaide Children's Hospital. *Medical Journal of Australia,* 1980, 2, 80–84.

Rotatori, A. F. & Fox, R. The effectiveness of a behavioral weight reduction program for moderately retarded adolescents. *Behavior Therapy,* 1980, 11, 410–416.

Rotatori, A. F., Fox, R., & Parish, P. A weight reduction model for mildly retarded adults living in semi-independent care facilities. *Journal of Advanced Nursing,* 1980, 5, 179–186.

Rotatori, A. F., Fox, R., & Switzky, H. A parent–teacher administered weight reduction program for obese down syndrome adolescents. *Journal of Behavior Therapy and Experimental Psychiatry,* 1979, 10, 339–341.

Rotatori, A. F. Parish, P., & Freagon, S. Weight loss in retarded children—a pilot study. *Journal of Psychiatric Nursing,* 1979, 17, 33–34.

Rotatori, A. F. & Rotatori, L. Behavioral weight reduction for the mentally retarded. *Journal of the American Dietetic Association,* 1979, 75, 46–48.

Rotatori, A. F. & Switzky, H. A successful behavioral weight-loss program for moderately retarded teenagers. *International Journal of Obesity,* 1979, 3, 223–228.

Rowe, N. R. Childhood obesity: Growth charts versus calipers. *Pediatric Nursing,* 1980, March/April, 24–27.

Rozensky, R. H. & Bellack, A. S. Individual differences in self-reinforcement style and performance in self- and therapist-controlled weight reduction programs. *Behaviour Research and Therapy,* 1976, 14, 325–364.

Rozin, P. Psychobiological and cultural determinants of food choice. In T. Silverstone (Ed.)., *Appetite and Food Intake: Report of the Dahlem Konferenzen.* Berlin: Abakon Verlagsgesellschaft, 1976.

Saccone, A. J. & Israel, A. C. Effects of experimenter versus significant other-controlled reinforcement and choice of target behavior on weight loss. *Behavior Therapy,* 1978, 9, 271–278.

Salans, L. B. Adipose tissue cellularity—An update. *Obesity and Metabolism,* 1981, 1, 48–53.

Salans, L. B. Cellularity of adipose tissue. In G. A. Bray & J. E. Bethune (Eds.), *Treatment and management of obesity.* New York: Harper & Row, 1974.

Salans, L. B., Cushman, S. W., & Weismann, R. R. Studies of human tissue:

Adipose cell size and number in nonobese and obese patients. *The Journal of Clinical Investigation,* 1973, 52, 929–941.

Salans, L. B., Horton, E. S., & Sims, E. A. H. Experimental obesity in man: Cellular character of the adipose tissue, *Journal of Clinical Investigation,* 1971, 50, 1005–1011.

Sallade, J. A. Comparison of the psychological adjustment of obese vs. nonobese children. *Journal of Psychosomatic Research,* 1973, 17, 89–96.

Sash, S. E. Weight reduction in obese schoolboys. In A. Howard (Ed.), *Recent Advances in Obesity Research,* vol. I. London: Newman, 1975.

Schachter, S. Some extraordinary facts about obese humans and rats. *American Psychologist,* 1971, 26, 129–144.

Schoenwetter, C. D. Case study: Weight control and retardation. *The Journal of School Health,* 1978, 48, 166–167.

Schwartz, F., van Gilst, M., & Rexwinkel, B. External factors causing childhood obesity. In E. Caccari, Z. Laron, & S. Raiti (Eds.), *Obesity in childhood,* London: Academic Press, 1978.

Schwartz, M. Z. Childhood obesity. *Surgical Clinics of North America,* 1979, 59, 995–1006.

Schwartz, R. P. & Sidbury, J. B. Childhood obesity. *Connecticut Medicine,* 1974, 38, 660–663.

Sells, C. J., Hanson, J. W. & Hall, J. G. The Summitt syndrome: Observations on a third case. *American Journal of Medical Genetics,* 1979, 3, 27–33.

Selph, A. D. & Street, B. G. *Alphabet soup.* Durham, North Carolina: American Printers Limited, 1975.

Seltzer, C. C. Limitations of height–weight standards. *The New England Journal of Medicine,* 1965, 272, 1132.

Seltzer, C. C. & Mayer, J. A simple criterion of obesity. *Postgraduate Medicine,* 1965, 38, A-101–A-107.

Seltzer, C. C. & Mayer, J. How representative are the weights of insured men and women. *Journal of the American Medical Association,* 1967, 201, 75–78.

Seltzer, C. C. & Mayer, J. An effective weight control program in a public school system. *American Journal of Public Health,* 1970, 60, 679–689.

Seymour, F. W. & Stokes, T. F. Self-recording in training girls to increase work and evoke staff praise in an institution for offenders. *Journal of Applied Behavior Analysis,* 1976, 9, 41–54.

Sgaramella, L. Z., Galante, A., Jayakar, S. D., & Pennetti, V. Obesity in a group of Italian elementary school children: Family structure. *Journal of Biosocial Science,* 1980, 12, 487–493.

Sgaramella, L. Z., Jayakar, S. D., Galante, A., & Pennetti, V. Obesity in Italian children: Regional differences in height, weight, and skinfold thickness. *Human Biology,* 1979, 51, 279–288.

Sharkey, B. J. *Physiological fitness and weight control.* Missoula: Mountain Press, 1974.

Shenker, I. R., Fisichelli, V., & Lang, J. Weight differences between foster infants of overweight and nonoverweight foster mothers. *Journal of Pediatrics,* 1974, 84, 715–719.

Shields, J. *Monozygotic twins brought up apart and brought up together.* London: Oxford University Press, 1962.

Shisslack, C. M. Naturalistic observations of eating patterns in humans: Relationships between obesity and eating style (Doctoral dissertation, University of Arizona, 1977). *Dissertation Abstracts International,* 1978, 38, 3416B. (University Microfilms no. 77–29, 355.)

Shukla, A., Forsyth, H. A., Anderson, C. M., & Marwah, S. M. Infantile overnutrition in the first year of life: A field study in Dudley, Worcestershire. *British Medical Journal,* 1972, 4, 507–515.

Sidury, J. B. & Schwartz, R. P. A program for weight reduction in children. In P. J. Collipp (Ed.), *Childhood obesity (2nd ed.).* Littleton, Massachusetts: PSG Publishing, 1980.

Siddamma, T. & Venkatramaiah, S. R. An index for measuring obesity in children. *Indian Journal of Pediatrics,* 1977, 44, 121–126.

Siervogel, R. M., Frey, M. A., Kezdi, P., Roche, A. F., & Stanley, E. L. Blood pressure, electrolytes, and body size: Their relationships in young relatives of men with essential hypertension. *Hypertension,* 1980, 2(Suppl. I), I-83–I-91.

Simić, B. S. Childhood obesity as a risk factor in adulthood. In P. J. Collipp (Ed.), *Childhood obesity.* Littleton, Massachusetts: PSG Publishing, 1980.

Simpson, J. W. Lawless, R. W., & Mitchell, A. C. Responsibility of the obstetrician to the fetus: II Influence of prepregnancy weight and pregnancy weight gain in birth weight. *Journal of Obstetrics and Gynecology,* 1975, 45, 481–497.

Sjöstrom, L. & William-Olsson, T. Prospective studies on adipose tissue development in man. *International Journal of Obesity,* 1981, 5, 597–604.

Skinner, B. F. *Science and Human Behavior.* New York: The Macmillan Company, 1953.

Skinner, B. F. Why I am not a cognitive psychologist, *Behaviourism,* 1977, 5, 1–10.

Skopec, H. M. & Cassidy, A. Sometimes our plans go awry. In LeBow, M. D. (Ed.), *Approaches to modifying patient behavior.* New York: Appleton-Century-Crofts, 1976.

Smiciklas-Wright, H. & D'Augelli, A. Primary prevention for overweight: Preschool eating patterns (PEP) program. *Journal of the American Dietetic Association,* 1978, 626–629.

Society of Acturaries. *Build and blood pressure study of 1979.* Chicago, Illinois: Society of Actuaries (208 So. LaSalle Street), 1980.

Spiegel, T. A. & Jordan, H. A. Effects of simultaneous oral–intragastric ingestion on meal patterns and satiety in humans. *Journal of Comparative and Physiological Psychology,* 1978, 92, 133–141.

Srole, L., Langner, T. S., Michael, S. T, Opler, M. K., & Rennie, T. A. C. *Mental health in the metropolis: The midtown Manhattan study.* New York: McGraw-Hill, 1962.

Staffieri, J. R. A study of social stereotype of body image in children. *Journal of Personality and Social Psychology,* 1967, 7, 101–104.

Staffieri, J. R. Body image stereotypes of mentally retarded. *American Journal of Mental Deficiency,* 1968, 72, 841–843.

Staffieri, J. R. Body build and behavior expectancies in young females. *Developmental Psychology,* 1972, 6, 125–127.

Stager, S. F. Externality, environment, and obesity in children. *The Journal of General Psychology,* 1981, 105, 141–147.

Stalonas, P. M., Johnson, W. G., & Christ, M. Behavior modification for obesity: The evaluation of exercise, contingency management and program adherence. *Journal of Consulting and Clinical Psychology,* 1978, 46, 463–469.

Stalonas, P. M. & Kirschenbaum, D. S. *Are changes in eating habits associated with weight loss?* Paper presented at the meeting of the Society of Behavioral Medicine, New York, November 1980.

Stanley, E. J., Glasser, H. H., Levin, D. G., Adams, P. A., & Coley, B. A. Overcoming obesity in adolescents. *Clinical Pediatrics,* 1970, 4, 29–36.

Stark, L. J., Collins, F. L., & Stokes, T. F. *Training preschool aged children to make nutritious snack choices.* Paper presented at the meeting of the Association for Advancement of Behavior Therapy, Toronto, November 1981.

Stark, O., Atkins, E., Wolff, O. H. & Douglas, J. W. B. Longitudinal study of obesity in the National Survey of Health and Development. *British Medical Journal,* 1981, 283,13–17.

Staugaitis, S. D. New directions for effective weight control with mentally retarded people. *Mental Retardation,* 1978, 16, 157–163.

St. Charles, A. An interdisciplinary model for the treatment of obesity in young girls. *Dissertation Abstracts International,* 1981, 42, 144-B–145-B.

Steel, J. M. Measurement of triceps skinfold thickness during the treatment of obesity. *Obesity and Bariatric Medicine,* 1977, 6, 20–22.

Steele, C. I. Weight loss among teenage girls: An adolescent crisis. *Adolescence,* 1980, 15, 823–829.

Stefanik, P. A., Heald, F. P., & Mayer, J. Caloric intake in relation to energy output of obese and nonobese adolescent boys. *American Journal of Clinical Nutrition,* 1959, 7, 55–62.

Stimbert, V. E. & Coffey, K. R. *Obese children and adolescents: A review.* Knoxville, Tenn: University of Tennessee, 1972. (ERIC Document Reproduction Service no. 30 Research Relating to Children.)

Stokes, T. F. & Baer, D. M. An implicit technology of generalization. *Journal of Applied Behavior Analysis,* 1977, 10, 349–367.

Stokes, T. F., Fowler, S. A., & Baer, D. M. Training preschool children to recruit natural communities of reinforcement. *Journal of Applied Behavior Analysis,* 1978, 11, 285–303.

Stollack, G. E. Weight loss obtained under different experimental procedures. *Psychotherapy: Theory, Research, and Practice,* 1967, 4, 61–64.

Straw, W. E. & Sonne, A. C. The obese patient. *Journal of Family Practice,* 1979, 9, 317–323.

Streja, D., Steiner, G., & Kwiterovich, P. O. Plasma high-density lipoproteins and ischemic heart disease: Studies in a large kindred with familial hypercholesterolemia. *Annals of Internal Medicine,* 1978, 89, 871–880.

Stuart, R. B. Behavioral control of overeating. *Behaviour Research and Therapy,* 1967, 9, 177–186.

Stuart, R. B. A three dimensional program for the treatment of obesity. *Behaviour Research and Therapy,* 1971, 9, 177–186.

Stuart, R. B. *Act thin, stay thin.* New York: Norton, 1978.

Stuart, R. B. & Davis, B. *Slim chance in a fat world: Behavioral control of obesity.* Champaign, Illinois: Research Press, 1972.

Stuart, R. B. & Guire, K. Some correlates of the maintenance of weight lost through behavior modification. *International Journal of Obesity,* 1978, 2, 225–235.

Stuart, R. B., Jensen, J. A., & Guire, K. Weight loss over time. *Journal of the American Dietetic Association,* 1979, 75, 258–261.

Stuart, R. B., Mitchell, C., & Jensen, J. Therapeutic options in the management of obesity. In L. Bradley & C. Prokop (Eds.), *Medical psychology: Contributions to behavioral medicine.* New York: Academic Press, 1981.

Stunkard, A. J. *The pain of obesity.* Palo Alto: Bull Publishing, 1976.

Stunkard, A. J. & Burt, V. Obesity and body image: II. Age of onset of disturbances in the body image. *American Journal of Psychiatry,* 1967, 123, 1443–1447.

Stunkard, A. J., d'Aquili, E., Fox, S., & Filion, R. D. L. Influence of social class on obesity and thinness in children. *Journal of the American Medical Association,* 1972, 221, 579–584.

Stunkard, A. J. & Mahoney, M. J. Behavioral treatment of the eating disorders. In H. Leitenberg (Ed.), *Handbook of behavior modification and behavior therapy.* Englewood Cliffs, New Jersey: Prentice-Hall, 1976.

Stunkard, A. J. & Penick, S. B. Behavior modification in the treatment of obesity: The problem of maintaining weight loss. *Archives of General Psychiatry,* 1979, 36, 801–806.

Stunkard, A. J. & Pestka, J. The physical activity of obese girls. *American Journal of Diseases of Children,* 1962, 103, 812–817.

Sveger, T. Does overnutrition or obesity during the first year affect weight at age four? *Acta Paediatrica Scandinavia,* 1978, 67, 465–467.

Swartz, H. & Leitch, C. J. Differences in mean adolescent blood pressure by age, sex, ethnic origin, and familial tendency. *Journal of School Health,* 1975, 45, 76–81.

Taitz, L. S. Infantile overnutrition among artificially fed infants in the Sheffield region. *British Medical Journal,* 1971, 1, 315–316.

Taitz, L. S. Overfeeding in infancy. *Proceedings of the Nutrition Society,* 1974, 33, 113–118.

Taitz, L. S. Obesity in pediatric practice: Infantile obesity. *Pediatric Clinics of North America,* 1977a, 24, 107–115.

Taitz, L. S. Weight gain and infant feeding. *Lancet,* 1977b, 2, 712.

Takahashi, R. Juvenile obesity and cardiovascular disorders. *Japanese Circulation Journal,* 1978, 42, 64. Abstracted in Information Retrieval (IRL), 1979, 4 (No. 1901–W4), 75.

Tanner, J. M. & Whitehouse, R. H. Standards for subcutaneous fat in British children. *British Medical Journal,* 1962, 155, 446–450.

Tanner, J. M. & Whitehouse, R.H. Revised standards for triceps and subscapular skinfolds in British children. *Archives of Diseases in Childhood,* 1975, 50, 142–145.

Tapper, D. Discussion on Anderson et al., 1980. *Journal of Pediatric Surgery,* 1980, 15, 881.

Thompson, J. K., Jarvie, G. J., Lahey, B. B., & Cureton, K. J. Exercise and obesity: Etiology, physiology, and intervention. *Psychological Bulletin,* 1982, 91, 55–79.

Thompson, P. D., Jeffery, R. W., Wing, R. R., & Wood, P. Unexpected decrease in plasma high density lipoprotein cholesterol with weight loss. *American Journal of Clinical Nutrition,* 1979, 32, 2016–2021.

Thompson, T., Kodluboy, S., & Heston, L. Behavioral treatment of obesity in Prader-Willi syndrome. *Behavior Therapy,* 1980, 4, 588–593.

Thomson, M. E. & Cruickshank, F. M. Survey into the eating and exercise habits of New Zealand pre-adolescents in relation to overweight and obesity. *New Zealand Medical Journal,* 1979, 89, 7–9.

Thorogood, M., Clark, R., Harker, P., & Mann, J. I. Infant feeding and overweight in two Oxfordshire towns. *Journal of the Royal College of General Practitioners,* 1979, 29, 427–430.

Turner, T. J. Obesity in children and adolescents. *Journal of Developmental and Behavioral Pediatrics,* 1980, 1, 43–47.

Tyler, V. O. & Straughan, J. H. Coverant control and breath holding as techniques for the treatment of obesity. *Psychological Record,* 1970, 20, 473–478.

Udall, J. N., Harrison, G. G., Vaucher, Y., Walson, P. D., & Morrow, G. Interaction of maternal and neonatal obesity. *Pediatrics,* 1978, 62, 17–21.

Ullman, R. Comments on Obesity study. *American Journal of Public Health,* 1976, 66, 906–907.

USDA. *Food and your weight.* Washington, D.C.: USDA (Bulletin No. 74), 1967.

USDA. *Nutrition*. Washington, D.C.: USDA, 1971.

VanBiervliet, J. P. & deWijn, J. F. Blood lipid values in obese children. *Acta Paediatrica Belgium*, 1978, 31, 27–34.

VanGelderen, H. H. Overgewicht en vetzucht bij kinderen. *Voeding*, 1976, 37, 208–212.

Vobecky, J., Demers, P. P. & Shapcott, D. Cited in "What's Being Written." *Obesity and Bariatric Medicine*, 1981, 10, 6.

VonVerscheuer, O. Die Vererbungsbiologische Zwillingsforschung, *Ergeb. Inn. Med. Kinderheilk*, 1927, 31, 35–120. Cited in Bray, G. A. *The obese patient*. Philadelphia: W. B. Saunders, 1976.

Voors, A. W., Foster, T. A., Frerichs, R. R., Webber, L. S., & Berenson, G. S. Studies of blood pressures in children, ages 5–14 years, in a total biracial community: The Bogalusa heart study. *Circulation*, 1976, 54, 319–327.

Voors, A. W., Sklov, M. C., Wolf, T. M., Hunter, S. M., & Berenson, G. S. Cardiovascular risk factors in children and coronary related behavior. In T. J. Coates, A. C. Peterson, C. Perry (Eds.), *Adolescent health: Crossing the barriers*. New York: Academic Press, 1980 in press.

Voors, A. W., Webber, L. S., & Berenson, G. S. Blood pressure of children ages 2 1/2–5 1/2 years in a total community: The Bogalusa Heart Study. *American Journal of Epidemiology*, 1978, 107, 403–411.

Voors, A. W., Webber, L. S., Frerichs, R. R., & Berenson, G. S. Body height and body mass as determinants of basal blood pressure in children—The Bogalusa Heart Study. *American Journal of Epidemiology*, 1977, 106, 101–108.

Vuille, J. C. & Mellbin, T. Obesity in 10-year-olds: An epidemilogic study. *Pediatrics*, 1979, 64, 564–572.

Wagner, M. K. & Schumaker, J. F. External-cue responsivity in obese children. *Obesity and Bariatric Medicine*, 1976, 5, 168–169.

Walike, B. C., Jordan, H. A., & Stellar, E. Preloading and the regulation of food intake in man. *Journal of Comparative and Physiological Psychology*, 1969, 68, 327–333.

Walker, A. R. P., Bhamjee, D., Walker, B. F., & Martin, A. P. Serum high-density lipoprotein cholesterol, glucose tolerance and other variables in obese black adolescent girls. *South African Medical Journal*, 1979, August, 221–224.

Wang, R.Y. & Watson, J. Contracting for weight reduction—making the sacrifices worthwhile. *The American Journal of Maternal Child Nursing*, 1978, January/February, 46–49.

Warner, K. E. & Balagura, S. Intrameal eating patterns of obese and nonobese humans. *Journal of Comparative and Physiological Psychology*, 1975, 89, 783–788.

WaterPik. *Countdown: The permanent weight-loss system*. (Advertising circular D27CD978) Fort Collins, Colorado: Teledyne, WaterPik, 1977.

Watt, B. K. & Merrill, A. L. *Composition of Foods* (Agriculture Handbook No. 8,

U.S. Department of Agriculture). Washington D.C.: U.S. Government Printing Office, 1975.

Waxman, M. & Stunkard, A. J. Calorie intake and expenditure of obese boys. *The Journal of Pediatrics,* 1980, 96, 187–193.

Weil, W. B. Infantile obesity. In M. Winick (Ed.), *Childhood obesity.* New York: Wiley, 1975.

Weil, W. B., Jr. Current controversies in childhood obesity. *The Journal of Pediatrics,* 1977, 91, 175–187.

Weisenberg, M. & Fray, E. What's missing in the treatment of obesity by behavior modification? *Journal of the American Dietetic Association,* 1974, 65, 410–414.

Weiss, A. R. A behavioral approach to the treatment of adolescent obesity. *Behavior Therapy,* 1977a, 8, 720–726.

Weiss, A. R. Characteristics of successful weight reducers. A brief review of predictor variables. *Addictive Behaviors,* 1977b, 2, 193–201.

Weninger, M., Widhalm, D., Strobl, W., & Schernthaner, G. Childhood obesity: Serum lipoproteins, glucose and insulin concentrations after an oral glucose load. *Artery,* 1980, 8, 185–190.

Wheeler, M. E. & Hess, K. W. Treatment of juvenile obesity by successive approximation control of eating. *Journal of Behavior Therapy and Experimental Psychiatry,* 1976, 7, 235–241.

Wheeler, M. E. & Hess, K. W. *Behavioral treatment of obese children: The first 100 cases.* Paper presented at the Meeting of the International Congress on Obesity, Washington, D.C., October 1977.

White, J. J., Cheek, D. Y. & Haller, J. A. Small bowel bypass is applicable for adolescents with morbid obesity, *American Surgeon,* 1974, 40, 704–708.

Whitelaw, A. G. L. Influence of maternal obesity on subcutaneous fat in the newborn. *British Medical Journal,* 1976, 1, 985–986.

Widhalm, K., Maxa, E., & Zyman, H. Effect of diet and exercise upon cholesterol and triglyceride content of plasma lipoproteins in overweight children. *European Journal of Pediatrics,* 1978, 127, 121–126.

Widhalm, K. & Schernthaner, G. Influence of hypocaloric diets on insulin and C-peptide secretion and lipoprotein composition in obese children. *Pediatric and Adolescent Endocrinology,* 1979, 7, 213–220. Basel: Karger.

Wilkins, L. *Diagnosis and treatment of endocrine disorders in childhood and adolescence* (3rd ed.). Springfield, Illinois: Charles C Thomas, 1950.

Wilkinson, J. F. *Don't raise your child to be a fat adult.* New York: Bobbs-Merrill, 1980.

Wilkinson, P., Parkin, J., Pearlson, G., Strang, H., & Sykes P. Energy intake and physical activity in obese children. *British Medical Journal,* 1977a, 1, 756.

Wilkinson, P. W., Pearlson, J., Parkin, J. M. Philips, P. R. & Sykes, P. Obesity in childhood: A community study in Newcastle upon Tyne. *Lancet,* 1977b, 1, 350–352.

Willems, E. P. Behavioral technology and behavioral ecology. *Journal of Applied Behavior Analysis,* 1974, 7, 151–165.

Willmore, D. W. & Pruitt, B. A. Fat boys get burned. *Lancet,* 1972, 23, 631–632.

Wilson, G. T. Methodological considerations in treatment outcome research on obesity. *Journal of Consulting and Clinical Psychology,* 1978, 46, 687–702.

Wilson, G. T. & Brownell, K. D. Behavior therapy for obesity: An evaluation of treatment outcome. *Advances in Behaviour Research and Therapy,* 1980, 3, 49–86.

Wilson, G. T. & Brownell, K. D. Behavior therapy for obesity: Including family members in the treatment process. *Behavior Therapy,* 1978, 9, 943–945.

Wilson, G. T. & O'Leary, K. D. *Principles of behavior therapy.* Englewood Cliffs: Prentice-Hall, 1980.

Wing, R. R., Epstein, L. H., Marcus, M., & Shapira, B. Strong monetary contingencies for weight loss during treatment and maintenance. *Behavior Therapy,* 1981, 12, 702–710.

Wing, R. R., Epstein, L. H., Ossip, D. J., & LaPorte, R. E. Reliability and validity of self-report and observers' estimates of relative weight. *Addictive Behaviors,* 1979, 4, 133–140.

Winick, M. Genetic and environmental factors in determining obesity. *Journal of the Canadian Dietetic Association,* 1978, 39, 100–104.

Withers, R. F. J. Problems in the genetics of human obesity. *Eugenics Review,* 1964, 56, 81–90.

Wolff, M. Social validity: The case for subjective measurement or how applied behavior analysis is finding its heart. *Journal of Applied Behavior Analysis,* 1978, 11, 203–214.

Wolman, P. G. The relationship between the introduction of solid foods in infancy and obesity in preschool children. *Dissertation Abstracts International,* 1980, 41, 1317B.

Woody, E. & Costanzo, P. The socialization of obesity prone behavior. In S. Brehm, S. Kassin & F. Gibbons (Eds.), *Developmental social psychology.* New York: Oxford University Press, 1981.

Wooley, O. W. & Wooley, S. C. The experimental psychology of obesity. In T. Silverstone & J. Finchman (Eds.), *Obesity: Pathogenesis and management.* Lancaster: Medical and Technical Publishing, 1975.

Wooley, O. W., Wooley, S. C., & Turner, K. The effects of rate of consumption of appetite in the obese and nonobese. In A. Howard (Ed.), *Recent advances in obesity research, Vol. I. Proceedings of the 1st International Congress on Obesity.* London: Newman Publishing, 1975.

Wooley, S. C. & Wooley, O. W. Women and weight: Toward a redefinition of the therapeutic task. In A. Brodsky & R. Hare-Mustin (Eds.), *Women and psychotherapy: An assessment of research and practice.* New York: Guilford Press, 1980.

Wooley, S. C., Wooley, O. W., & Dyrenforth, S. R. Theoretical, practical, and social issues in behavioral treatments of obesity. *Journal of Applied Behavior Analysis,* 1979, 12, 3–25.

Worsley, A. In the eye of the beholder: Social and personal characteristics of teenagers and their impressions of themselves and fat and slim people. *British Journal of Medical Psychology,* 1981a, 54, 231–242.

Worsley, A. Teenagers perceptions of fat and slim people. *International Journal of Obesity,* 1981b, 5, 15–24.

Wright, P. Development of feeding behavior in early infancy: Implications for obesity. *Health Bulletin (Edinb.),* 1981, 39, 197–205.

Yeung, D. L., Pennell, M. D., Leung, M., & Hall, J. Infant fatness and feeding practices: A longitudinal assessment. *Journal of the American Dietetic Association,* 1981, 79, 531–535.

Ylitalo, V. Treatment of obese schoolchildren. *Acta Paediatrica Scandinavica,* 1981, (Suppl. 290), 1–108.

Zack, P. M., Harlan, W. R., Leaverton, P. E., & Coroni-Huntley, J. A longitudinal study of body-fatness in childhood and adolescence. *The Journal of Pediatrics,* 1979, 95, 126–130.

Zakus, G., Chin, M. L., Cooper, H., Makovsky, E., & Merrill, C. Treating adolescent obesity: A pilot project in a school. *The Journal of School Health,* December 1981, 663–666.

Zakus, G., Chin, M. L., Keown, M., Herbert, F., & Held, M. A group modification approach to adolescent obesity. *Adolescence,* 1979, 14, 481–490.

Zegman, M., Lamon, S., Dubbert, P., & Wilson, G. T. *The role of exercise in the behavioral treatment of obesity: Multivariate analyses of posttreatment and follow-up results.* Paper presented at the meeting of the Society of Behavioral Medicine, New York, November 1980.

Zuti, W. B. *Effects of diet and exercise on body composition of adult women during weight reduction.* Unpublished doctoral dissertation, Kent State University, 1972.

Index